Praise for the National Best Seller
Parenting Your Premature Baby and Child: The Emotional Journey
by Deborah L. Davis, PhD, and Mara Tesler Stein, PsyD

" . . . an invaluable resource."—William Sears, MD, co-author of *The Premature Baby Book*

"With a caring and compassionate voice, this book guides parents through the complex and ever-challenging emotional journey of parenting a premature infant."
—Dianne I. Maroney, former NICU nurse, co-author of *Your Premature Baby and Child*

"This book is full of knowledge, hope, wisdom, and reflection, and goes far beyond available books for preterm parents."—Heidelise Als, PhD, psychologist, Harvard Medical School and Children's Hospital, Boston

"Deborah Davis and Mara Tesler Stein have created a gentle and safe haven for the entire family. . . . It is evident that the authors both deeply and sensitively recognize all that is lost through this experience, but much more importantly, all that is gained."—Liza G. Cooper, CSW, neonatal social worker

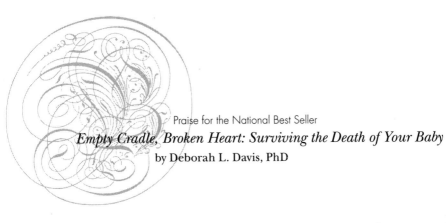

Praise for the National Best Seller

Empty Cradle, Broken Heart: Surviving the Death of Your Baby
by Deborah L. Davis, PhD

"*Empty Cradle, Broken Heart* is written with great awareness and sensitivity. Deborah Davis gets it just right."—Sheila Kitzinger, author of *The Complete Book of Pregnancy and Childbirth*

" . . . there is comfort in these pages."—*Mothering* magazine

"Davis speaks directly to the emotional and physical needs of bereaved parents." —Judith Lasker, author of *When Pregnancy Fails*

"The best book on this subject. I did a huge amount of reading after I lost my baby, and I can tell you that this book is head and shoulders above anything else I've read on this subject. Thank you, Deborah Davis."—A. Douglas, Canada

Intensive Parenting

Surviving the Emotional Journey through the NICU

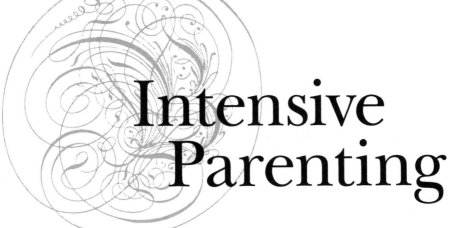

Intensive Parenting

Surviving the Emotional Journey through the NICU

Deborah L. Davis, PhD
& Mara Tesler Stein, PsyD

FULCRUM
GOLDEN, COLORADO

Also available from these authors:

Empty Cradle, Broken Heart:
Surviving the Death of Your Baby, Revised Edition
by Deborah L. Davis, PhD

Parenting Your Premature Baby and Child:
The Emotional Journey
by Deborah L. Davis, PhD,
and Mara Tesler Stein, PsyD

The information contained in this book, although based on sound medical judgment, is not intended as a substitute for medical advice or attention. Please consult your doctor or healthcare provider for individual professional care.

Library of Congress Cataloging-in-Publication Data

Davis, Deborah L., 1955-

 Intensive parenting : surviving the emotional journey through the NICU / Deborah L. Davis and Mara Tesler Stein.

  p. cm.

 Includes index.

 ISBN 978-1-55591-744-9 (pbk.)

1. Premature infants--Care. 2. Parent and infant. 3. Parent and child. I. Tesler Stein, Mara. II. Title.

 RJ250.D37 2013

 618.92'011--dc23

                    2012025224

Printed in the United States of America

0 9 8 7 6 5 4 3 2 1

Design by Jack Lenzo

Fulcrum Publishing

4690 Table Mountain Dr., Ste. 100

Golden, CO 80403

800-992-2908 • 303-277-1623

www.fulcrumbooks.com

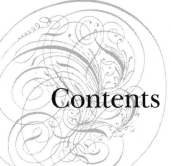

Contents

Preface

This book rides on the crest of a new wave in neonatology. The modern Neonatal Intensive Care Unit (NICU) now provides more than just state-of-the-art medical technology. NICU policy is becoming *relationship-centered* rather than technology-centered, and in tandem, individualized *developmentally supportive* care is increasingly provided to babies—and to their parents. While the NICU is often an unavoidably stressful environment, these new models of care are comprehensive and compassionate and can successfully reduce infant suffering, parent distress, and caregiver fatigue.

Relationship-centered care focuses on nurturing the relationships between everyone, including the medical staff, family members, and the patient. Relationship-centered care is an expansion of patient-centered care or family-centered care, as it values not just the patient and family but also the medical practitioner. This new model of care attends to the specific support each person needs in order to thrive, whether it's the patient achieving the best possible quality of life, the family coping and adjusting, or the medical practitioner collaborating with teammates and forming therapeutic relationships with each patient and family.

In the NICU, relationship-centered care means that the parent-infant bond is considered paramount and parents are welcomed as integral members of their baby's collaborative care team. Parents are encouraged by the team in their efforts to be close to their baby and coached in caregiving, so they can become attuned, responsive, and sure with their little one. Parents are informed and communicate with the team about their baby's conditions and treatments, so they can advocate for their baby's needs. Parents are supported emotionally by the team, so they can be more emotionally available and nurturing to their baby. By cultivating relationships, NICU policy not only promotes optimal caregiving but also accommodates and even reinforces the positive, connective emotional experiences between parent and baby that contribute to optimal infant development.

In concert with relationship-centered care, developmentally supportive care attends to the specific developmental needs of each patient and family. Care is responsive to each infant's sensitivities and thresholds and includes close physical contact with the parents in a muted, gentle, nurturing environment that mimics the womb. For parents, developmentally supportive care honors their need to get physically close and feel emotionally connected to their newborn and become confident in caregiving. In other words, developmentally supportive care tries to give babies and parents what they've been promised.

Renowned researcher Dr. Heidelise Als, champion of relationship-centered care in the NICU and founder of the Newborn Individualized Developmental Care and Assessment Program (NIDCAP), has repeatedly shown that for "very low birth weight" premature babies in particular, developmentally supportive care results in fewer complications, shorter stays in the NICU, lowered family stress, enhanced parent appreciation of the infant, and better neurological and neuropsychological outcomes that last beyond early childhood. (Go to www. nidcap.org for more information.)

Last but not least, a focus on relationships and developmental support benefits practitioners as well. Ongoing training, institutional backing, and collaborative relationships with colleagues can allow each practitioner to acquire and fine-tune comprehensive professional skills—including technical, interpersonal, and developmental expertise—building confidence in the ability to provide optimal care. In a relationship-centered workplace that provides developmental support, NICU practitioners are more attuned and able to provide relationship-centered, developmentally supportive care to babies and families.

How to Use This Book

When your newborn baby* requires intensive care, this is more than a medical crisis. It's a family** crisis. Besides facing your baby's medical condition, you must also adjust your expectations, cope with your feelings, and learn how to parent your baby in the Neonatal Intensive Care Unit (NICU).

There are many good books that explain your baby's medical conditions, developmental diagnoses, treatments, and procedures. This book is different. It focuses on your experiences, feelings, and relationships around the hospitalization of your special newborn.

This book does not try to tell you how you should feel or what you must do. Rather, it strives to describe and affirm the wide range of experiences and emotional reactions that occur in the NICU and to offer strategies for coping with your baby's condition and hospitalization. It focuses on how you can deal with the challenges you meet so you can revel in the pleasures of nurturing and cherishing your little one. With factual information and the words and insights of other parents, you can also establish realistic expectations for yourself. You can also gain reassurance that you are not crazy; you are not the only one who feels betrayed, terrified, or guilty. You are not the only one to be wary of the tiny creature in the incubator, to wait and worry for the arrival of each new milestone, or to compare your child to both

---

  * It can be awkward to accommodate singleton and multiple babies in the same sentence, so most of the time we will simply refer to *your baby* or *your child*. If you delivered twins, triplets, or more, please know that whenever applicable to your situation, *your baby* or *child* means "your babies" or "children."

 ** This book embraces all types of families, and it strives to honor your relationship to your baby and your relationship with your baby's other parent(s). As a result, we typically use the word *parent* unless *mother* or *father* applies due to the gender or biological differences described. We also use the term *partner* to apply to any relationship between co-parents.

fellow NICU babies and his or her healthy peers. Whether your baby was born recently or long ago, or spent days, weeks, or months in the hospital, you will find yourself reflected in these pages. Whatever your child's condition, complications, or outcome, you will find support.

You may find yourself wondering about the parents and babies who appear in this book. You may want to measure your experiences against theirs and compare medical conditions, complications, gestational ages, lengths of hospital stay, development, or medical outcomes. But this book does not dwell on details, which vary widely, because that's not where you will find yourself or your emotional journey. Instead, you will see yourself reflected in the emotional nuances of these parents' experiences. This emotional common ground is where you will find orientation and kinship with other parents and the comfort of truly knowing that you are not alone.

So for the parents quoted here, when you wish you knew the rest of the story, keep in mind that you are reading about the most important parts of their journeys—the emotional, wrenching, life-enriching, deeply meaningful parts, many of which may resonate for you. And what matters most down the road is that these parents are continuing on their journeys, and they've survived. You will too.

☙❧

It is not necessary to read this book through from start to finish. As you weave your way through the book, you can also peek ahead into the future for preparation and reassurance or review the past for validation, affirmation, and to make sense of where you've been and where you are. Take in whatever seems helpful and pass by whatever isn't. Return to the passages that are particularly comforting and try reading other parts later.

Even if you do read it cover to cover and then put it away, we encourage you to revisit this book from time to time. You'll notice that what you need will stand out every time, and what you need will always seem to be different. This book is meant to be your companion, and it will follow your lead.

If reading this book moves you to cry, try to accept this reaction. These are healing tears of grief and joy, courage and strength that mix with those of other parents. You are not alone.

Time is too slow for those who wait,
Too swift for those who fear,
Too long for those who grieve,
Too short for those who rejoice.
But for those who love,
Time is eternity.

—Henry van Dyke

1:

An Unexpected Journey

We'd seen the NICU on a tour when I was first pregnant, and I had thought it was for the very sick, deformed children, babies that weren't going to live. I told myself I would never be there. I'm going to have normal, healthy children. Why wouldn't I? Everybody does—except those people, those poor, poor people. So when I found myself in the NICU, I just couldn't believe it.—Vickie

When you find out you are pregnant, you are anticipating so much more than just a baby. You may hold optimistic expectations for a smooth pregnancy, an uncomplicated birth, a healthy baby, and an easy adjustment with your newborn. You may start forming a picture of the expanded family you're creating and the future you're building. You imagine being a certain kind of parent to a certain kind of baby.

But now your newborn lies in the Neonatal Intensive Care Unit (NICU), and many of your hopes and expectations come crashing down. Even if your baby stabilizes quickly, his or her need for intensive care is incompatible with your ideas of how and where newborns are meant to be.

The day we left the hospital without the baby, my husband and I sat on our sofa and sobbed all night long. We felt empty and exhausted. We realized we had been in shock and still were. I was feeling great loss. I rely heavily on tradition. I'm a planner. This was not how it was supposed to be, not how I had planned it.—Laura

As you peer at your infant surrounded by tubes, wires, and buzzing machinery, you may wonder how to parent this small creature; how to best stroke your baby's soft, perhaps fragile skin; how to comfort and come to know your child. You may wonder when you will be able to take your baby out of the hospital and somehow find your way back to the path you had planned.

But you're not experiencing a mere misstep, you're embarking on a new journey through uncharted territory. You may feel lost, terrified, bereft, and unsure. How will you find your way? How can you relinquish old dreams, adjust to what is, and dream new dreams?

When expectations are shattered, nothing feels right. It's difficult to imagine that you will ever adjust or recover your happiness. This is a jarring, harrowing experience, and with dread you may sense that there's no turning back.

Finally, we got the call saying we could go up and see our son. I was put in a wheelchair, and we entered the NICU, the artificial womb that we all would live in for a while.—Laurie

I focused more on their baby-ness than on their medical condition. They were little and helpless and mine. But I also had a sense that this was the beginning of a dramatic step that I couldn't undo and that would change our lives forever.—Dwight

Hopes and Expectations

I had always known I wanted to be a mom. I wanted a peaceful pregnancy where I could enjoy all the pregnancy symptoms and watch my belly grow. I wanted to bond with my child as soon as he was born. We dreamed of having this little boy who would become our world. A little one to make our family whole.—Corin

During pregnancy, it is natural for you to revel in the wonder and anticipation of it all. You may envision gently welcoming your baby into the world. You may dream of nuzzling and nursing your little one, and you imagine a newborn who is cute, tranquil, and fits nicely into your arms. You naturally anticipate bringing your baby home after a day or so, to the congratulations of friends and family. Picturing your healthy, robust infant, you see a bright future.

I had every hope and dream imaginable for an idyllic pregnancy, birth, and baby. I had waited so long that everything was bound to be perfect! I immediately took on the role of mother-to-be—I ate well, slept, and took good care of myself and this baby of mine.—Sara

These visions are not just enjoyable daydreams. They are an important psychological preparation for your future as a parent. Having certain expectations lets you make plans and feel some measure of control. Positive assumptions give you confidence and hope. You invest in your future as you imagine it.

I read everything I could get my hands on about pregnancy. My husband, Chris, and I wanted a natural childbirth. We practiced the Bradley Method every night together. He was a wonderful coach, and I envisioned him there with me as we welcomed our new baby into the world without drugs or machines.—Rebekah

When I found out Cyndy was pregnant with twin boys, I had dreams of big, strapping football players—the first twins in the NFL. I dreamed of the things we would do together, running, biking, watching the games on Sundays.—Rich

During the pregnancy, I was not afraid of anything—I just took for granted that everything always goes smoothly. . . . It never once occurred to me that things do go wrong.—Jodi

You may also have expectations about how life is supposed to work, such as doing all the right things during pregnancy will guarantee a healthy baby. You may believe that nothing bad happens to good people, and especially to their babies. Even if you feel a sense of uneasiness or if your pregnancy is identified as high risk, it may be hard to believe that bad things could really happen to *you*.

But as events begin to unfold in unexpected ways, your anticipated path starts changing. Whether your baby receives a firm diagnosis during the pregnancy, you launch into preterm labor or experience other problems, or your baby is unexpectedly whisked away from you after birth, you are confronted with the possibility that your future will be different from the one you had imagined.

When the Unexpected Happens

In many cases, problems are detected during pregnancy. If there are maternal complications or if the baby has a medical condition, you may feel stunned, distant, confused, or inept. You may struggle to comprehend what the doctors and nurses are telling you. With your baby tucked away inside the womb, you may not comprehend the magnitude of the problem. At first, it's tempting to tell yourself that the warning signs are not ominous or that after some monitoring you'll be sent on your way.

During a routine Level II Fetal Ultrasound, my doctor looked at us and said, "Mr. and Mrs. ——, I found an anomaly with the fetus." I felt like the rug had been pulled out from under my feet. Barry and I were being told that there was a good possibility our baby had a fatal genetic issue and, even if she didn't we were looking at a huge undertaking following delivery. To say that I felt like crying would be an understatement.—Dina

I'll never forget that first night in the hospital, being poked by those interns. I couldn't sleep at all. I kept thinking it was just a mistake and that when the "real" doctors came to examine me, they would set it all straight and send me home. But, of course, that didn't happen.—Rebekah

There I was, flat on my backside. How was I going to make it through the next three months? Of course, I was sure I'd carry the baby at least close to term. I had no sense of urgency, as I should have had. I still feel guilty about that.—Cindy

For me, it was the first time in my life that I was living completely in the moment. I was too terrified to think of what would happen next, so I just learned to be completely grateful for each minute I stayed pregnant.—Susan B.

If you have weeks or months of monitoring or bed rest, you may walk that fine line between hope and despair or vacillate between them. You may deny the possibilities or try to protect yourself from the worst by withdrawing emotionally from this baby. Detachment mixed with terrible fear make for a bewildering roller coaster of emotions during the rest of your pregnancy. It can be a very difficult time.

There were so many emotional ups and downs. That was perhaps the hardest thing. One day they talk about sending me home, and the next there's a fetal monitor strapped around my belly indefinitely.—Rebekah

I had been very excited about the baby and had begun preparing for the arrival from the start of this pregnancy. Now, I wouldn't let myself get my hopes up. During the two months between the first hospitalization and the delivery, I imagined frequently what it would be like for the pregnancy to end without a baby.—Shaina

I began preparing myself, subconsciously, for what might be the death of both my babies. I guess I thought that if I detached myself from my feelings for them, it wouldn't hurt so much if I lost them.—Sara

All I could think of was *I just want this to be over.* So I had two sides of the coin—the side where I'm fighting for the life of this baby and the other side where I just wanted to give up.—Vickie

When the doctors finally prepped me for my cesarean, I felt some relief. My five weeks in the hospital had been full of close calls, and I was exhausted—emotionally and physically. I wanted it all to be over.—Rebekah

Sometimes complications lead to imminent delivery and the shock of emergency birth. As a father, you may feel removed and unlike yourself in the midst of this crisis. As a mother, you may be bereft and filled with dread.

In forty-five minutes we went from "We're having twins. Isn't that great?" to a shocked, crying, sad, and frightened "We're having them now—we're going to the hospital." So here we are, scared. We have no idea. We know squat about what's going on. I'm in my own world, and Debbie's in her world.—Mitch

When I called the doctor that morning at 2:00 AM, he said to bring Lauren to Labor and Delivery. I was so upset driving the twenty miles to the hospital that I could hardly keep the car on the road trying to see through my tears. When I got to the hospital, I drove up and down the street three times looking for a Delivery sign. I'm lucky that they didn't have a Delivery sign, or I would have left Lauren at an empty loading dock while I went to park the car. After I had circled the hospital one more time, Lauren had sense enough to tell me to just go to the Emergency Room and they would get her up to Labor and Delivery on the third floor. Actually, I'm glad that the doctor did not tell me on the phone that Labor and Delivery was on the third floor, or I might have tried to drive my car up the stairs.—Michael

I tie on my papery surgical mask and wonder how life is about to change. Wondering how I'm going to screw up this kid. Wondering if I'll get the chance. Wondering.—Jeff

The first feeling when the doctor said that I was going to have a C-section right away was *No—I'm not ready!* I wanted to be pregnant for a couple more weeks!

Then I was afraid to face my son, to really see how he was. . . . I wasn't ready to face the truth if it wasn't a happy one.—Inkan

The whole time they were prepping me and doing the C-section I was crying. They told me to stay calm—like that was possible! I just kept thinking, *If I lose my baby, I will die.*—Dusti

Neither boy cried. There were so many people in the delivery room—doctors, neonatologists, specialists—it was chaotic. I felt lost and that my body had failed me again.—Jody

When the baby is expected to do poorly outside the womb, the birth is an intense and watchful period. With the NICU team present, everyone holds a collective breath, hoping for the best and wondering how the baby will respond to being born. Tracy remembers, "The silence that followed his birth was the loudest thing I have ever heard."

When I saw [the babies] for the first time, it was a relief that the trials and tribulations of trying to hold on to the pregnancy were over. Now we had new trials and tribulations to work on, and that was Riley and Banning.—Pam

If your pregnancy was uneventful, the unveiling of your baby's condition after birth may be gradual, or it may be swift and shocking. Either way, it can feel awful to realize that you've taken a terrible detour.

The labor and delivery went very smoothly. I remember it being a very beautiful experience and being so excited to meet my little boy. When he was born he let out one cry, and she held him up for us to get a picture. After a couple of minutes, she called in some doctors, and they took him away. I was told he was having signs of distress and needed "a little help to get started." Since he was my first and I didn't know what was normal, I was still oblivious that anything was seriously wrong for a while. After about an hour of not being able to see or get an update on Gabe, I began to panic. A doctor finally came in to tell me the diagnosis and that he was very sick and needed to be transferred to a larger hospital. Almost two hours after he was born, they brought him in a transport incubator covered in wires and tubes. I was able to touch his hand briefly and say good-bye as they quickly whisked him away to transport to another hospital. It was heartbreaking, scary, and confusing. I had no idea what to expect or what was happening.—Corin

After birth, Kit did not do well on her Apgar test and almost immediately her little chest started caving in due to the stress of trying to breathe. She was like a wet noodle, according to the nurse, and after her initial cry would only whimper. She also turned very pale very quickly. No one got to hold her but me and it was very brief, maybe a minute, and I had to keep an oxygen mask up to her face. The boys and my husband just got to look at her.

It was magical, then scary—the fear really hit me because I could see she was not breathing well at all and the look on the nurse's face was that of worry.—Jennifer E.

This was not at all what I imagined our birthing experience would be. Jeff and I had signed up for parenting, breast-feeding, and childbirth classes. None had started. We were not prepared. I really felt I was apart from my emotions and this experience.—Sandy

Whether you had advanced warning or not, as you watch the doctors and nurses work on your newborn, you may anxiously look for signs of survival and spunk from your baby. For many parents, hearing the baby cry is a powerfully welcome and reassuring sound. As Sharon remembers, "I was afraid that he would die, but once I heard his little squeak of a cry, I knew he had the will to survive." Encouraged, you may be able to rejoice in the moment.

There were so many people in the room, it was like a minyan—that means ten adult male Jews, enough to have full prayers. There was a neonatal team for each kid. An awful lot of people. And then Daniel was born, and he was cute—I remember seeing his little hand—and he was whisked away immediately and intubated, and that was the last I saw of him for a while. After some manipulating, Shayna was born too, and it was a little exciting—there was actually some happiness. We'd just became the parents of twins, and for a little bit, it was kind of okay.—Mitch

You may also look for signals from the medical team. They might bring your baby to you for a peek and maybe a kiss before the move to the NICU. Dare you touch such a fragile infant? Indeed, some parents fear that they are being asked to say good-bye to a baby who may die.

After three pushes he was out, and he didn't look good. He was purple. When they went to clean his nose and his throat, there was so much blood, it was scary. . . . I was afraid. My husband lost control. He had to leave the operating room, and I could hear him in the hallway, punching the walls. And the baby didn't cry. They were doing CPR on him, resuscitating him. And finally, the neonatal resident went out in the hall and got Tom, and at that point I had just about convinced myself that the baby was dead. And they brought Tom back and said, "Here, you can see your son." And Tom looked down and said, "Oh, wow, he's pink, he's pink, he's pink." After being born so blue and purple and scary, he was pink, and he was okay. Then the nurse brought him over to me and said, "Here, you can hold him." And I held him for just a little minute, kissed him, told him I loved him, and she took him back and he was on his way. But I wasn't sure why she had handed me him and not my daughter. I was convinced that they thought he wouldn't make it and wanted me to be able to see him. After all this time and a happy outcome, I'm sitting here bawling about it.—Pam

The nurse brought Ryan over, hurriedly, telling me to give my son a kiss. I took this to mean, "You may never have another chance. Better kiss him now," and I was resistant. I brushed the top of his little head and said I'd see him *soon*. They brought Elizabeth over and put her head next to mine for a picture. I felt removed still, and I wavered between *How dare you think my baby will die* and *I can't love them, they might die.*—Sara

I remember wanting so bad to hold her because I knew they were going to take her away from me. But I was unnaturally calm.—Jennifer E.

I don't think anything in the world can prepare you for the sight of your premature baby. I only saw her for a moment before she was whisked away to the NICU. She did not appear in any way to be human.—Renee

Shocked and distressed, some parents still hold out hope for a healthy baby or speedy recovery. But when you see your baby truly struggling, another layer of expectations tumbles down.

On Gabe's second day of life, I remember staring blankly at the doctor as he told me that Gabe was very sick. It was like a bad dream. I felt like I was outside of the situation, watching it happen. I kept waiting and praying I would wake up. It wasn't until we made it to the NICU at the second hospital where I had time to talk to the doctors and nurses and *see* him hooked up with all the machines that I started to understand how sick he was.—Corin

The first forty-eight hours after birth were a nightmare. The hospital we were at simply was not equipped for her, but they tried. We were told she was having some trouble breathing and that was expected, and her lungs were wet, but that usually clears up over a few days, and she should be fine. They had put her in an oxygen tent at the back of the tiny NICU. We can see her soon. This was heart-wrenching. I thought she would have some oxygen via a mask and that we could hold her like they show on all the shows on TV. It was awful.—Jennifer E.

If your baby looks nothing like you'd imagined, or if you're recovering from complications and numbing drugs, you may have a hard time feeling connected and struggle to relate to your little one. Jody recalls, "It's sad to say but it was terrifying to see him. He was so small."

Seeing a premature baby is so very different from anything you could ever imagine! The things you have come to consider normal just aren't there! There is no fat at all on these little peanuts. Their ears are like pieces of paper, moldable to any shape, depending on how they were positioned. Their heads look monstrous in comparison to that teeny body. Could anyone possibly see their newborn baby looking like this and not be shocked, scared, and saddened?—Sara

Initially, I felt disconnected from my baby. He was hooked up to tubes and oxygen and didn't look particularly cute. He looked more like ET, and I found it difficult to bond with him. I went through the motions and held him but was sort of relieved when it felt like I had spent enough time with him.—Liza

My heart broke at how tiny she was, yet she still didn't seem real to me. I was concerned that the nurses would think I was unfeeling, but I just didn't know how to react or feel about this baby. All I knew was that one moment I was pregnant and looking forward to my final trimester, and the next moment found me in a NICU, staring at a creature that did not look, act, or sound like a baby.—Renee

A Different Path

He was so small at the beginning. You're almost scared to touch them and pick them up when they're so tiny. And then it takes you a little bit to get comfortable, and then you have to learn how to give them a bath, which is a big thing. You gave baths to your two other kids, no problem, but this is really a big thing, to feel comfortable. So I guess I had to learn how to be a mom again—a new kind of mom or a different kind of mom—to a different, new sort of baby I had never experienced before.—Gallice

Naturally, parenthood transforms you. Even before this crisis, you may have experienced a wide range of feelings triggered by pregnancy, birth, and welcoming a new baby. But having a baby who needs intensive care brings tribulations and opportunities beyond those typically faced by parents. The NICU experience challenges your emotional coping, your developing parental identity, your relationship skills, and your ability to adjust. Coping, parenting, relating, adjusting—these are the central tasks you face in the NICU and beyond. Here is an overview of the journey.

Emotional Coping

Up to this point in your life, you've probably encountered a number of painful losses and challenges and managed to get through them. But when your baby needs intensive care, the associated losses and challenges likely reverberate through every cell of your body and touch the deepest parts of your being. As your journey unfolds, you may be overcome by grief and anxiety, and you might need to acquire new coping skills to manage your feelings and the intensity of this experience. You can learn to observe and accept your pain so that you can move through it, instead of being afraid of it or becoming immobilized by it.

Developing Your Parental Identity

Over the years, you've probably absorbed general knowledge about how to take care of a new baby, but much of this knowledge doesn't seem to apply to your newborn. If your baby arrives early, you may feel psychologically and logistically unprepared for parenthood. If your baby's delivery is a medical emergency, you miss some of the classic milestones of parenthood such as a joyful birth and close contact with your newborn. If your baby experiences unexpected distress after birth, your joy turns to shock and fear as your baby is abruptly taken from your arms.

The NICU is an unwelcome intruder, derailing you from the typical parental tasks. How can you assume your parenting role when your baby is inaccessible to you? NICU policy, practitioner viewpoints, and your baby's medical condition can create barriers that keep you from even feeling connected to your little one. As you learn caregiving skills that you didn't even know existed, at first you might feel utterly unable to take care of your newborn. Under these conditions, it's challenging to feel like a real mother or father. But with time and practice, you can soon feel connected, confident, and competent with your baby.

Managing Your Relationships

The NICU can be an emotional roller coaster, and this heightens your need for understanding and support. Unfortunately, you've embarked on a journey that is foreign to most people, and many of your friends and relatives won't understand or know how to support you. When you don't feel up to the task of explaining, or if they run scared, this chasm can strain your relationships. Even your relationship with your partner can become rocky as you both enter unfamiliar terrain. In addition, your relationships with NICU nurses and doctors will require a level of collaboration and communication that may be new to you. This journey is an opportunity to hone your relationship skills, and as a result, your friendships and partnerships can deepen and become more rewarding.

Adjustment and Healing

You may find it reassuring to remember that even a routine pregnancy and the birth of a healthy newborn are never "perfect." All parents have to face the new reality and adjust their expectations. Granted, having a baby in the NICU can be intense, frightening, disappointing, and demanding, requiring far more adjustment than usual. But parenting this baby is a journey that's just as legitimate, worthy, and meaningful as parenting a typical baby. As you get to know your baby, you can modify your expectations and some of your goals and become the kind of parent you want to be with this child.

As you look around the NICU and learn more about your baby, you become wiser. You begin to realize that you will always do everything you can for your child, but there are things you cannot know and cannot control. Your perspective shifts. You take nothing for granted. As a result, watching your baby grow brings you some unexpected gifts. The joy of a smile, the appreciation of even small developmental steps, or respect for your child's unique path makes parenting an even richer experience than it might have been. Even as you acknowledge what's been lost, you can move forward with what you've gained.

This isn't the journey you planned on, and though chaotic and distressing at times, it can ultimately be a healing journey. Indeed, your baby's time in the NICU is an opportunity for growth—for all of you. Simply put, your baby's arrival has set you on a different path, and you can learn to travel it well.

Points to Remember

· *Your vision and expectations for your pregnancy and your baby represent important psychological preparation for your future as a parent.*

· *Your baby's need for intensive care is a profound loss and a violation of your natural, heartfelt expectations.*

· *Just as your baby is beginning a new journey, you are too. Your main tasks are emotional coping, developing your parental identity, honing your relationship skills, and adjusting to this new path.*

· *The challenges you meet, the strength you develop, and the steps you take will be unique to your journey.*

· *Becoming a different kind of parent to a different kind of child is full of unique challenges, certainly, but also full of unique joys and opportunities for your own growth as a parent and as a person.*

The Tapestry That Reflects Your Emotional Journey

Throughout your life, you are weaving a tapestry that reflects your emotional journey—where you've been, how you've changed, and what you've learned, lost, and acquired all along the way. The threads you are weaving are the threads of feelings, the threads of your identity, and the threads of your relationships.

In this tapestry, different parts of your life are represented by varying textures, colors, and patterns. Some woven sections are smooth, others are coarse. There are vibrant colors and muted tones. Some sections are crisp or solid, and in others there is a blending of colors or textures. Some blendings are messy or clashing, and some are more harmonious.

When crisis hits, the tapestry that you've been weaving abruptly changes. The threads become rough and unwieldy, and you're not sure what to do with them. They are still the threads of feelings, the threads of your identity, the threads of your relationships, but they are no longer the ones you are familiar with, no longer the ones you have become comfortable weaving. Instead, they have become more complex, more intense, more painful, and more challenging to work with. You feel unprepared. You can no longer weave the pattern you'd planned. Your tapestry is not what you thought it would be. Instead, you must improvise.

Tentatively, you begin to weave those unfamiliar strands. At first your weaving seems messy and discordant, but as you become more adept and at ease, you begin to appreciate the surprising and creative aspects of your weaving. What you thought was messy, ugly, or clashing can become quite special and meaningful because it is hard-earned. You've adjusted in ways you never dreamed of. When you step back, you can see how this weaving fits into the bigger tapestry you have been creating your whole life. In fact, your tapestry has become richer, more interesting, and more beautiful. And so have you.

Along with an orientation, a map, and a compass, this book also offers you a weaving guide of sorts. It is a guide that informs, supports, and empowers you to improvise. It describes and affirms the changes in your tapestry and shows you how to value them. It encourages you to see this transformation as a reflection of your healing.

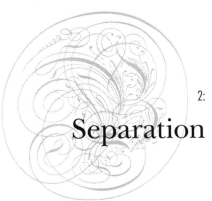

2:

Separation

I felt so bad because my new baby was all alone in the big world. His mommy was only able to spend short amounts of time with him.—Cynthia

The postpartum period is a time of intense focus on the infant. The baby on the inside becomes the baby on the outside, and parents devote care and attention to their little one.

Throughout pregnancy, the mother's direct physical connection with her baby spurs her emotional bond. After birth, she is primed for nurturing her baby in myriad ways, including feeding, holding, soothing, swaddling, and cleaning. The father may feel less of an emotional bond during pregnancy, but after birth he experiences *engrossment*, or a surge of pride, confidence, and commitment when he first lays eyes on his child. He is also primed for caregiving as well as supporting the mother in her efforts.

When your newborn needs intensive care, you are still primed for nurturing your infant, but you face the heart-wrenching disruption of medical crisis. Your devotion and your distress both run deep.

I was very afraid that the split-second glimpse I had had of my baby alive would have to last a lifetime. I was afraid my baby would not make it to the first time I would be able to visit him in the NICU. I was happy about being a mom . . . but I was not happy with how quickly and unexpectedly it had happened. I hurt. I ached for my baby.—Misty

The worst day in my entire life occurred in my daughter's second week, when she had a collapsed lung, and we thought we might lose her. . . . By this point I had totally bonded with her and would have been in incredible pain if we had lost her.—David

When I left the hospital the first night of the boys' life in the NICU, I was confident that they would be fine. They were small, to be sure, but I was reassured by the feeling that they were in very good hands. That night, at around midnight, the phone at my home rang, with the caller ID showing the name of the hospital. I was informed that Justin (the two-pounder) had low platelet levels and would probably need a blood transfusion. I was further told that it was a fairly routine thing and not to worry. However, given that they needed my authorization to perform it, I inferred that it was anything but a routine procedure. I hopped in the car and drove the thirty miles to the hospital at 1:00 AM. Although I was told to remain home, there was no way I was going to let my poor little boy go through this thing alone. During the ride, I kept repeating to myself "You'll be okay, buddy, you're a fighter, my boy's gonna make it," through tears. I don't think I will forget that ride—it is the moment in which I most feared that perhaps Justin would not make it. As it turned out, when I arrived, they informed me that they did not need to do the transfusion after all (although they would do two of them in later days). The NICU nurses also told me that they had a bet going with each other over whether or not Dad would come down to the NICU after that phone call, even after being told not to bother, for such a routine procedure. I won somebody some money and, in the process, realized for the first time just how much I cared for my boys.—Craig

You are also met with the tough challenge of being separated from your little one. Instead of eagerly tending to your baby, you are fearful of what's happening and what lies ahead. Instead of being able to protect and soothe your baby, you are helpless to make it all better.

We waited for the call from the NICU that would say we could go see the baby that we had just had. The longer the time stretched, the more anxious we became. We had been told that it would take time to get Thaddeus set up and evaluated, but we became afraid that something was wrong. I tried to make conversation, but half my mind was up three floors with the baby I didn't yet know.—Laurie

I was terrified to see them. I'm not sure what I expected, but I thought they might die between the time I left my room and got down to the NICU.—Susan B.

I would stand by their warming beds looking down at their limp, still bodies and sob. The only thing I could think to say was that I was so, so sorry. I felt as if I had failed them on the most fundamental level.—Rikki

Separation from Your Baby

The neonatologist said, "We have to transport. We have no equipment to deal with this here." And I'm just saying, "But I want to see my baby again, I want to see my baby again, I want to see my baby again." And they said, "You can't."—Beth

When a baby is admitted to the NICU immediately or soon after birth, the father can usually accompany his baby whereas mother cannot, as she requires a period of physical recovery. This initial separation can feel monumental and like a cruel tearing apart.

He was taken down the hall to the NICU, but I felt as if he were a million miles away.—Jenny

Being away from your baby at the very time when you had expected to be close, watching over, counting fingers and toes, can be particularly anxiety provoking. Not only is your baby far from you, but strangers in scrubs are performing mysterious and (hopefully) miraculous treatments that you can't be a part of, things you don't yet understand. It's disorienting and dislocating to be in a hospital bed when your little one needs intensive care. Your parental instincts may be on high alert.

Nicholas was just taken downstairs, but it might as well have been in another world for all the access I was allowed at first. They kept telling us that we would be able to go right down and see him . . . but then they wouldn't let us. The longer they made us wait, the more frantic I got—thinking that something really horrible was happening to him and I couldn't be there.—Sterling

It may be hours or even days before you are able—or can even think about—seeing your baby. Particularly if your baby's birth is by cesarean section and/or accompanied by maternal complications, or if your baby is transferred to another hospital, you may experience a prolonged separation. Until then, all you may have is a photograph of your little one taken in the NICU. This tantalizing glimpse of your baby may leave you with mixed feelings.

They showed me David right after I gave birth then whisked him away. Since I was still pregnant with Derek, I didn't get to go to the NICU and only saw photos and videos my husband took. That was very hard because I felt that David needed to know I was there for him.—Jody

I got the proverbial Polaroid photos the next morning from our social worker and was completely ambivalent. I played the role I thought I was supposed to—the doting mother telling this stranger how cute my babies were—but as soon as she left, the photos went in my drawer, and I didn't look at them again.—Sara

The NICU nurses sent up a Polaroid photo of my daughter with a nurse's hand next to her for perspective. I think that helped prepare me a little for the technology overload of the NICU.—Susan B.

The picture was dark and fuzzy. He looked like a sick monkey. But suddenly I was less fearful of seeing him.—Laura

When you finally go to the NICU, you may feel relieved at how babylike your infant appears—or you may find it hard to believe that this unfamiliar being is your own child. If you're ambivalent about your baby's appearance, you may feel both repelled and drawn toward your infant. You may find it difficult to envision this vulnerable baby's growth or future. You may still be too exhausted or medicated to care.

The first real look I had was a day after the C-section, when I was able to sit in the chair beside the incubator. His eyes were closed, and I felt like I wasn't really sure this was my baby . . . and I looked for signs of problems more than looking at him, I suppose.—Inkan

He looked like a little old man. I couldn't believe this was a living human being. I couldn't imagine how they put so many tubes in such a small baby.—Susie

The first time I saw James he was lying in his Glad-Wrapped warmer bed, splayed like a frog, surrounded by machinery, and covered in tubes and monitors and leads. My only feelings for him at that time were that he was going to die. I turned and left that NICU ward and returned to my room convinced that my son was as good as dead. I will never forget those feelings.—Leanne

The first thing I said when I saw him was "What is wrong with his head?" I feel horrible about that now, but it was so misshapen that I thought something was terribly wrong with him. Then he let out a little wail, and I broke down. The doctors assured me that that little noise was a very good sign—but it was so hard to believe.—Sterling

There is no way anyone can ever be prepared for that first look at your baby in this condition. I had never seen anything so small in my life. . . . He looked like a tiny roast. Lying there in his big square plastic pan covered with cellophane, looking all shiny and greased up, with the heat lamps glaring above him. He honestly looked like he was being cooked. I couldn't look at him anymore. I went to my room, curled up with Jon, and cried myself to sleep.—Ami

He was lying on a flat sort of raised crib, and his little chest was all depressed, and he was sort of panting. It was really strange, but I had no emotion at that time. I was glad it was finally all over. I really didn't care if I saw him or not, which was really sad, especially when the neonatal nurse told me he wouldn't last the night. The next couple of days were a blur of pain-relieving drugs.—Amber

When I first saw Selina, I was still having a hard time getting out of the anesthesia. It never really occurred to me that she was my baby. I was shocked to see her. She looked like a toad that I had killed and that had been sitting in the sun for too long. I had never seen anything like that in my life.—Jodi

Going into the NICU for the first time was such a surreal experience to me. It was almost as though I was going to see someone else's baby. It didn't feel real. It couldn't possibly be real.—Angie

Sometimes a mother is in such a fog that she cannot recall her first sight of her baby. Cindy says: "I remember the trip to the neonatal unit, but I don't remember the first time I saw her. I felt numb—like I was there physically but not mentally." For others, the image is burned into their minds.

I was terrified of her and for her! I never thought something so tiny could possibly live, and I kept apologizing to her. It still, after nineteen years, brings tears to my eyes to remember looking at her in that incubator.—Janet

I was in love and in shock all at once. I saw this beautiful, tiny little infant who looked like a baby bird who had fallen out of his nest too soon. He was hooked up to all sorts of machines, had a vent tube, numerous IVs, and an umbilical catheter. He was red and wrinkly. His head was very large for his short body. He reminded me of what Frankenstein must have looked like! I cried, and all I could think was *What did I do wrong? Why is my baby suffering so?*—Jayna

My first feeling was that I wanted to rip all of those machines off him and hold him and make everything all right.—Jennifer A.

Whether you think your baby appears beautiful or strange (or both), seeing your newborn covered with wires and tubes and surrounded by beeping equipment can be overwhelming. The intensive care setting can be disturbing and the medical technology distracting. You may be painfully struck by how your baby should be encircled in your soft, watery womb or cradled in your loving arms, not surrounded by medical technology and strangers in scrubs. If you have twins, triplets, or more in the NICU, you may worry about their separation, not only from you but also from each other.

I will never forget the first time I saw him. . . . It was the most horrifying, pathetic sight I had ever seen. He lay there covered in tubes and wires and was fully ventilated. I almost screamed, and I vividly recall putting my hand over my mouth to stop myself. I'd had a "perfect" baby just two years earlier, and now this. I kept on thinking what a terrible introduction to life—he had come from a nice, warm, harm-free environment to this. It really hurt me.—Amber

Seeing both boys in the NICU was hard. They were on the oscillating vent and had tons of cords and IVs. I kept thinking that they should be inside me, not here fighting for their lives.—Jody

I hated the fact that they were about three feet away from each other and not together. For their short life in the womb, they had been together and were probably wondering what had happened to their other half.—Rosa

As the father (or mother's partner), you can usually stay with the baby, but your natural desire to be with both mother and baby is thwarted. Even when the mother insists that you go with the baby instead of staying with her, this can feel difficult to do. You may wish you could bend the space-time continuum and be both places at once. Yet going with your baby lets you play a singular and vital role. Typically the mother really does want at least one of you watching over your little one. Even if she envies your ability to be with your newborn, she longs for the news you bring and is grateful that you're brave and willing to make those solitary treks to the NICU. Taking on this "job" can also help you orient to the situation and build your confidence.

The first day I visited Chris in the NICU, I was lucky enough to get some advice from a neonatologist, who told me that I had a unique opportunity as a father in this crisis. I could do something better than anyone else could. I could be the link between Chris and my wife, Lauren, who was in a different hospital. I could help Lauren believe that she really had a baby, and I could help her to get to know Chris despite the ten miles between them.—Michael

The first day, Laurel wasn't going anywhere, so I was the one to describe Buddy, take pictures, relay weight and length, make phone calls, and so on. But that also gave me a purpose and something to do.—Ed

It was amazing to me how the babies responded to Tom, even turning to his voice. It was almost twenty-four hours later that I got to see them, and he was down there every two to three hours with them so they knew him.—Betsy

Particularly if there have been maternal complications during the pregnancy or the first days following delivery, it is normal for you to fear more for the mother than the baby. If the mother is recovering from a difficult or surgical birth, her safety may be foremost on your mind.

Not to sound too terribly callous, but I didn't know these unborn kids, nor did I have any understanding of what was really going on. All I knew was that my wife was in the hospital, and I was not thinking about any unborn children; I was thinking about my wife's health. In retrospect, I guess it's kind of silly. Debbie wasn't at risk for anything. The only risk was losing the kids, but I didn't realize that. I was thinking, *My wife is in some sort of trauma right now,* and I was very concerned about her.—Mitch

It is also common for the mother to feel more distressed than the father about leaving her baby behind when she is discharged from the hospital. Because her physical connection was well-established during pregnancy *and* her postpartum hormones make it an imperative to hold her baby close, this separation feels especially cruel to her.

I was discharged the same day Gabe was transferred to be put on ECMO. I remember thinking that this was supposed to be the time we packed up the car and brought him home; instead we were rushing to the next hospital to see him. The empty car seat in the car was a heavy reminder that everything was not okay.—Corin

I was able to stay in the hospital for four days after their birth. Going home was the hardest thing I think I've ever done, even though we lived only three miles away. I went home, showered, and came right back.—Susan B.

Leaving the babies behind in the hospital was uglier for Debbie than it was for me. . . . I suspect that's a typical dad response. I was much more concerned about Debbie's state of welfare than I was, certainly, about my state of welfare—and also I sort of felt as if the kids were in the best possible hands. Whatever happens, happens. I'm an eternal optimist, and I figured that they'd kind of be fine. But Debbie was in horrible shape, and I was concerned. I was preoccupied mostly with her distress. I was completely on call to calm her.—Mitch

I was very tired and not overly concerned with the separation as much as the uncertainty for the future—a lot of concern for the future, not knowing how it will turn out, but hopeful.—Chip

Whether your baby is in a NICU down the hall, across town, or in another city, separation from your baby often extracts an emotional price. For many parents, separation leads to feelings of detachment, especially in the early days after birth.

Feeling Detached from Your Baby

It took me some time to feel connected to my baby. I wasn't ready for him to be born. I wasn't ready to be a mother yet. I was expecting another three weeks to prepare mentally.—Liza

After recovering from delivery, I was taken back to my room. It was dark, probably midnight, and it felt creepy. I was numb and empty. I knew the girls were in the NICU, and I couldn't even imagine a way to get to them. They were simply inaccessible to me. It didn't occur to me to ask. I was just this empty, powerless creature on the bed.—Rikki

I knew she had just been removed from my body, but it still seemed unreal to me. While I was in recovery, my husband saw the baby in the NICU and returned crying. My parents saw her and returned crying. I remember feeling afraid to go to the NICU. When I finally went, my reaction was still one of unreality. Of course, she did not look at all like the baby I had envisioned. My dreams met reality that night in the NICU, and I just could not reconcile the two.—Renee

After the birth and hospitalization of their infant, many parents feel emotionally detached from their baby or the situation. There are many sources of this detachment, including disorientation, isolation, exhaustion, denial, a sense of loss, and, of course, separation from the baby. In short, feeling distant isn't evidence of failure but a natural reaction to this crisis.

Disorientation

When your baby needs intensive care, you make an abrupt transition from expectant family to parents of a critically ill newborn. It can be difficult to change gears rapidly enough to absorb the details of this reality. Many parents report feeling disoriented or, as Sandy remembers it, "feeling as if this was an out-of-body experience. How could this be happening?" It can seem as if you have been dropped, all alone, in the middle of the ocean without a boat. Shocked and disoriented, detachment ensues.

The first time I saw Jake, I was being wheeled back from the recovery room. I was still somewhat in shock from how quickly everything had happened. I was about as frightened as I had ever been in my life. I couldn't believe that was my baby.—Susie

All I remember is the activity in the operating room and the calm reports from the doctors. . . . Numbness set in quickly as I looked at the two tiniest faces I had ever seen gazing out at me as if in confusion. "Show her the baby," my doctor said as each one was examined and prepared for transport to the NICU. "Kiss her," she said each time to me, the stunned and paralyzed mother. That was the last I saw of them until 2:30 that morning, when I finally thought to ask if I could go to see my babies.—Rikki

They called me and said it was a boy, and I could see him through the window. He wasn't crying or anything, just kind of lying there, very small. It was like I was in a dream—this really wasn't happening; my wife's still pregnant in another room somewhere, but here, my son's lying here all hooked up to wires and stuff like that. That was a real, real drag.—Charlie

Many parents also have faith in modern medicine and assume their baby will recover easily and come home on schedule. Even when you know your baby is critically ill, it is disorienting if your baby struggles a lot more than you expected.

When they called at 5:00 AM and said Travis was getting sicker, I figured I'd get there, they'd work on him a little bit, and he'd be back to normal, you know, just like on the TV shows. I didn't know what was going on.—Charlie

I needed to think that they were just young, born early. Then a neonatologist said to me, "They are so sick," and I went ballistic. I told everyone, "I don't want her talking to me! It's a preemie thing; they are not sick. Don't say that to me!" I couldn't handle it.—Rikki

Isolation and Exhaustion

After delivery, when attention turns to the baby and all the action is in the NICU, the mother may feel suddenly abandoned and out of the loop. Michele recalls, "Plenty of times I wanted to pull out the IV and run to their sides. I didn't have the strength to do that, or I would have!" At the same time, pain and exhaustion can leave you numb and depleted. You may feel hesitant to go to the NICU, fearing what you'll see. And as mentioned earlier, medication side effects, your own recovery from birthing, or delivery complications can compromise your ability to be with your newborn. Diana remembers, "I was very tired and didn't want to deal with the situation."

Once the afterbirth was taken care of, I was left all alone in the room. That was the worst part. I didn't know anything. No one was there to calm my fears and hold my hand. Of course, everyone was concentrating on the baby—rightly so. Thankfully, they drugged me heavily. I had three transfusions as a result of blood loss. I don't remember a lot about the next few hours. Actually, that's about the time I began blocking a lot of things.—Cindy

After T.J. was born, he was quickly whisked off to the NICU. The respiratory team did stop by my bedside so that I could peer into his incubator and offer him my finger. He wrapped his little hand around my finger and squeezed. That was precious, but I longed to hold him and touch him. I remember feeling an incredible sense of loneliness when he left my womb and was immediately taken to the NICU. Most of all, I was exhausted both physically and emotionally.—Claire

Suddenly everyone was gone. I wanted to go too and was very frustrated when the nurses wouldn't let me get up to go to the nursery. I felt fine. Looking back on it now, I wasn't all right; I was in physical shock from the delivery and emotional denial from the whole event.—Andra

Postpartum was rough due to lack of sleep and a high level of stress. I don't ever remember being so exhausted in all my life.—Jennifer E.

I was on morphine for the next two days and was very foggy about a lot of things. I had a fever and was not allowed to go see the baby. Privately, I was thankful. I was terrified of seeing him. I had no idea what to expect. At the same time, I was terrified that he would die before I got to see him.—Laura

Fathers can feel isolated as well, detached and disbelieving.

Things aren't supposed to happen like this. One of the tougher initial feelings was in the recovery room after the C-section. My wife was still under the anesthesia. There were four couples in the room, and the other three had babies. It was a very separating and isolating feeling. I'll never forget it.—Preston

Denial

During a crisis, denial is a necessary and normal protective mechanism. Sudden, traumatic events and frightening information can be simply too much to take in all at once. Denial lets you hold out hope that everything will turn out okay. Detachment gives you a chance to recuperate and rebuild your emotional reserves. Disengagement from your baby lets you maintain objectivity and absorb difficult information at a reasonable pace.

I wanted to be there, but—and I don't know if I was finding excuses not to be there or if I had to go back to pump in my room—there was always something that made me not be there. It was too much to handle in the beginning.—Gallice

Life takes on a surreal quality as you gradually comprehend what is happening and start to envision what might lie ahead. You may appear to be taking things in stride because the enormity of it all hasn't hit you yet.

Looking back, you may remember just going through the motions without much feeling—or with overwhelming emotion hovering just beneath the surface—especially early on. As Michelle B. remembers, "I just wanted to curl up and cry." It takes time to wrap your mind around the situation—and reengage with your baby.

I was in denial of the whole experience, so I thought that the staff was out to make my baby look sicker than he actually was. I just laid there and told myself that he was going home in the morning. I told myself that every day for the next thirty-two days. I felt as if someone had ripped out my heart and given me a piece of paper with some baby's footprints on it in return.—Jenny

Just before Daphne was taken from the delivery room, Barry and I asked when we could next see her. In response we were told, "Even though your daughter looks stable now, she isn't. I have seen many children with her problem expire suddenly, so I give you no promises. We'll have someone tell you as soon as you can visit her." Again, I felt helpless. There was really nothing I could do about Daphne except pray that she wouldn't die. So I tried to emotionally detach myself from what was going on with her and instead tried to concentrate on what was happening with me.—Dina

My coping mechanism of choice was denial. I didn't think it was particularly serious that he was there. I acted as if he was there for observation and thought it would be a couple of hours. Only, the hours turned into days, and he was breathing with an oxygen tube and eating through an NG tube.—Liza

A Sense of Loss

If complications deprive you of a term pregnancy or a typical birthing, and when intensive care deprives you of your baby and your role, you feel a sense of loss. Instead of feeling connected and well-equipped to respond to your baby's needs, you feel bereft and uncertain. It takes time to adjust your expectations about parenthood and what will be asked of you as a mother or father. (For more on this sense of loss, see chapter 3; for more on coping and adjustment, see chapter 4.)

We glanced at him really quickly, my husband took a couple of pictures, and then he was gone. It's so strange because you just lie there and the room is so quiet and you're wondering what's happening, what's going on? It's a huge letdown because you're expecting more from the delivery of your baby.—Vickie

It took me about a week to get a grip on the fact that I had actually had a baby. I kept feeling as if I'd never been pregnant—or as if my baby had died. It just wasn't right to come home without your baby after giving birth. It probably wouldn't have been so bad if I'd been able to hold him.—Ami

The minute I was conscious after my twins were born, I wanted to be pregnant again. Even though I'd been sick beyond all imagining, even though I'd nearly died on more than one occasion, I wanted desperately to be pregnant again. The state of pregnancy had come so hard to me, it was so precious, so incredible. I couldn't believe it was over. I felt so empty, so ordinary.—Susan C.

It takes away the fairy tale. You know—you have a baby, everyone's happy, you pass out cigars, and the baby goes home and goes to sleep and you just give them your life.—Charlie

Separation

Naturally, you feel detached when your baby is taken away from you and placed into the care of strangers. After months of being intensely connected to the child in your womb, you are now barred from being present or involved in what's happening until you can make your way to the NICU.

If your baby must be transported to a distant NICU, this is an especially surreal and detaching aspect of your experience. The more prolonged the separation, the more detached you may feel. If more than a few hours pass before you can see your baby, you may feel as if you do not have a baby at all.

How could I have these negative feelings? How could I not want to see my baby? There were a lot of feelings of being cheated, and I stared at that picture [of the baby] a lot.—Kathy

When I was still pregnant, I knew firsthand what was going on with the babies, and the doctors had to go through me to monitor them. And then suddenly, I was all alone, and it didn't matter anymore. It was out of my hands. I had no more influence. I wasn't included because they were now completely separate from me. And I no longer held that illusory power to protect them. It felt horrible.—Rikki

It is a moment I'll never forget, lying in my hospital bed with Joe standing nearby listening to the helicopter taking Leo away. Joe and I just looked at each other and said, "What just happened? Are we really parents? Do we really have a son?" It was all very unreal.—Mindy

I had very severe complications after her birth and was in ICU for a long time myself. I guess that the first time I actually did get to see her without my mind being hazed out by drugs was when she was three weeks old. Even then I felt terrified and still denied that she could possibly be mine. My idea of babies was that they were big, seven to eight pounds, and healthy—not two pounds and struggling to live.—Jodi

Being discharged from the hospital without your baby can feel like the most devastating separation yet. Even if you knew your baby was likely to need special care, you probably didn't envision leaving the hospital with empty arms.

Going home without her was about the toughest thing of all. . . . You get this disconnected feeling, as if part of you isn't fully there. It's hard to describe.—Linda

It was weird to return home without my baby. I felt as if everything had changed, but when I returned to my apartment, it seemed as if everything was the same. I was at a loss. It was painful to look at the empty crib—I so longed to have it full.—Claire

Coming home was especially difficult. I knew I was leaving the most important piece of my life in the hospital. Some friends had decorated our house with It's a Boy decorations. . . . I don't know if that made it easier or harder. It was very depressing.—Misty

Going home was the worst. Instead of leaving the hospital in a wheelchair holding my baby—like you see in the movies, and like I saw every day when I went to visit my son in the NICU—I left in a wheelchair by myself. It was almost like I didn't have a baby or like my baby had died.—Sally

I can't even begin to tell you how terrible it is to have to go home without your child, not knowing if you'll ever see him again.—Dawn

You may feel strange entering your home without the baby who has accompanied you everywhere for months. Instead of carrying a baby in your womb or in your arms, you are carrying a heavy emotional burden.

I firmly believe that leaving the hospital that day (and I stayed as many days as they would allow me) was the hardest thing I had to do. I was discharged with three other mothers, all of whom had their babies with them—big, healthy, fat newborns—and mine was still upstairs hooked up to machines that he couldn't live without. And I was being forced to leave him. I can't think of anything that was as hard.—Sterling

Even though I knew my chances of having the babies in the NICU were about 95 percent, I hoped throughout my pregnancy that I would take them home with me. When I went home without them, I didn't feel like a good parent. I felt like I was leaving them behind. I felt great guilt rather than the joy I had anticipated.—Jill

Debbie was being discharged the day after the kids were born, and it was very ugly because here, you're carrying twins, you give birth to your twins, and you come home with nothing. . . . We had the feeling of, like, a close family member had died—it was like coming home after a funeral instead of coming home after giving birth.—Mitch

Your discharge may also bring you some relief. After all, your home is probably more comfortable than a hospital room. Especially early on, when the NICU is so overwhelming and you don't feel at ease with your baby, being able to retreat to your home for rest and respite may not be all bad. It is normal both to wish for more closeness with your baby and to appreciate your freedom to leave the hospital. Separation can be both agony and a relief.

I was discharged just thirty-six hours after his birth. It was so hard to tear myself away from that warming table. I knew that as soon as I left, he would go downhill again. I didn't want to leave, but I didn't want to stay.—Jayna

Going home was almost okay because I had spent about ten days in the hospital. I couldn't stand to see mothers and babies going home together. It hurt. So I yearned [for the babies] from the safety of my home. I was still too emotionally drained to think too much about anything else. I only rolled with what life was throwing my way.—Rosa

As you reorient, recover your strength, grasp reality, and adjust, you will be able to spend more and more quality time in the NICU. You can reengage with your little one—even though it'll be in ways you never imagined—and feelings of detachment will naturally fade. As you become acquainted, you will learn how to respond to your baby's cues and carry out many caregiving tasks—and enjoy the accompanying feelings of devotion and pleasure. Your confidence will grow, which in turn will reinforce your bond. (See chapters 5, 6, and 7 for more on adapting to the NICU, feeling like a parent, and getting close to your baby.)

Until then, dare to get close to your little one, so you can bask in even the faintest glimmers of connection that exist between you and your baby.

The first time I was watching him, I recognized all the little baby movements that were inside of me just a short while ago, and I got excited because I could tell he was my baby.—Ruby

I think he looked better than I expected him to look because, of course, I was very scared of finding him disgusting and repulsive and of not being able to get attached to him. The first time I saw him, I thought he looked so tiny and skinny, but he was not repulsive, not at all. The first day, I already found him cute and good-looking, and I was in love with him right away.—Gallice

We didn't get to hold him for a few days, but I remember sticking my hand under that plastic wrap and stroking him and touching him and just seeing how beautiful he was. And just—he was mine. That's what I couldn't believe, mostly. I felt like a parent when I could see him—not after I delivered and not while in that hospital room. That's the most empty thing, when you can't see that baby. What does it is going to the baby and sitting by that baby's bedside in the NICU. You just want to tell all the other parents, "This is my baby!"—Vickie

Points to Remember

· *When a newborn needs intensive care, parents are still primed to focus their devotion and care on their baby. That's why separation feels so heart-wrenching and disruptive.*

· *Whether you ache to have your baby with you or feel detached and wish you didn't, you are grappling with the painful feelings of separation that come with having a baby in the NICU.*

· *Feeling detached is a natural result of disorientation, isolation and exhaustion, denial, deprivation, and, of course, separation from your baby.*

· *As you reorient, recover, and adjust, you will be able to get to know your little one, feel closer, and form a meaningful connection.*

3:

The Emotional Landscape

I thought, *He's actually alive. Now what?* I had tried desperately to prepare myself for my son's simultaneous birth/death. But he was alive, and I was incredibly shocked and horribly scared. I felt terrible for not having the faith in my son's strength to live but was incredibly fearful of the impending outcome/pain he would endure.—Andrea

When your baby needs intensive care, you experience many emotions. You fear for what will be, and you mourn for all that might have been.

Grief is at the emotional core of this journey and encompasses all your painful feelings, including sorrow, detachment, fear, frustration, and regret. You may even begin to grieve before your baby is born: anticipatory grief is a normal reaction to the uncertainties that surround high-risk pregnancy, preterm labor, or prenatal diagnosis. Your grief may persist after you bring your baby home, when your parenting experience does not match the one you had envisioned. Many parents continue to be affected by this rough start whether their child is or not.

Fortunately, grief isn't the only element of this experience. Love, joy, and hope are also at the emotional core, and you can have many times of delight, wonder, and devotion. As such, you are likely to experience wildly opposing emotions as sadness and happiness mix with other profound feelings.

Understanding this emotional landscape of grief and joy gives you a context in which your feelings and reactions can make sense to you. Although facing your feelings means confronting your pain, it also allows you to experience your pleasure and boosts your coping, healing, and growth.

A Mix of Emotions

I saw my baby for a split second. It was the happiest and saddest moment of my life. I was the proudest mother in the world; I was also so scared for this poor, innocent little baby who needed so much more time in his mother. My husband and I glowed . . . but it was a sad glow.—Misty

She was so tiny. I was just sitting there looking at her. I was thinking, *Oh, my God, that's my baby.* I was just really afraid. . . . She didn't look like a real baby but like a medical experiment gone awry. She looked absolutely horrible. She wasn't moving at all, except for her chest going up and down. But she was also really beautiful. I liked the way her mouth and chin looked. It was just so cute.—Brooke

Bewilderment comes to mind. I couldn't quite get my mind around the fact that he was finally here. I couldn't quite take in that he was so fragile. I couldn't figure out the turmoil of emotions rolling around inside. I was wrung with tenderness for this little delicate creature. I wanted to hold him to my face and feel his skin and envelop him with kisses. I wanted to smell his skin and stroke his face while I studied his features. I wanted to play with his hands. I wanted to experience his presence and I couldn't. I was numb and I was on fire at the same time. I was panicked and exhilarated. I was living a paradox of emotions.—Laurie

You get this honeymoon, the first twenty-four hours [after delivery], and the kids are coasting on all their juices from mom, and they're doing pretty good. They're intubated, but we were told that they were doing fine and there was a little while of joy. And then that wore off, and it wore off quite quickly. By that evening, things had definitely become sad. I had a cot in the room where Debbie was staying, and I'm not real big on crying, but I remember lying there crying because I knew—and I don't know how I knew or what I knew exactly—that surely we were in for some serious trouble. And so it was really hitting me at this point. So this joy we had, this joy over the excitement of having twins, lasted for an hour before it came to an end, and then it was bad.—Mitch

Even though intense feelings of disappointment and fear can overcome your hopes and dreams, your hopes and dreams are still there, and so you vacillate. Should you celebrate or mourn?

Many people had a hard time facing the babies; they didn't look like babies. And people didn't know what to do. We didn't get cards or gifts or flowers. I was shocked by this lack of acknowledgment about the birth of my babies. My mom explained that friends and families didn't know whether to say "Congratulations" or "I'm sorry." They were afraid to send gifts or cards in case the worst happened before the present arrived. My husband said to my mom, who was our point of contact with the outside world: "You tell everyone one that Isaac and Molly are here. This is the one and only life they will ever have, and whether they live for ninety days or ninety years, we intend to celebrate." From that point on, everything seemed to make sense, at least to us.—Susan B.

This situation calls for both celebration and mourning, but feeling such opposing emotions can be unsettling, confusing, and exhausting. For instance:

- You may fear the worst, but being too frightened to consider the possibilities, you try to remain positive and hopeful.

- You feel confident everything will turn out okay, but your worries make you uncertain.

- Your feelings of joy upon your baby's birth and survival are coupled with sadness for what you and your baby have lost.

- You may feel guilty that *somehow* you must have contributed to your baby's current condition, even though rationally you know you are not responsible for it.

- You may want to be in charge of overseeing your baby's care yet feel powerless to control what happens in the NICU.

- Although you long for your baby, you may resist going to the NICU because you dread what you will see or fear how you will react.

- You may feel devoted to your baby's best interests but feel emotionally detached.

- You may resent the NICU or certain medical professionals yet feel eternal gratitude for the technology and the skilled and dedicated staff who are working to save your baby's life.

- You may pity the families whose babies are doing worse than yours and envy those whose babies are doing better.

- You may love your baby but hate the situation.

Although seesawing between divergent emotions can be jarring, you're experiencing a normal, naturally complex reaction to a complex situation.

I saw Daphne for only a few moments right after birth. Once she was in the hands of the doctors, in one way, I felt somewhat relieved because my job was over. I had done all I could for my daughter. At the same time, though, I felt very anxious because I did not know what was going on and I did not know whether, despite all my efforts, my daughter would even survive. Finally, I remember feeling very tired and wishing that I could just go to sleep, which I didn't because of my fear for my daughter.—Dina

It is also normal to experience discordant reactions, where the intensity of your emotions does not match the intensity of the situation. For example, especially early on or during sudden crisis, instead of feeling alarmed you are likely to feel numb.

It all happened so fast, really, that I couldn't keep up. My thoughts, my reactions, my emotions—I just couldn't swallow it all. It almost seemed like a dream sequence. The neonatologist visited me while I was in labor to inform me of what circumstances we would be facing. He told me there was a fifty-fifty chance she would die and, if she lived, a fifty-fifty chance she would be severely damaged in some way. I just couldn't get my mind around it. I was devastated, but it all seemed so unreal. It was so sudden and unexpected.—Renee

During the ultrasound, I could tell immediately something was wrong. My funny, fun-loving doctor was serious and straight-faced. I thought the worst. Then he said, "I am not finding a flow in the umbilical cord of baby A." My heart sank. I was quiet, waiting for him to say something. He just kept looking and looking. I said, "What does that mean?" He said that the flow was diminished and the baby was not getting enough nutrition. I honestly thought that no flow would have meant the baby had died and was getting no oxygen. I was being incredibly calm, now that I look back at it.—Pamela

I zoned out. I went numb and stayed numb for a very long time. I was dealing with the most traumatic event of my life. . . . I had feelings, but looking back . . . I was a zombie.—Misty

You may look back in disbelief or embarrassment for being so naive, so in shock, so in denial. But even NICU doctors and nurses, when their own babies are admitted to intensive care, report utter disbelief and uncertainty, and they grieve like any other parent in the NICU. No amount of medical experience or knowledge can spare a parent from the emotional trauma. Dianne, a highly skilled neonatal nurse practitioner, describes her reactions:

I was terrified, along with my husband. Things happened very quickly. Our baby cried, we cried, and the journey began. Her delivery was late at night, and I was drugged, so I didn't see her until the next day. I woke up very distraught and cried uncontrollably while answering the phone calls from friends and family. . . . I'll never forget when I saw the name tag over her bed with our last name on it—I wasn't sure if I could withstand the fear, sadness, and guilt I felt, still trying to comprehend how this could be happening to me. What will tomorrow bring?—Dianne

Soon enough the shock starts to wear off, and throughout your journey you may alternate between numbness and feeling overcome with emotion. Sometimes a seemingly insignificant event will trigger a flood. If you're the mother, your postpartum hormonal fluctuations may contribute to your sense of emotional instability.

On the third day, I was wheeled down to the NICU. I didn't notice any of the thirty other babies I passed. I was in a haze. But when I saw my son, I immediately fell in love with him. I cried, but I don't know why. I just remember being very hot and weak and woozy.—Laura

When they were born, I refused to leave the hospital. I thought they would die, so I wanted to spend every moment they were alive with them. (At least I think that's what I was feeling. I just know I couldn't leave them. They needed me, and I needed them.) After many days, my mother-in-law and mother talked me into getting some fresh air. Of course, what we saw as we walked outside were new parents video-taping taking their new baby home. I lost it at that moment, and maybe for the first time, I was really able to cry.—Stephie

Emotional storms and calms are a normal part of weathering your baby's complicated start. It is normal to feel crazy amidst the chaos, but you won't feel this way forever. Here are some initial coping strategies. (You'll find lots more in chapter 4.)

· *Find out what happened.* Knowledge has a healing effect as it helps you understand and make sense of the situation. If you don't have clear memories, ask your obstetric team and your baby's medical practitioners to fill in the gaps. Request medical records: the written play-by-play can clarify what you and your baby have gone through. Knowledge restores your feelings of control and mastery in the face of the unexpected.

- *Learn about your baby's condition.* Another way to seek mastery is to learn everything you can about your baby's condition and treatments. In fact, you may feel an obsessive need to immerse yourself in the medical literature or parent blogs and Listservs. This is normal and a way to assuage feelings of powerlessness.

One thing that did help was information. I was fortunate (or stubborn) enough to find doctors who gave me information about Stephen, and I looked up everything about him. It was as though the more I knew, the more I felt some sense of control in the completely uncontrollable situation.—Tracy

- *Let your numbness work for you.* Detachment gives you the time you need to absorb and comprehend traumatic events.

- *Accept the wide range of your emotions.* This is a complicated journey that calls for a number of feelings and reactions.

- *Take care of yourself physically.* If your body is strong, your ability to cope becomes stronger too. Attention to physical needs is especially important to ensure the mother's recovery from pregnancy and birth.

- *Accept your partner's reactions.* Expect them to differ from your own much of the time. Your emotional highs and lows are also likely to be out of sync. Still, you will experience many of the same feelings as you navigate this emotional terrain.

The remainder of this chapter focuses on your sense of loss and your grief, illuminating the emotional landscape of the NICU journey.

A Mosaic of Losses

On the second night of my stay in the hospital, I was lying in bed, trying to sleep. On either side of me, I could hear babies crying and the enthusiastic "Oh, he's so cute" from nurses and families. Alone in my bed, I felt my hand stray to my stomach, so recently purged of its little occupant. I felt then that I had lost on two planes: my baby was no longer inside me, but he wasn't physically near me either.—Claire

Having a baby in the NICU is associated with many complicated losses. Perhaps you've lost the last weeks of your pregnancy, that time you were counting on to prepare for the arrival of your baby. You may not be able to experience the gentle birth you were wishing for. You lose the precious moments you may have fantasized about for months—meeting, cuddling, and nursing your newborn. You lose the pride, glory, and celebration that usually accompany the birth of a baby. Instead, you find yourself going home with empty arms. As Gallice notes sadly, "It is so hard to leave without the baby. You're broken—just broken."

I felt like I had lost my pregnancy. I had just started to show and had recently bought new maternity clothes that I never got to wear. I was looking forward to looking pregnant. It was my turn to be pampered and doted on. I didn't have a baby to bring home either. Not that we were ready for a baby. There had been no shower yet. There was no baby's room.—Laura

I really grieved the loss of the normal birth experience. I wanted desperately to know what it was like to have a baby placed on my chest after Ayla was born. I wanted to know what those first moments should feel like and be able to put a baby to my breast and know that instant love and joy everyone associates with the miracle of childbirth. I missed that bonding experience that you expect to get those first few days.—Corin

I lost the beautiful birth at home that I had in mind. I lost the first two weeks of my son's life.—Ruby

I think I missed out most on breast-feeding. While my baby was in the NICU, they wouldn't let me nurse him because he was on oxygen. I grieved for that the most.—Liza

I got in the car and cried all the way home. My husband tried to console me, but all I could think of was that I had just left my only son in the hands of strangers, and he was less than one day old. We got home, and I greeted my two daughters with little enthusiasm, even though I hadn't been home with them in almost a month. All I could think of was getting Ricky home with us. It consumed my every moment, even the few that I slept.—Jenny

Returning to the hospital to gaze at your infant through the barriers of incubator, tubes, tape, and wires, you may wonder how you can possibly comfort and get to know your tiny, often unresponsive baby. You may also grieve for what you perceive to be your baby's losses: the loss of the warmth and safety of your womb, the loss of your touch, the loss of innocence that results from being poked and prodded under bright lights. You may feel helpless to ease your baby's struggles.

After I was in the recovery room, they wheeled me into the NICU, and I saw him for the first time—I saw him the way I would come to know him. He was so tiny and frail. I started to cry. I was terrified. A nurse came over to tell the doctors or me that he was doing good, but I didn't even hear her. I was in my own little world. I just wanted him to be a "normal" baby.—Lori

Brand-new babies aren't supposed to need intensive care. Parents' arms are supposed to be enough.—Rikki

Losses big and small can accumulate over the days, weeks, or months your infant spends in the NICU. You might feel a loss of community because your friends and other new parents don't understand what your baby is going through and what this experience is like for you. Holidays and family occasions can be painful because they aren't the way you had imagined them to be.

You may also keenly miss the chance to be consistently involved in your little one's everyday life, both the ordinary and the special. You may feel as if the nurses are stealing such milestones as the first bath or diaper change. However insignificant particular milestones may seem to others, they can be immensely important to parents in the NICU. Whatever activities and opportunities you hold central to the parenting role, those are the ones you'll miss the most.

I noticed one day that a nurse had clipped his fingernails. I felt angry that it wasn't me clipping his nails and that I had lost that time to do those things for my son.—Ruby

I feel like I missed out on a lot of things. I couldn't hold my baby right away. I couldn't do kangaroo care early on, even though all of the parenting books said it was really important for a child's development. I missed out on bonding with her sooner (better) and on using any of the 0–3 month clothing I had for her at home. I missed out on participating in a religious naming ceremony for her.

I grieved over not being able to put Daphne to breast right away so that she could benefit from the colostrum in my milk. Instead, I had to use an electric pump for months to keep my milk flowing at an adequate level. I grieved over having to struggle to bond with my daughter when, in normal circumstances, there would have been no issue if I could have just held her, stroked her, nursed her, and loved her the way a mother should from day one.—Dina

Furthermore, you've lost your innocence. This experience can undermine your beliefs about life, safety, goodness, and health. You may question your religious convictions, your faith in medical technology, or your trust in medical practitioners. You may struggle with feelings of vulnerability as you come to realize that you don't have as much control over your life as you once thought you did. Your sense of confidence or grounding can be shaken as you peer into an uncertain future. Eventually, you will modify your philosophies and adjust your expectations. But in the beginning, losing your sense of safety and control can be most unnerving. If you've experienced traumatic loss in the past, you may have especially strong feelings of dread ("Oh, no, not again") or hopelessness ("There's nothing I can do to fix it").

I did not see any change in my role as a father, but what did come out of it was a recognition that the medical establishment does not necessarily do things for the benefit of the patient, nor is it as scientific as I had previously thought.—Marco

Since the birth, I have felt tremendous loss in many areas. "How it's supposed to be" is rather broad and covers all of the losses. But that's it in a nutshell. We lost "how it's supposed to be."—Cindy

Whatever your situation, you have a long list of losses to acknowledge. Pinpointing your losses can make your grief seem more manageable, as you can understand why you are grieving and feel entitled to your reactions.

To most parents, newborn babies elicit thoughts of soft blankets, sweet-smelling skin, spit-up, diapers, cooing and giggles, and lack of sleep. My newborn memories include hours watching my tiny son paralyzed by drugs, aware but unable to respond, to avoid the expenditure of calories he could ill afford to waste kicking his legs or waving his arms. I remember learning about pulse ox and brain bleeds and perforated bowels. My newborn memories include medical discussions of how to wean my morphine-addicted infant once the painkiller was no longer required. While other new parents learned to change diapers, we learned to change the adhesive bag covering his ileostomy.—Susan C.

The Grieving Process

Grieving is the process of acknowledging your losses, letting your feelings and reactions flow, and seeking comfort and meaning. Throughout this process, you can gradually let go of what might have been and adjust to what is. Grieving is ultimately how you can adjust to your baby's hospitalization and challenging start. As you cope and adjust, you heal.

Grief encompasses many painful feelings, including sadness, anger, guilt, fear, worry, and powerlessness. You may also experience physical symptoms, such as fatigue, sleeplessness, sighing, poor appetite, crying spells, shortness of breath, tightness in the throat or stomach, clenched jaw, and heart palpitations.

When our baby was in the NICU, my predominant emotion was anxiety. It was hard not to worry. I felt guilty initially, wondering if I should have gone to the hospital sooner, and so on. I also felt a little angry that my doctors hadn't hospitalized me when the bleeding didn't stop. I mostly felt bad for my daughter, feeling that she had done nothing to deserve this, and here she was, put in this terrible situation.—Mary

I cried my eyes out. I felt faint, extremely scared, and guilty for bringing such a small, frail, innocent child into this situation that I really had no control over. I was so scared to love her because I truly felt that she would not make it. She was so tiny. Her skin was almost transparent. There were so many machines, tubes, IVs, beeps, and buzzes. She was so small that I thought there was absolutely no way she could survive without the grace of God. She was so helpless looking. I even questioned myself about why I didn't have an abortion at the beginning of my complicated pregnancy. I felt like a complete failure. I questioned why I could not have a normal pregnancy and birth like other women. I felt cheated and very hurt, but above all I felt the greatest sense of fear I have ever felt in my whole life!—Jillian

Grief is a fluid experience that follows no predictable order or timetable. There is no right or wrong way to grieve, and you may experience a wide range of feelings and physical symptoms or a narrow range. Your reactions will ebb and flow, and as the initial shock wears off, you will probably feel worse rather than better for a time. This can be disheartening, but gradually the ups will become more frequent and the downs fewer and more gentle.

You are also likely to experience anniversary reactions. Early on, you may feel most unsettled or sad at certain times of the day or week. Later on, you may notice that you feel especially blue at certain times of the month or year. It's as if your body remembers and associates certain conditions with your pregnancy, your baby's birth, and the

NICU stay. Acknowledging these anniversaries can help you make sense of your reactions.

Eventually, you'll reach a point where you can accept what happened and acquire a sense of peace. Even if your child has ongoing challenges, you can still get to this place of contentment. Your sorrow doesn't completely disappear, but as you get to know and love your baby, joy can become more prominent. Whatever the outcome, your bond with your baby can be a source of comfort and healing.

I have good days and I have bad days. It is nice for me to know that as time goes on, the bad days are fewer and farther between. I felt more numbness while it was going on than I do now. Sometimes the flashbacks and intense feelings of it happening again are more than I can handle. I am so thankful that my husband is as understanding and open about this situation as he is. I think about everything much more than we talk about it. The week after I got home was a very tough week for me. Everything hit. Then there was a time soon after Alison was discharged that I just wanted to forget about the whole thing and for no one to talk about it. I had a desire just to go on with life. I still find myself looking at Alison and wondering how we both made it through this and saying a prayer of thanksgiving that we did. Everything took its toll, but it is getting easier as time goes on.—Stacy

As you travel this path, you may survey the emotional landscape and wonder how you'll ever make it through. When your grief knows no bounds, peace feels so far away. But even in the depths of your despair, you are gradually letting go of what might have been and adjusting to new realities. Even though you may repeatedly revisit painful feelings, you are not in the same place. Each time, you'll grieve in different ways, from different perspectives. It may feel like regression, but it's actually a healing progression. Even as you grieve, you are healing. (See chapter 11 for additional insights on healing and transformation.)

Common Feelings of Grief

Typical feelings of grief include:

- Shock, including numbness, denial, confusion, detachment

- Sadness, including sorrow, hurt, anguish

- Fear, including worry, anxiety

- Yearning, including longing, wishing

· Guilt, including regret, responsibility

· Failure, including incompetence, inadequacy, defeat

· Powerlessness, including hopelessness, vulnerability

· Anger, including envy, resentment, frustration, irritability

You may feel overcome by some or all of these painful feelings associated with grief. Parents in the NICU especially struggle with emotions associated with yearning, worry, guilt, powerlessness, and anger.

Although you may feel discouraged by this long list of painful emotions, you can also feel affirmed. Having a baby in the NICU poses a number of exceptional challenges, and your feelings and reactions are natural responses to a distressing situation. The following descriptions can help you recognize and acknowledge the emotions that make up your grief.

Shock
As discussed earlier, particularly immediately after hearing bad news, you may feel as though you are numb with shock. The full scope of reality may not sink in for several days or longer. As your disbelief, confusion, and denial fade, you can get a handle on the situation, and other painful feelings of grief will arise. Still, throughout the following months—or longer if your baby has ongoing medical problems or emerging developmental challenges—it is normal to have occasional brief periods of shock and the associated detachment. (For dealing with persistent numbness/detachment, see chapter 5.)

I was on automatic, I think. People would come in, and I would laugh and joke with the nurses and the doctors. But it wasn't really me. I wasn't feeling anything. I would go down and look at my daughter, and talk to her doctor and find out information, and file it back into my brain without letting it go through any emotions first.—Brooke

I didn't know what I was supposed to do, how I was supposed to feel, or even what I felt. I wanted to hide, to run away, and yet I couldn't. I wanted to cry and scream and keen, yet the tears wouldn't come. I wanted to mourn and grieve, but no one had died, nothing was gone, except my dreams—and how could I sob for lost dreams when my baby was fighting for life? I was lost and alone.—Leanne

Sadness
You may feel overcome with sorrow for what you've lost and agonize

over what you and your baby must endure—hospitalization, prolonged separation, and perhaps a perilous medical course.

As soon as the doctor left the room, I began to cry. Not because I was scared but because I knew that my girls would literally have to fight for their lives. I knew deep down that I should have been expecting the worst. Instead, I tried to think positive and hope that nothing would go wrong. The nurse assistants kept telling me not to worry, but I wasn't worried, only sad. Sad that they would not have a good chance.—Rosa

I can remember the day, going in to see him all hooked up to the vent. My wife about passed out, and I just fought it back, but the tears welled up inside me. Geoffrey recovered and was out a few months later, but every time I think back I realize just how he almost did not make it and how short his life could have been. . . . One thinks of our children as being invincible, and to see a young baby who has so much of his life to look forward to teetering on the edge of life was very difficult for me.—Shaw

Fear

When your newborn is in the NICU, it's only fitting that you should be anxious for your baby's well-being. What you may be unprepared for is the intensity of your worry. If your baby remains in critical condition, fear is a constant companion. As you peer at your baby surrounded by the wonders and coldness of medical technology, you may feel alternately grateful for what medicine can do and fearful for what it cannot.

I hated every time the phone rang for fear that the hospital was calling with bad news.—Susan B.

I was most afraid of losing myself in my fear. I was afraid of any and all of the complications we were told to expect. I was afraid of how difficult it would be to have my daughter in the hospital for at least 2 to 3 months after delivery, assuming everything went well. I was afraid of what the stress of losing a child after fighting so hard to have her would mean to me, my marriage, and my son.—Dina

I was afraid of death. I remember walking around the mall, looking at doll clothes, and thinking what I'd have to bury my babies in. The thought that I might have to do that was just, really, really unbelievable.—Stephie

There are few guarantees in the NICU. If you tend to be a worrier, or if you are uncomfortable with uncertainty or loose ends, the unknowns will be doubly hard for you to bear. If you mistrust the care your baby is receiving or modern medical technology itself, this is likely to heighten your anxiety. That's why early on, before you've come to know and believe in the nurses or the treatments, you may feel compelled to stand guard over your little one. If developmental or medical problems persist beyond the NICU, your worries will persist as well.

Yearning

You may yearn to recover your hopes and expectations, to go back to the path you'd planned. Longing to hold your baby close is a natural aspect of parenting, but when your baby's fragile condition or NICU's policies thwart this desire, this longing becomes another source of grief.

I didn't want more drugs [painkillers after delivery], I just wanted my baby. I spent most of the day crying and staring at the pictures of him.—Tracy

I was terrified . . . and so sad. I wanted to hold him, but at the same time I didn't. But I do know that when they wheeled him out of the delivery room, it felt as if they were tearing off a piece of me as they left.—Sterling

Guilt

I just knew I had to have done something to cause this to happen. It had to be my fault because I'm his mommy and my job was to protect him from everything. And if I couldn't even protect him before he was born, how was I going to protect him now?—Ami

Feelings of guilt arise from your normal sense of parental responsibility. Intense helplessness can be triggered when it's not possible to protect your baby from everything. But rather than lose yourself in what might be overwhelming and frightening helplessness, you may instead wonder what you did or didn't do that contributed to your baby's plight.

I had these immense feelings of guilt as if somehow I had failed her. She had to come out before she was ready, and I should have done something to stop it. Those feelings are still there. I just cannot shake the thought that maybe I could have stopped my labor. She has endured so much pain, and there was nothing that I could do to stop it. Had she been born at the right time, she would have been saved all this trauma.—Moni

There's this guilt that will probably never leave me. That's so big at the beginning. You just can't help feeling guilty, so guilty. This guilt that you're the mother and you weren't able to keep him inside. You're the only one to blame because—well, actually you're not the only one to blame, but at that point, you think you are the only one to blame. It takes a long time to get over that.—Gallice

It is particularly common for the mother, despite assurances to the contrary, to feel responsible on some level when her baby is born early or with problems. You may wonder, *Why didn't I know something was wrong?* Or, *What kind of a mother can't protect her baby from harm?* You may wonder what role you, your decisions, or your body played. Even fathers wonder about their own contributions.

I felt guilty because although Barry and I were told over and over that CDH can happen for no apparent reason at all, I still felt like it was somehow my fault that this was happening. Maybe there was something wrong with me. Even if there wasn't, Barry and I now had to face this challenge because when I had lost pregnancy after pregnancy, I never took the hint that maybe I shouldn't keep trying to get pregnant.—Dina

As a dad, I often wondered if I had wished too hard for a son. I had gotten my wish, yes, but look at the situation he was in. I felt guilty about that.—Shaw

You may agonize over what you could have done differently. Even if you know in your heart that you took the best actions and made the best decisions you could, lingering beliefs about your responsibility can spawn feelings of guilt. You may blame yourself for your child's suffering or outcome.

I felt a lot of guilt that my children were born so early. Intellectually, I knew I had done everything possible to give the girls a chance, but emotionally, I still felt the guilt.—Kimberly

We both lived in guilt. [My husband] for being a doctor and not seeing that my pregnancy was in trouble and not getting me help when I needed it (even though he is not an ob-gyn and could not have known). Mine for "allowing" myself to give birth so early.—Raquel

Many parents also feel directly responsible for exposing their baby to the harsh conditions of the NICU. There's just no comparison between where your baby is and where your baby is supposed to be. If your infant's prognosis is poor or uncertain, you may face life-and-death decisions and feel especially responsible for the outcome. Guilt can accompany any regrets you may have. (For more on difficult decisions and regrets, see "Advocating for your Baby" in chapter 5 and "Making Medical Decisions in the Gray Zone" in chapter 9.)

You go to the hospital to have a baby, and then you come home without your child. . . . All I remember is crying all the way home and feeling guilty as I left my baby behind. It seemed to me as if I was abandoning her.—Jodi

We didn't spend much time in the NICU following the baptism because I was overcome with sheer exhaustion, and it was suggested to me that I go up to my room and get some rest before it was time to say good-bye to our daughter. I have turned that decision over in my mind: why didn't I insist that I spend every second I could by my little girl's side? Especially knowing that we had such a short time with her. Why didn't I push through the exhaustion and just stay with her?—Angie

Guilt is the agony of anger and blame turned inward and is often accompanied by feelings of failure. Guilt is a way to hold onto the illusion that you have control over the uncontrollable. It's a way to try to make sense of the senseless.

I felt like I hated everyone, but mostly myself. I had let this happen to my baby. How could I be so helpless?—Jenny

I felt extremely guilty. I had no one to blame, so I blamed myself. Then I blamed the doctors, my husband, even God. I just couldn't make sense of any of it.—Jayna

I felt both guilty and like a failure. What did I do to cause my baby's early birth? He has to go through so much, and I didn't even feel pain from delivering. I still wonder if I did something wrong.—Cynthia

Failure
Related to guilt, feelings of failure arise from the belief that you should be able to accomplish the tasks of pregnancy and birthing a healthy baby. Like many mothers, you may feel a sense of failure when you have a complicated pregnancy or birth or bear a baby who needs intensive care. If you're the father, you may believe that your fragile newborn is a

sign of your paternal incompetence. Your fatherly pride and confidence may feel deeply wounded over your belief that you failed to safeguard your family, adding to any perception of "second-rate" fatherhood.

We were having a little boy. I was a proud papa-to-be. A son at last. Well, the night Linda went in to premature labor, I thought that pride would be dashed. I knew the chance of survival was slim. . . . Small and so frail, he fought with everything he had. To see him all hooked up—translucent skin, so tiny—it really hurt.—Shaw

I remember a lot of the nurses congratulating me for the birth of my son, and I just didn't get it. . . . It didn't feel like I should be congratulated; I felt like I had completely failed as a mother.—Corin

I felt like such a failure as a mother. I had failed to protect them. I also had two other children who were crying at home for me as well. I felt so torn. I didn't want to leave either place.—Miriam

Feelings of failure often arise in the NICU as you struggle to find your place as your baby's parent. You may wonder if your baby's need for intensive care is a reflection of your incompetence or a sign that you don't deserve to be a mother or a father. As you watch medical practitioners provide for your baby, you may feel inadequate and incompetent, which in turn can contribute to feeling detached from your little one. Naturally, feelings of failure can be intertwined with feelings of responsibility and guilt.

The biggest thing I felt was inadequacy. Every time one of his alarms beeped, I felt as if I had done something wrong. I was petrified that I was holding him the wrong way or that he would stop breathing on me. Once, I was holding him while he struggled to come back from an apnea. I was devastated because I couldn't help him and felt as if it was my fault that it had happened. It was a stressful situation, different each day.—Claire

I felt like I had failed, like I was a failure. I'd tried so hard, but I didn't get it right; I didn't get to finish it. The sense of loss and incompletion was overwhelming. I didn't think I could become pregnant again, knew that I would never undergo infertility treatments again, knew I would never have the joy of telling people I was carrying twins again. I was mourning all of this at the same time that I was mourning for my tiny, wounded boys. I can't possibly explain the grief and guilt I felt—I still feel—at not being able to protect them, to keep them inside and away from the incredible pain they were suffering because I wasn't strong enough, because my body failed them. I desperately wanted to have another chance to get it right.—Susan C.

Powerlessness
I never felt as if I had control over my body with respect to the pregnancy. It controlled me.—Cindy

I wonder what kind of father would allow this to happen to his family.—Jeff

As your baby's arrival spins out of your control, you are likely to feel entirely powerless. The NICU is disorienting with its technology. The unfamiliar medical terminology can render you helpless. There's so much you've yet to learn about your baby's condition. Even as you adjust to the NICU, you may feel powerless as a parent, unable to step in and meet your baby's complex needs. When you experience your newborn only through the porthole of intensive care, it is natural to feel discouraged. You may be reluctant to exert what little control you have, not realizing that you have a significant say in your baby's care and can have a profound impact on your little one's recovery.

You may also feel powerless to protect your little one from invasive or painful medical procedures. These treatments are necessary, but they seem so rough. During intense crisis, you cannot step in as a protector, the most basic of parenting jobs.

At the age of three weeks, Seleste coded for the first time. . . . Within a minute or two, they started doing CPR—and I've never seen anything so brutal in all my life. . . . There were two things on my mind: One, *I've got to stay under control so they don't kick me out of here. I want to be here.* And two, *Stop, stop, you're torturing her!!!* It just looked so inhumane.—Suzanne

You may also feel powerless in the face of so many uncertainties. There is no way for you to ensure that your baby's hospital stay will be short and without crisis and that he or she will emerge normal and healthy. If your child continues to need hospitalization, therapies, surgeries, equipment, or special-education services, you pass through one foreign land after another. With each new challenge, it is natural to feel helpless initially. Mastery takes time and practice.

The worst part is that you have absolutely no control over anything. You do not make decisions about how your own child sleeps, eats, dresses, and so forth. But most of all, you cannot just wave a magic wand and make it all go away. You simply do not have that choice.—Jen

I had no expectations left. Every dream that I had was ruined.—Stacy

Even if your child's hospital course, health, growth, and development are relatively uncomplicated, you may still feel vulnerable and unsure. The initial separation and the losses it brings can leave you shaken even if no additional traumas follow.

Anger

Anger often accompanies feelings of isolation, powerlessness, fear, guilt, and failure. You may be angry that no one understands, upset that there's nothing you can do to improve the situation, distressed about your baby's prognosis, frustrated at the uncertainties, and, if you're the mother, mad at yourself or your body. Your physical fatigue, stress, or illness can also make you more irritable and postpartum hormones make you even more vulnerable to fluctuations of emotion. Even as you hope for the best and try to cope with this turn of events, you have every right to be hopping mad. You, your family, and your baby do not deserve this.

Nothing seemed real as I lay in the bed in the labor room, waiting for Jon and my mom to get there. I was scared and nervous, and really, really mad. I couldn't figure out what the hell (sorry) I had done to deserve this happening to me, to my baby.—Ami

As it happened, I was only confined to bed for five days. But those five days were very long. I was angry that I had to submit to the rules. Perhaps I was actually angry that control had been taken away—a big issue with me.—Cindy

Having a preemie ended the fairy tale. The fairy tale is over. I walk around in anger because this is not what I signed up for.—Raquel

I remember feeling really mad at my cervix for failing me, just really mad at it. But it was like it was not part of me. It wasn't me that I was mad at, it was this part that had failed and had done something really bad, and I was mad at it.—Stephie

Anger is a powerful and compelling emotion that may consume you at times. You may feel angry at invasive medical technology, upset at the breast pump, or fuming about your separation from your baby. You may be furious with the injustice dealt by fate, God, or Mother Nature. You may feel as if you paid your dues, and yet you were cheated of a healthy baby. Your baby is cheated of a healthy start. You may envy other parents in the nursery whose babies are doing better than yours or resent friends who have uncomplicated deliveries and newborns in their arms. It's all so unfair. To your dismay, you may find yourself even feeling angry with or disappointed in your tiny baby.

I was thinking, *If you have one problem, that should protect you from having one of the other possible problems.* I know, of course, that this isn't true, but I had gone through all that infertility stuff and then how cruel that I should also have to have a preemie! I felt as if I had spent all that time and money and I wasn't getting what I had paid for, as if there was a contract or something!—Nola

I felt this jealousy when I knew I wasn't going to have a natural delivery, and my best friend would visit me with her son, who I saw born into the world. My loss was already potent, not being able to look forward to this [gentle birth]. I felt this jealousy when I was in the NICU with my son and the little girl next to him, who was also born at the same gestation, was off the vent and growing. Or when the woman next to me was pumping full bottles of breast milk, and I couldn't get even a half ounce after two months of pumping, so my son was now on formula. I felt this jealousy when my friend had her home birth, and, as much as I wanted to be there, I couldn't handle it. I was overjoyed with her, even though it killed me to think of her little boy being cuddled in her arms in bed for twenty-four hours after his birth, just nursing and sleeping peacefully.—Maren

If you believe you received inadequate care, you may be furious at the practitioners who discounted the severity of your symptoms or minimized your concerns. Someone may suggest that you file a lawsuit, but most parents can see that this won't get them what they really want—a normal birth and a healthy newborn.

In the NICU, you might feel aggravated by a lack of information or forthrightness, or any failure to include you in decision making for your baby. You may be frustrated that you are not adequately supported in your desire to breast-feed or to pump and provide breast milk, to be more involved in caregiving, or to have adequate opportunities for privacy or holding your baby close.

I was desperate to pump some more milk for my son, but the nurse on duty wouldn't help me. She said okay and then never showed up, so I kept calling her to help. Finally she told me that she was waiting for the lactation specialist to come in at 10:00 AM. I was mad and shot her a dirty look. I don't think she realized how important it was to me to get some more milk to my son. I am still mad about it four months later. I was also mad at the NICU people who fed my son formula because they didn't have any of my milk. Didn't they realize that I had plenty of it but that I just couldn't get it to them? Why didn't they come get my milk—I was only a few corridors away? If my milk is so much better than formula, then why??? The more I think about it, the madder I get!!—Ruby

If he was hungry, they wouldn't call me, they would just feed him formula. I was down the damn hall.—Linda S.

Particularly if you have more than one baby in the NICU or other children at home, you may feel irritated by the fact that there just aren't enough hours in the day to tend to everyone's needs or to have much time to yourself.

While grief with its myriad feelings is painful to endure, it is a natural part of adjusting to your baby's need for intensive care. Your feelings are normal, and you are not alone.

I had such hopes and dreams when I was pregnant with my first child. I'd lie in bed and wonder what my baby would be like. I thought about the birth, the first cuddle, hearing that first cry, the first breast-feed, first bath, all of these things, and more. And then in the space of a day they were all gone—all my dreams, all my hopes, my desires, gone, changed, forever different. There was no celebratory champagne, no moments of rapture as we gazed upon this wondrous child snuggled at my breast, marveling at what we'd created, no quiet kisses, no tears of joy, no laughter, no counting of toes and fingers, nothing. There was instead pain and fear, tears and confusion, anger and shame, panic and agony, emptiness and terror, dread and heartache. Instead of trying to grapple with nappy pins and grow suits, night feeds and burping, I quickly learned about ventilators and oxygen, CPAP and IVs. Questions about NEC, ROP, and IVH, blood transfusions, and lung damage replaced those normal newborn thoughts. Instead of wondering whom he looked like, I wondered if he would live. Of course, mere words on clean white paper can never convey the absolute hopelessness of that day. Nor can words ever accurately describe the feelings as you are wheeled into an operating theater, to have your baby ripped from you, months before he should be, begging the staff surrounding you to save him and seeing the look of pity in their eyes as you realize that it might already be too late. There is no way to explain the feeling of having a mask placed over your face and feeling your baby move and wondering if that might be the last time you feel him alive. My dream had become a nightmare, and there was nothing that I could do. Part of me wanted to run, run far, far away, and keep on running until it didn't hurt anymore, and then another part of me demanded that I stay by this scrap of humanity, this tiny, bruised boy that my body had failed to keep safe. I wanted to scream, but what could I say?—Leanne

Couples and Grieving

Initially, my husband didn't want me to inform people that we had had a baby because he was afraid the baby would die. Whereas I was in denial about the severity of our son's condition, my husband was catastrophizing. That was extremely difficult for me.—Liza

With your baby in the NICU, you and your partner will likely share much common ground. But you will also experience some different perceptions, feelings, and viewpoints. How you grieve can be affected by your inborn temperament, personality, socialization, philosophies, personal history, and postpartum adjustment. The losses associated with pregnancy, childbirth, and the newborn period hit each of you in a singular way. You assign a unique meaning and framework to your experiences and follow a unique process of grieving, coping, adjusting, and healing.

For example, perhaps you dive into the core of your pain, while your partner takes in small doses so that it feels more manageable. Perhaps you are more adept at compartmentalizing your grief, putting it away so you can accomplish other things. Maybe you tend to be action oriented, preferring to get something done, while your partner would prefer to sit with her feelings and talk about her experience. For one of you, the grieving process may seem delayed or take longer or be more roundabout than the other's.

He's never cried over this, never once, which I wish he would do. He looks at me now and says things like, "It's over with, they're fine, why should I cry about it?" I still don't completely know how he dealt with it or how he felt. Like the first week after they were born, his dad and his brothers took him golfing—like okay, let's get his stress out. And I was kind of ticked because I was left visiting the babies and dealing with all the people coming back and forth, and I was like, how could he be golfing? We have these sick little babies. But I guess his family was thinking, *Let's get his mind off it. This will help him feel better.*—Stephie

You and your partner may also experience some typical gender differences. For example, it is natural for the mother to feel a more intense grief over the disruption of her close physical connection with her newborn. Many moms tend to focus on feeling and sharing emotions, while many dads tend to focus on taking action.

I would say—and this is coming from a guy's perspective—that the delivery was relatively uneventful because, after all, these kids weren't much bigger than a sandwich. Even though they were twins, it was not such a big deal.—Mitch

I never felt guilt or pained by the fact that my daughter was there [at the hospital] instead of at home because I felt confident that the nurses were giving her good care. Whereas, my wife definitely felt a sense of loss that my daughter would not breast-feed, and needed to be bottle-fed; as a man, I never had that expectation. I expected to be able to hold, hug, clean, caress, play with, and talk to my daughter, and I could do all of those things on a daily basis. That I did these things in the hospital instead of at home really didn't make a big difference to me.—David

Dwight was action-oriented and very pragmatic. He just wanted to spend time with them, which was great, and he just didn't worry. Everything that happened hurt me and made me sad and worried. He was able to just focus on their baby-ness.—Rikki

The mother and father often take on different roles as well. While the mother's experience is unique due to carrying the baby during pregnancy, her postpartum adjustment, and perhaps her desire and ability to breast-feed, the father's experience is unique due to his natural desire to protect and provide for his family. For example, your fatherly pride may take a hit by the way the NICU limits your access to your baby. You may resent being expected to ask permission to do even those things you might already feel competent doing, such as bathing and diapering your baby or changing the dressings. You may feel embarrassed by how frail your infant appears and concerned about the financial, emotional, and physical burdens of care. You may worry about appearing selfish, weak, or unable to provide for your family if you share these kinds of concerns or your feelings, even though you're quite entitled to have them. For most fathers, the worst aspect is feeling helpless, unable to fix the situation.

I'd always been a pretty optimistic person before this. If I got in a bind, I always figured I could find a way out or work my way out of it. But this was something totally different, you know? Nobody knew—and that was probably the most upsetting thing, that nobody knew and nobody could tell you what you could do, what I could do or what anybody could do, to fix it. And as it turned out, there was no fix.—Tim

You know us men. I had to be the big tough one, the alpha male, if you will. I fought it back and fought it back. So that my wife would not see, often after she went to bed, leaving me alone at my computer screen or in front of the TV, I would just lose it. Particularly on those tough days when Geoffrey was fighting for life. I would sob and cry and would just sit there until weariness would take over and I would be falling asleep. Then and only then would I wander off to bed.—Shaw

Many men also find it difficult or unnatural to verbalize their thoughts and feelings. As Charlie said during his interview, "I'm not much of a sharer." It's hard to find the words, and many men exhibit a narrow range of emotions, seek and accept little support, and are not eager to express painful feelings and talk about their babies. In addition, many fathers believe they can't afford to get emotional, as they are the ones who must continue going to work and running the household while the mother recovers from childbirth and focuses on her infant. Is gender disparity due to living in a society that values male stoicism or due to the fact that males are neurologically different from females? Culture or biology? It's undoubtedly both.

I think the experience of the NICU really does impact us, but I think it's tough to put into words, and it's tough to go back to and look at. Sometimes you're just trying to get through another day of supporting your family.—Ed

Not only was my son in the hospital, but she was too. I had to hold it together for all of us. . . . I had to keep it together so it wouldn't affect my judgment while at work as well.—Hugh

I found it tough at times to balance the expected strength of being male and the sadness and fear of being the father to a baby who was struggling for life in the NICU.—Shaw

It's hard for me because men don't really talk about it. They just kind of skim over it and try to get on to the next subject. So at times it's kind of hard because I don't really have a best friend to confide in. I have a lot of friends, but I'm sure Janet's friends ask her, "How are you doing? How are you doing?" But men just don't do that. My brother sent me a nice card, but you just don't speak about it. That's just the way we were raised.—Tim

Jill asked me if I was mad, and I told her no. I walk and walk and walk, and I know that I'm pretty sure I lied.—Jeff

As it is, grieving is very much a solo journey, and most parents take turns experiencing grief's intensity. When one partner is having an especially hard time, the other may put grief aside to hold down the fort and tend to life's day-to-day demands. At times, partners may feel miles apart.

Your differences can make it easy to fall into the trap of judging each other: "Since he buries himself in his work, he must not care about the baby" or "She'll never get over this if she doesn't stop worrying about the baby and crying." This attitude only widens the gap between you. It is hard enough to find each other as it is. Instead, focus on the fact that you are different individuals and no two people grieve alike. When you accept your partner's feelings, you acknowledge that each of you is entitled to whatever feelings you have. Curiosity is the antidote to judgment and resentment, so maintain a curiosity about your partner's perspective and experience. You may not share your partner's feelings or understand his or her reactions. You may even feel anxious or disappointed. But by accepting each other's silences and tears, you provide the kind of support, reassurance, and understanding that promotes healing and affirms your commitment to your partner.

At times, I really feel like I lost the first month of our [family's] life together because we weren't able to be together twenty-four hours a day. My husband looks at it like we were able to get her early and get to know her before she was even due!—Stacy

I would suggest more wives and moms ask their husbands and partners what it was like for them and just listen. Don't compare, don't judge, just listen to what it was like. And it may take more than once. That's just my buck twenty-five.—Ed

Multiple Birth and Multiple Realities

If you are in the NICU with twins, triplets, or more, you may feel excited, blessed, proud—and overwhelmed. Even as your joy is multiplied, so are your worries, losses, and grief.

If your newborns cannot share bed space, whose side do you sit by? You may also mourn for your babies' separation from each other. And how will you take care of more than one fragile infant? Rarely do multiple babies have identical medical courses. You may have more than one series of complications to deal with. Your babies may not be able to come home at the same time. *This is not what you were wishing for.*

Your babies' differences in the NICU can render your emotional landscape more complex. When you are facing multiple realities, you will react and respond to each one differently than if you had to cope with just one reality. You need to find people who can understand and listen to all of your experiences with each baby. This will help you celebrate each triumph and mourn each defeat. Remember that the realities you are enduring would be considered overwhelming for a family to deal with over a number of pregnancies and several years. You are experiencing them *simultaneously.*

With multiples, you also have the added challenge of finding the time and energy to attend to your own needs. Particularly if your babies experience poor outcomes, you may not feel you can afford the luxury of self-care. It may well take you many years to adjust and heal. It is especially important that you be patient with yourself and your feelings.

What I've come to realize is that I haven't ever had a time to indulge (I don't mean indulge in a patronizing way, I really mean indulge) in grief or the grieving process. Through each situation, there have always been so many other demands on my time that I am never able to focus on grieving. Now I am a busy mom of two preschoolers, working more than full time, and not able to just pull the covers over my head for a few days, which I think would do me good. This isn't making me feel sorry for myself, though. I am glad to have my kids and my company and my life now. It does make me feel a little kinder toward myself, a little more patient that I am still slogging through all this even five years down the road. It helps me to understand that I wasn't able to properly grieve, and though that wasn't my fault, the outcome is definitely my reality.—Susan C.

Points to Remember

· *Having a baby in the NICU is a journey that entails a mosaic of losses, emotional storms and calms, and a confusing mix of emotions.*

· *Grief is at the emotional core of this experience, as are love, joy, and hope. In spite of your grief, you can still have times of delight, wonder, and devotion.*

· *As part of your adjustment to your baby's NICU stay, you may experience many feelings of grief, including shock, sadness, yearning, fear, anger, guilt, failure, powerlessness.*

· *Even though no two parents follow the same path, you are experiencing many of the same emotions and reactions as other parents in the NICU.*

· *Although you and your partner may hold different perspectives and can expect to grieve differently, you can tolerate, accept, and not be threatened by these differences. They are normal and natural.*

· *If you have multiple babies in the NICU, even as your joy is multiplied, so are your losses and your grief.*

· *Even as you grieve, you are adjusting and healing.*

4:

Coping and Adjustment

When it comes to coping with grief, many people admire stoicism. They'll say, "She's handling it so well," often meaning that she doesn't talk about the situation, look sad, or act upset. However, "handling it" does not mean avoiding grief or habitually bottling up feelings. Suppressing grief only sabotages your happiness by keeping you stuck, blocking not just your sorrow, but also the return of your joy and contentment. Coping means acknowledging your pain and letting it move through you so you can stay open to the potential for joy.

As your shock and numbness wear off, remaining open to all your emotions enables you to form a strong emotional bond with your baby, which benefits you both. Unencumbered by stifled feelings, you can feel more confident and competent as a parent, and your baby thrives under your responsive care. You get to experience the affectionate, satisfying, and happy feelings that are also central to your journey. Facing all your emotions also helps you uncover their true sources, freeing you to see your baby, yourself, your partner, and others in a positive light.

Still, this is a tall order. At times, you may wish you could avoid your emotional pain and feel only joy and optimism. But to appreciate or even feel the positives, it helps to get a handle on the pain. It also helps to view grieving not as your enemy but as your ally—the process that moves you toward healing and harmony.

This chapter contains a number of coping strategies that can foster your adjustment and healing.

Meeting Your Physical Needs

I don't remember thinking too much about how I felt, only that the longer I slept, the faster I would get better and the sooner I could start being a mother to my girls.—Rosa

When you foster your physical well-being, you also foster your emotional well-being. After all, having a healthy brain and body will boost your mood, stamina, and ability to cope with the stress of having your newborn in intensive care.

Whether you're a mother or a father, taking the time and effort to tend to your physical well-being can pay high dividends. You will have your own priorities and unique needs, but in general you might find it most helpful to practice relaxation techniques, get enough quality sleep, eat healthy foods, and move your body every day. Nurturing yourself is key to being able to nurture your baby. (For a related discussion with regard to breast-feeding, see "Enhancing Your Milk Supply" in chapter 8.)

Do not suggest we get some sleep. If we could sleep, we would sleep.—Jennifer E.

Granted, tending to your physical well-being is easier said than done. When you're overwhelmed and bereft, you may lose your appetite, struggle to find the time to prepare healthy meals, put off exercise, or suffer from insomnia. With your baby in the NICU, sleep may feel like an abandonment of your parental duty to remain vigilant. At times, staying by your baby's bedside or waking during the night to pump or call the hospital may be your highest priority. The trick is to find the balance that works best for you, keeping in mind that many parents, in hindsight, agree with Jody who says, "If I could go back in time, I would tell myself to be in the NICU as much as I could but also to take care of myself."

Recovery from Childbirth and Any Complications

Depending on any complications you might have experienced, you may need a long recuperation before you can turn your full attention toward your baby. Besides being physically compromised, you may be emotionally compromised due to medications and your body using its energy to repair itself. When you can finally be with your newborn, it's only natural to feel emotionally overwhelmed.

The first day, I was so sick that I did not want to see her. I can hardly believe that now!! The second day, I wanted to see her, but I knew that I would be way too weak to hold her. By Saturday, after everyone I had talked to had asked if I had seen her yet, I was ready, and very upset—crying hysterically—because I had not seen my baby yet.—Stacy

If you feel strongly about wanting to be with your baby in spite of being physically compromised, trust your intuition about how to balance your physical needs with your emotional needs as a new mother. For some mothers, the emotional benefits of being with their baby seem to facilitate physical healing. *Do what feels right for you.*

One of the hardest things was leaving him. I was there most of the time during the day, but I was still in the hospital, post–C-section, and the nurses just kept saying to me, "You have to take care of yourself. You are post-op yourself. You've got to take care of yourself. Get out of here. We are kicking you out of here. For three hours we don't want to see your face." Then I'd go to leave him, and he would start crying. It was so hard to leave him because at that point it was clear to me that he knew.—Micki

I was taking longer to heal, and I had some complications afterward. The nursing staff would tell me, "You know, maybe you should stay home, take a day and just rest, do some things for yourself, go have your hair done, or whatever." And what I really wanted to hear was somebody saying, "Good for you. What you're doing is so important." That's really what I wanted to hear because there was no way I was staying home. There was no way. I wasn't going to have my hair done. And rest? I had to get up every three hours to pump anyway. I wasn't getting any rest. I might as well be at the hospital. There's no way anybody was going to talk me out of being there.

Do whatever you need to do. Don't let anybody talk you out of it. I went every day. It took me longer to heal, but I healed. It was more important that I was there with him.—Marcia

Postpartum Adjustment

Mothers have the added challenge of hormonal postpartum adjustment. After delivery, hormone levels plummet as they readjust to nonpregnant levels. Most mothers experience baby blues, a transient cluster of symptoms appearing during the first two weeks postpartum that can include

- mood swings,

- sadness,

- anxiety,

- feeling overwhelmed,

- crying spells,

- loss of appetite, or

- trouble sleeping.

If you have the baby blues, these symptoms won't be severe, won't require treatment, and will disappear on their own within two weeks after delivery.

More serious is postpartum depression, which can include intensified and longer-lasting symptoms (above), thoughts of hurting yourself or your baby, or having predominantly negative feelings or little interest in your baby. Postpartum depression can begin any time during the first year and it can also compromise your ability to manage everyday life.

I didn't have a sense of joy regarding Emma for most of her ICN stay. Just sadness and fear and guilt and more sadness.—Diane

To some extent, after your baby's birth, your emotional sensitivity, tearfulness, and anxiety are due to postpartum hormonal adjustment. Add the extra distress posed by your baby's condition and hospitalization and you can expect a more taxing postpartum period. Certainly, if you develop any intense or bothersome postpartum symptoms, don't delay telling your doctor or midwife. Treatment can boost your bonding and parenting confidence. You don't have to endure being incapacitated.

I felt torn in half. Like there was a part of me that wanted to be in bed with them, taking them back in, but at the same time I was so incredibly knotted up with terror and sadness at their condition that it got in the way of any natural instincts I might have had to know what each of them needed. [For instance,] I didn't feel confident picking up Hannah after a blood draw when she was screaming. I couldn't push past the anxiety, fear, and sadness, to Yes, you pick up a crying baby. I know this. It's like it was an effort to remember that it was loving and a good thing to pick up a crying baby, that it was allowed, that's what mothers do, and to not be looking over my shoulder, wondering if I'd get in trouble or hurt her.—Rikki

I was miserable; I ended up in a deep depression. I didn't get the bonding time I would have liked, and with postpartum depression, I felt disconnected for a very long time—until he was almost two. It was horrifying. I knew something was wrong. Nobody bothered to inquire about this, and I didn't get help until much later.—Linda S.

Accepting Assistance

Naturally, you can expect to feel more overwhelmed than the typical new mother or father. If you feel disappointed with how little you seem to accomplish, remember that your main job right now is to be a parent. Especially if you're the mother, taking care of yourself, perhaps pumping breast milk, and especially spending time with your baby—whether your baby is still in the NICU or is at home now—are all *essential tasks* that you are completing. If you accomplish anything else, *you are overachieving.*

A neighbor who had one-year-old twins invited me to join her twins group. These women were ecstatic if they got to take a shower before dinner.—Susan B.

So when friends or family offer to help, delegate household chores, including cooking, cleaning, yard work, and errands. Doing so reduces your load and gives them a sense of accomplishment and kinship.

For the father in particular, this kind of social support is immensely helpful, as it temporarily relieves him of his protector/provider role. This kind of support doesn't require you to share emotions, and it shores you up, reduces the pressure, and lets you know that others care.

We were renting our home, and the front yard was a mess. The lawn was getting long, there were spiderwebs and stuff left over from the fall and winter. It wasn't really bad, it just needed attention, and it was the easiest thing to put off, but it was also the thing that was apparent every day when I pulled up in the driveway. Since we would go see Buddy on Wednesdays and Saturdays, and I tried very hard not to work on Sundays, the lawn just kept getting worse and worse.

Well, one Saturday we headed up to the hospital, and Buddy was probably either recovering from a surgery or getting ready for one. It was that time in his stay when his intestines were having a really hard time. We wanted to stay as long as we could, but we knew we had to get home to pick up our daughter, and there were things to do around the house.

When we arrived home, things looked very different. The lawn was mowed, the leaves were raked and piled, even the shrubs were trimmed. There were things done that I wouldn't have thought to do, even if Buddy hadn't been in the hospital. And I had no idea who did it. I suspect I do now, but I'll likely never be sure. When I saw it, I cried. Huge sobs of relief and gratitude. Not because it was a confirmation of all I couldn't do, but because someone had finally done something I really needed. I didn't need dinners and lunches or extensions on assignments. I needed my home and my family to be unaffected. I needed something normal looking. I needed not to have to ask or beg for help. I was asking for help with everything else: school, church, bills, employers, hospital staff. Someone looked, found a need, organized it, and did it. All I could do was just say thanks.

And I could go in the house and relax and not feel guilty because I wanted to catch five minutes of a baseball game or play with my daughter, and it would be at least two weeks before it had to be done again. It freed me not only for that day, but for days to come. Since it was done anonymously, there also wasn't anyone I owed anything to either. No one to pay back. It meant everything to me. I was given time to take care of me without some task pounding on the door demanding my attention.—Ed

Getting Close to Your Baby

I was able to touch my baby and hold him. It was wonderful to do the kangaroo care. . . It made a huge difference in terms of getting to know my baby and feeling connected. I also felt more connected when I gained confidence in feeding and changing him and felt more comfortable with the nurses in the NICU.—Liza

No matter what the future may bring, finding ways to get close to your baby will help you move toward emotional healing. Nurturing your baby builds your confidence as a parent and is a way to do something positive in a difficult situation. Research shows that being included by your baby's medical team and participating in your baby's care reduces stress in you *and* your baby. Your involvement also supports the development of your parental identity and your bond with your infant.

Assume that your baby's medical practitioners are trying to boost your attempts to be close to your little one. Ask them to teach you how to do things for your baby. You may discover that by seeing the medical team as your teammates, you become more aware of and open to their ongoing attempts to encourage and include you. (See "Joining Your Baby's Care Team" in chapter 5.)

Also, practice doing what you can for your baby. Don't fall into the trap of thinking you can't learn how to take care of your little one.

Like any skill, taking care of a baby in the NICU requires experience and time to acquire. Practice builds competence—and confidence.

When you cannot be with your baby, dwelling on your little one is a natural result. Your thoughts can always be with your infant, even when you can't. (For more on finding your place in the NICU, feeling like a parent, and building a relationship with your baby, see chapters 5, 6, and 7.)

Letting Your Grief Flow

When intense feelings are rising, do your best to acknowledge them. Of course, this is easier said than done. Grieving is hard work. It takes time and energy. It can make you feel broken, discouraged, and overwhelmed. You may fear that if you open up, you'll never be able to pull yourself back together. But you will. Falling apart is always temporary and can help you to rejuvenate and regain control over your life.

When you open yourself to grief, your painful feelings can flow through you. Being open to grief doesn't mean nonstop pain. There is a natural ebb and flow, moments of intensity diffused with respite. By facing and experiencing the depths of your grief, you can release powerful feelings. Far from a show of weakness, it is the brave, strong, smart thing to do. Over time as grief is dispersed, you'll discover that you can think back on your experiences and your baby's ordeal without being overcome with emotion.

In contrast, if you suppress your grief, the effort continually drains your energy and demands that you spend precious resources avoiding, ignoring, and dismissing the feelings that warrant expression. As feelings stay mired in you, you stay mired in grief rather than move along a path of adjustment and healing.

Here are a few general coping tips that can help you face your grief, open up, and let it flow:

- *Remember that grief is normal* and you share common emotional ground with other NICU parents.

- *Identify your feelings individually, as well as their sources.* For example, you might acknowledge feelings of anger, fear, helplessness, frustration, and sadness. Perhaps you feel angry about what you consider to be heartless hospital policies, which is different from your natural feelings of helplessness over your baby's hospitalization, which is different still from your fear that your baby won't ever recover, which is apart from the frustration over the sad but necessary lack of free access to your newborn. Identifying the terrain of your emotional landscape lets you address the challenges indicated by your feelings instead of simply feeling overwhelmed by a massive wad of pain.

· *Voice your fears and concerns.* Practically speaking, identifying your worries enables you to ask pertinent questions and get the information or reassurance you need. Emotionally, airing your fears also keeps them from devolving into anger and adding fuel to the fire. By being mad at what's maddening and scared of what's scary, you're less likely to get stuck in rage. Then instead of putting up an angry guard, you can face your fears and move through the vulnerability, disappointment, and hurt—hurt that this happened to your precious child and family. Your hurt lies at the bottom of your grief, which in and of itself can be scary, but hitting bottom ultimately lets you bounce up toward healing. (See also "Dealing with Fears" in chapter 6.)

· *Have realistic expectations for your grief.* Certain sights, smells, sounds, and situations can prompt your grief anew. Rather than combat it, accept that ups and downs are a natural part of the ebb and flow. Even years from now, antiseptic smells, beeping sounds, or songs you heard on the radio can transport you back to those difficult days in the NICU. Just driving in the direction of the hospital might give you flashbacks. This return of grief can be discouraging—but it is normal and more fleeting as time passes.

· *Find books, articles, blogs, and videos* on coping with a NICU stay and the medical, emotional, or spiritual issues you face, which feature personal accounts by parents of NICU babies. These resources can offer insight, opportunities to release painful feelings, and the comfort of knowing you're not the only one to go through this experience.

· *Engage in creative or athletic endeavors.* These activities can encourage the expression of emotions or the release of tension and can offer you a sense of accomplishment.

· *Appreciate the joy, hope, pride, delight, confidence, and love whenever and wherever you find it.* You deserve the respite that happy moments offer. Over time, as you and your baby adjust, it is those positive feelings that will govern your lives.

· *Trust that you can adjust and heal.* Know that in time you can let go of what you lost and move forward with what you gain.

Whether you talk about your feelings or keep them to yourself, whether you set aside time to reflect or keep a busy schedule, whether you can find the words or not, be true to your process and your needs. Know that the bottom line is that you face the situation and your feelings, and find ways to cope and adjust that work for you.

I remember that the social workers would come and talk, even if just to ask how the girls were doing and whatever I would want to talk about. They kept asking me, "Are you doing okay?" Then I started to feel really bad for doing okay. I thought, *Why? Shouldn't I be?* I began to question myself. Should I be feeling bad? I almost felt guilty. Then I realized that I was okay and that I was strong enough to deal with life's challenges. I had been so prepared with the possibilities of things that could go wrong that when they did, I was ready. I have always told myself, "Why cry over spilled milk? Instead, clean it up and move on." I am not the type of person who worries over things that are out of my control.—Rosa

No one can tell you how you should feel or what you must do. You will discover the answers for yourself.

Practicing Reframing and Mindful Acceptance

Reframing and *mindful acceptance* are cognitive techniques that can boost your coping. They are based on the idea that how we think about a situation affects how we feel about it. For instance, you've probably noticed that when all you can think about is how terrible this NICU stay is, all you can feel is terrible. But whenever you can think about how being in the NICU also gives you the opportunity to nurture your baby in the ways he or she truly needs, you can feel some joyful anticipation. Likewise, if you chastise yourself for feeling terrible—or get down on yourself for feeling okay when your baby isn't—you're only adding to your distress.

Reframing involves countering distressing thoughts with positive ones. For example, if you are preoccupied with what a challenging blow this is, try resting on how much love you hold for this child. If you're focusing on how little you can do in the NICU, focus on the nurturing activities you *can* do, such as soothing your little one with your simple presence. You can also draw your focus to what's going well with your baby or turn your mind toward other slices of your life that are blessings or still enjoyable. This doesn't mean becoming a Pollyanna or denying reality. You aren't trying to banish your painful thoughts. You're simply adopting other perspectives and finding a balance that is less agonizing for you. Whenever you are feeling over-run by distressing thoughts and incapacitated by misery, focus on the positive and you can find respite.

I always kept a thought, tucked away in the back of mind, that things could suddenly go really bad. Each time this thought crept into my consciousness, I made a distinct effort to resist even allowing the concept to remain in my thoughts for very long. I would think *No, no, no, just don't think of it . . . so what football games are on this weekend?* or something else to immediately divert my mind to other things. This occurred about three or four times a week for the eight weeks they were in the NICU.—Craig

To help me cope, I tried to concentrate on the positive—she was alive and stable for the time being. And knowing, even before my baby was born, that I was doing everything physically possible to make sure she would have a chance to grow up to be the best person she could be.

In the beginning, I focused on other things. I knew that the doctors and medi-cal staff in the NICU were doing everything they possibly could for Daphne. I tried to tell myself that the weeks or months she was in the NICU would give me time to recuperate from my postpartum surgery and the ability to catch up on sleep and to much better prepare for Daphne's homecoming (which I hoped would be sooner rather than later). I also told myself that, even though Daphne wasn't healthy enough for me to hold her yet, I was nevertheless still doing so much for her like keeping her company in the NICU and pumping constantly to ensure enough breast milk for when/if she was ever able to ingest it. I participated in a scrapbooking support group that encouraged me to chronicle Daphne's life no matter how things turned out. And I prayed often for her full and speedy recovery.—Dina

The cognitive technique of *mindful acceptance* involves paying attention to what's going on inside you and around you, in the moment, nonjudgmentally. You can observe your thoughts and feelings, however positive or negative, and accept them as a natural part of your experi-ence with this child. In fact, the previously listed tactic of letting your grief flow is an example of mindful acceptance, in that instead of fight-ing or avoiding grief, you embrace it.

This memory lives on in infamy in my mind—I remember leaving the hospital, sitting at an intersection, just thinking to myself. At that point I must have realized that Deb-bie's fine and that these kids are about to be born, and maybe all the warnings [about the complications of prematurity] from the neonatologists were playing in my head, and I realized that these kids were at risk. And I remember sitting there thinking that if this is the hand of cards that I've been dealt, so be it, I can deal with it. It's kind of interesting that that's the kind of hand that I was dealt, but that's all right, we can do something about that. No one told me this, but I had an expectation that my kids were going to be mentally retarded and somehow physically handicapped. I just thought, *I am going to get some really sick kids who are going to live, and that is going to be my lot in life, to be a father to these kinds of kids.* And I was just thinking, *Okay, that's what you're getting, and you're going to rise to the occasion, that's what you're going to do, and you're going to take care of these kids. Maybe that's not what you would have ordered, but you don't order your kids from L.L. Bean, and so that's what you're getting.* They didn't turn out that way . . . but I remember thinking that, and it was a pretty heavy thought. That thought has actually come back to me hundreds of times in the three years since then—seeing myself sitting in the car, I can see what the dashboard looked like, thinking, *That's the hand that I was dealt.*—Mitch

Aside from the obvious fear that I would lose my wife and son, after the initial shock I couldn't dwell on his prematurity. It may sound cold, but I looked at it as either he'll make it or he won't. I kept hoping that he would make it but felt that if he didn't, I'd cross that bridge when I came to it.—Hugh

Facing and embracing reality can be a significant key to survival. It's your choice whether to acknowledge what has happened or cling to old expectations. You can decide to empower yourself by embracing this experience, or you can limit yourself by trying to hide, flee, catastrophize, or protest. When your baby's life is on the line, there are clear advantages to facing and embracing, remaining mindfully in the present moment.

If there was going to be any chance of saving my daughter's life after her birth, I simply didn't have time for denial or anger. I needed to accept that I had to get certain testing done as soon as possible to confirm the prenatal diagnosis of CDH. Then meeting with various specialists who had expertise dealing with these children and touring the NICU; then seeing what happened to Daphne immediately after she was born.—Dina

As you can see, the power of any cognitive technique is that even though the situation doesn't change, you can change the way you view it. Cognitive techniques help you be more psychologically flexible and therefore resilient in the face of stress. You can also acquire a sense of peace about your journey, sooner rather than later.

Becoming proficient in cognitive techniques requires practice, particularly if you are changing deeply ingrained habits, but you may see results quickly. Many suggestions throughout this book have cognitive aspects to them. You can also practice these techniques in other areas of your life.

Addressing the Emotional Trauma

Periodically, I resolve to meet my challenges from a positive, upbeat point of view. Intellectually, cognitively, I understand that's the right way, the best way to look at things. But there is something else at a darker, deeper emotional level that won't cooperate with my resolve. I wake up in the middle of the night aware of terrible danger. I don't know what will happen or when, I just sense it out there. And I lie awake, trying to think of how to keep it from coming, what to do, how to protect.—Susan C.

Emotional trauma can result from any ordeal that entails shock, distress, fear, and suffering. There's no question that having a newborn sent to Intensive Care is traumatic for parents. The degree of trauma can be related to the severity of the infant's condition and the duration of the NICU course, but the key is how shocking, distressing, frightening, and painful it is for the parent. So whether your baby is admitted briefly for observation after troubling signs or struggles mightily for months, the disbelief, agony, and strain take their toll.

While the vast majority of parents are traumatized by at least some aspects of the NICU experience, some parents develop posttraumatic stress disorder (PTSD) as a result of their experiences.

I really think I have PTSD from this experience. Every time I see a Children's Hospital ambulance, I cry. Every time I see their billboard, I remember the NICU. Every friend or family member who has a new baby, I remember the NICU.

In my mind there is Kitquin now and there is Kitquin in that oxygen tent at the first hospital, and they are both very real. I get flashbacks to that day where all I could do is look at her and cry, and it's like I'm right back there and she is right back there fighting to breathe. In reality, she is sleeping peacefully in her bed in the next room over.—Jennifer E.

It's as if I am walking through my life and the path I am on, and all I can see to my left contains all the blessings and wonderful possibilities for my family and our lives and our future. When I look to the right, I see a terrible cliff dropping off into disaster. The cliff was always there, is always there for everyone. Anything can happen. But before the losses we have experienced, I was able to concentrate on the path I was on and all that lies to the left. Since my experiences, I spend a lot more time conscious of and worrying about the abyss. I don't feel safe anymore, even though that safety was always at least potentially an illusion. I really miss the ability to live with that illusion.—Susan C.

PTSD can develop as a result of enduring overwhelming stress while being fearful and helpless to affect an often life-threatening situation. The essential, persistent features of PTSD include:

- Reexperiencing the trauma through recurrent, painful, and intrusive memories, flashbacks, or dreams, which can be triggered by smells, sights, sounds, or other situations that resemble or symbolize the trauma

- Diminished responsiveness, including detachment from others, reduced interest in previously enjoyed activities, continuing emotional numbness, and detachment from the original traumatic experience

- Hyperarousal, including outbursts of anger, difficulty concentrating, insomnia, and excessive vigilance, which is indicated by hyperalertness and an exaggerated startle response

On the second or third day, after I was getting around pretty good on my own, I waddled over to visit her in her original incubator parking spot. I knew she was doing well, had been fine the night before, but when I walked in, she was gone! That cold fear feeling you get when you have a close call with disaster came over me. I can't really describe it other than chilling! On the outside I appeared calm, but my insides were mush. . . . I asked someone, and that's when they told me about moving her to the transitional nursery. Whew!—Linda

After experiencing this crisis, if you have another child down the road, you are covering similar terrain and it's normal to be hyperaroused. If you unfortunately experience another crisis, you may feel transported back in time and react intensely. Corin had this experience during the birth of her second child.

Ayla ended up stuck in the birth canal. They were able to get her head out with suction but couldn't get her shoulders out for quite some time. They called in the NICU team, and I remember watching the look of fear on the doctor's face. I began crying hysterically, knowing something serious was wrong. When they were finally able to force her out with manipulation and other tools, she was blue, limp, and didn't cry. They intubated her next to my bed, and I remembering watching it all in horror, screaming, "It's happening again!" I thought I had lost another one of my babies. It was one of the worst moments of my life.—Corin

PTSD has a strong biological component, with changes in brain chemistry and function. Treatment options include psychotherapy, medication, group therapy, and a unique treatment called EMDR (Eye Movement Desensitization and Reprocessing). EMDR utilizes the brain's innate ability to process information and transform the memory of disturbing and traumatic experiences to more adaptive, healthy recollections. If you are interested in pursuing EMDR, look for a mental health practitioner who has received specific training in this technique (www.emdr.com).

Having some or even many of these symptoms doesn't necessarily mean that you have full-blown PTSD. You can be traumatized by an experience without being disabled by it. What is important is that your symptoms count, however mild or severe, and they are related to trauma. If you feel unable to function, definitely seek help. But you needn't be diagnosed with PTSD to benefit from addressing your emotional trauma with tailored treatment, which may include teaching you ways to calm your body and reprocess your memories. Addressing the trauma can enhance your healing.

Do not assume that just because a child only spends a few weeks in the NICU that it was not a traumatic experience. People think that since she is normal and healthy now that I should be fine. It doesn't work that way.—Jennifer E.

Dealing with Burdensome Emotions

Some emotions are agonizing, such as yearning to hold your newborn, sorrow at your separation, and the heart-wrenching distress of seeing your baby struggling in the NICU. Other emotions such as guilt, inadequacy, and powerlessness are burdensome in that they wear you down and sap your confidence and faith. Guilt, inadequacy, and powerlessness all stem from the belief that you are personally responsible for your baby's plight. This can be a horrifying burden to bear.

I did find myself going over the day before his birth, over and over again. I tore myself apart wondering what I could have done differently. If only I hadn't done this, if only I had done this . . . That sort of thing.—Claire

I was so afraid of failing as a mother, not being able to care for them the way they needed medically, doing something wrong.—Michelle B.

Each day, I felt more like a parent, but I often felt completely helpless and useless. Maybe all parents feel that way, but it's more pronounced in the NICU.—Susan B.

To cope, reframe your thinking so that you can shape the burdens of guilt, inadequacy, and powerlessness into more manageable and appropriate feelings of parental responsibility. Try on the following perspectives:

· Feelings of guilt and inadequacy arise out of your devotion to your child and your desire to be a competent parent.

· Even though you're not at fault, taking on the burden of guilt can feel more manageable than the terror of helplessness.

· *Feeling* guilty is not the same as *being* guilty.

· Recognize that you never acted with the intention of making your baby need intensive care.

· Instead of being disappointed in yourself, be disappointed that medical science doesn't fully understand or prevent pregnancy complications, fetal anomalies, or neonatal illness.

· You are not responsible for knowing everything. You made the best decisions you could based on the information and support available.

· *Under the circumstances, you are doing the best you can to nurture and protect your baby.* If you fear that you didn't speak up enough, be aggravated that the NICU staff didn't encourage more parental input. Instead of regretting your decisions, regret that you had to decide without benefit of sufficient information, time, or support.

· You cannot always avoid tragedy or know the right course of action. No one can.

- You may have made heartfelt promises to your unborn child, but no parent can offer a guarantee. Alas, there is much that is beyond your control.

- If this appeals to you, embrace the idea that your child's fate is determined not by you but by what serves his or her higher good.

- Don't expect yourself to make sacrifices at the expense of your own basic needs. Depleting yourself also depletes your ability to be an effective parent—you can't nurture your children if you don't nurture yourself first.

- When others criticize your parenting, they are really expressing their beliefs about what they would do in your situation. That isn't necessarily an educated opinion nor what you should do. Nor is it necessarily what they would actually do should they ever find themselves in your shoes. Listen to others who can reassure you that you are not to blame.

- Feelings of guilt, inadequacy, and powerlessness are normal and natural parental reactions that can subside over time as you let go of what might have been and embrace what is.

There was a time when I really wanted to know exactly what had caused Vincent's IVH [intraventricular hemorrhage] and whether there was anything else I should be blaming myself for. As time goes on, the reason seems to matter less.—Anne

I think most of us, if we are honest with ourselves, have confessions relating to guilt and our little ones. Please know that you are not alone. When I was placed on home bed rest, I was told to stay down absolutely as much as possible, but that I could get up to grab a very fast snack or use the washroom. I remember standing at the stove making pasta over and over (it was my craving at that time), and even now I feel guilty and even embarrassed that I may have brought on my full-blown labor because of my insatiable need for rotini. What was I thinking, hanging out in the kitchen for twenty minutes at a stretch with a cervix that was soon halfway to delivery? I just didn't know the consequences, and I was all alone.

Then, in the four days I was hospitalized before Cailean was born, I was given medication to help prevent his birth. He suffered complications at two days of life that studies later potentially linked to the prenatal use of that medication. Oh my. Now I had not only brought on his preterm labor/delivery, but because of the meds they offered and I accepted, I had perhaps caused his neonatal crises as well. Years later, two years after my younger preemie was born, diagnostic studies revealed I had a condition that became the attributable cause of my obstetric complications. (Sigh.) Now I knew with some certainty that my body had been engineered all along to basically reject these little loved ones of mine. . . .

Now that my boys are four and six years old, much of that guilt has eased, and when I think back, I'm more inclined to be proud of all that I did do to help continue, support, and prolong my pregnancies. What does remain is an enormous sense of responsibility, and it helps me raise my sons with great care and vision for what they can become.—Maureen

By shaking off the belief that you are and should remain in total control of your baby's destiny, you are unfortunately now faced with the reality that you and your baby are vulnerable to tragedy. Life may seem so unpredictable now, and you may feel betrayed and even more powerless. Although feelings of vulnerability are frightening at first, it is also quite freeing to learn to live with the knowledge that you cannot, nor should you try to, control everything that occurs around you. It's not that you are powerless, you just need to find that balance between controlling what you can and feeling okay about letting go of the rest.

I felt helpless. My first thought was, *Why us? What had I done wrong?* I now know that it is not me that did anything wrong—it just happened.—Jodi

You can still hope and dream. But instead of seeing your expectations as guarantees or demands, you can prevent needless suffering by surrendering your wishes for a specific outcome and hold onto a wondering frame of mind: wonder what will happen, and trust that whatever unfolds, you can find meaning and treasures.

Surrendering also means taking each day as it comes and cherishing what you have. You no longer regret the past, and you fear less for the future. What will be, will be. You can learn to worry less, not more.

But how can you trust the world again? Many parents simply come to accept that difficulties and detours are a part of life. Coupled with an enhanced appreciation for any good fortune, you realize you can manage whatever the future brings, and even prevail. So can your child.

A couple hours after they took Ayla away, I was able to go into the NICU and see her. They had just extubated her and she was perfect in every way. I was able to hold her for the first time, and it was an indescribable feeling. I cried knowing how lucky I was to have her in my arms . . . *alive.*—Corin

Telling Your Story

Talking about her really helped make her a lot more real. All my coworkers would ask me, "How's she doing?" and they didn't understand half of what I was saying, but they still asked.—Brooke

Telling your story over and over can be tremendously therapeutic. You can correspond with friends and relatives, updating them with your baby's progress as well as on how you're doing. You can talk about your baby and your experiences with your partner, close family, supportive friends, a therapist, and anyone else who asks and *really* wants to know. Some parents find it helpful to post updates on free blogs sponsored by websites such as www.caringbridge.org.

By telling your story, you process and make sense of your experience. The resulting empathy and encouragement you receive from others can ameliorate your distress. Sharing anecdotes can also help you feel like a parent to your baby. Bringing up your little one in conversation integrates him or her into the family and can lend a sense of normalcy and even lightness, as Susan B. recalls.

I'd tell stories about their little triumphs to our close family. I would call my dad and say, "They're huge. They gained two grams last night." He would laugh and say, "Yeah, really huge. A dime weighs more than two grams."—Susan B.

Although you may prefer to keep your experiences and emotions private, doing so might make you feel isolated and alone. Try to find at least one person (besides your partner) who can listen and empathize. For the most personal parts of your story, you might keep a journal where you can record your deepest thoughts and feelings.

It would've been a help to be able to sit down with somebody. I've never really sat down and really talked about all of it because who wants to listen to it? And Bill doesn't. We don't want to dredge it all back up again. But it would've been very helpful to be able to get it out and to talk about it with someone who either had gone through it or understood it a little bit or even just truly wanted to hear. Talking about these things is so important and so incredibly cathartic. You can talk about it ad nauseum, but now I know it's so important to get it out and talk about it, at least in my case. So yes, I think that if I had talked to somebody and gone through the entire thing, it would've really kind of let me let go of some of this sooner than I did.—Jaimee

Keeping a journal was helpful. I had been alone a lot of those scary times, so I could write about what I was thinking. Sometimes I couldn't even sort out my thoughts, but if I wrote them down, somehow they made some sense, or things came out that I didn't even know I was thinking about. It gave some sort of routine to my life when it was so chaotic. Plus, finding people to talk to who were going through the same thing at the same time. I just talked to everybody.—Stephie

I kept a journal for each baby during their stay. At first the idea was just to try to keep straight everything that was going on. It soon morphed into a daily pep talk from me to them (or more likely, from me to me). I talked to my parents by phone daily.—Susan B.

I continue to scrapbook my daughter's life, which has helped me both confront and sort through my feelings about what has happened so far.—Dina

Some people may believe that the quicker you can forget about the trauma and move on, the better off you'll be. But you never forget, and, in fact, processing the details makes moving on possible.

Seeking Emotional Support outside the NICU

The twins support group probably saved my sanity. They helped me feel like a mom, even though my babies were still in the hospital. All had a unique perspective on parenting that was refreshing at a time when parenting had become a competitive sport.—Susan B.

At the time my son was in the NICU, I sought out support from friends and brought them to the hospital to see my son. That was extremely helpful. I was also touched by unsolicited support from other people who have had children in the NICU. I was amazed to learn of so many people who had children in the NICU, and it was helpful to hear their experiences and feel like someone understood.—Liza

Your baby's NICU may provide excellent emotional support to parents, but it can be important to find additional support outside the NICU. You may strike up new relationships, join a support group of other NICU parents, or already have people in your life who can listen well or reach out to you. You can continue to rely on this support after your baby's discharge.

Your first challenge is finding people who can be responsive and compassionate. Friends and family generally mean well and want to be helpful, but many do not know how. There is a lot of ignorance, not only about what intensive care means for a newborn, but what it means for the parents. People may make comments like these: "Lucky you. You can go home and get some sleep." Or, "I wish my baby had been born small like that. I'll bet delivery was a snap." Or, "Aren't you over this yet? Your baby is home and doing fine!" Worse yet, they may judge you or your actions, wondering about your contribution to your baby's condition. In addition, people may try to ignore, belittle, or erase your grief in an attempt to fix it. They may believe they are being supportive by avoiding the topic or encouraging you to look on the bright side. Unfortunately, these tactics are likely to have the effect of shutting you down.

Never tell anyone "It's God's will." There is no circumstance where that phrase helps, even if it is meant well. Don't tell a mother of multiples that having two babies fourteen or fifteen or sixteen months apart is just like having twins. It's not. Other stupid things people say: "Maybe it would have been better if they had died right away." "The money it's costing to keep your babies alive would provide a lot of healthcare for people who really need it." I could go on, but I try not to remember those comments.—Susan B.

Don't tell parents, "They are just tiny babies," "They are fine now that they are out of the NICU," "My cousin's friend had a thirty-weeker and he's fine now." I really don't want to hear about almost full-term babies. Micropreemies are not anything like thirty-plus- or even twenty-nine-weekers! Don't tell parents, "Everything happens for a reason," "At least you didn't get stretch marks" (I really loved that one), "You are being too overprotective," "What did you do to cause their early birth?" (That's another great one). Just listen and let them vent/cry/complain to you. Offer to do their laundry, clean their house, make meals, drive them to the hospital.—Jody

When other people said to me, "You should have taken better care of yourself during pregnancy," or, "Maybe this wouldn't have happened if you had been stronger in your faith," I took it to mean that these people believed that either my negligence put my daughter in the NICU or it was G-d's punishment. It's not for others to judge me or any other NICU parent. They are not G-d and have no divine authority to proclaim that my daughter's being in the NICU was anyone's fault, especially mine.—Dina

In the past, you too may have offered these platitudes or passed judgment, but now you know how isolating and hurtful this can be. Forgive your friends' and relatives' ignorance, just as others have forgiven yours. Educate the people you trust most about what you need. Tell them, write them a note, or give them this book to read. After all, they *want* to know how they can support you.

You may find it especially comforting to turn to other NICU parents. Garnering the support of others who have walked your walk also circumvents the challenge of educating folks. You don't have to explain yourself or hide the truth. You can talk about your baby without worrying that you'll shock these people or, worse, have to comfort *them* about your situation. You can grieve openly without having to fend off clichés, embarrassment, or efforts to "fix" you.

I may not have had the exact same feelings as someone else, but I have certainly had my share of feelings that made me uncomfortable, even shocked me. Lots of feelings that I certainly wished I never had and I was ashamed to admit to others. That is what allows me to connect with and empathize with the feelings other parents express, even if I haven't felt the particular feeling. For me, shame is the most destructive emotion, and bringing our nightmares out into the light of day often takes the power out of them.—Kris

A support group, whether online or in person, can help you feel less isolated, give you opportunities to develop supportive friendships, and offer hope for the future as you observe how others have managed. Find the avenues of sharing that work best for you.

The CDH support groups I joined have also been helpful sources of inspiration. One of the groups sent me a package shortly after Daphne was born that included a story likening having a child with special needs with a couple planning a trip to Italy but ending up in the Netherlands. That story helped me see past my daughter's difficulties and experience the beauty that my daughter adds to my life.—Dina

Talking about the experience is helpful to me. But it's got to be someone you trust and who cares about you above their needs. Especially for dads. . . . Fortunately I had the [Internet] list to speak my piece at times, people whom I still trust a great deal. They didn't seem to mind if it was heavy and at times seemed to reinforce or reward open and honest expressions of the shared difficulties, as well as the unique.—Ed

Navigating with Your Partner

The stress of everything can ruin a marriage. It has affected my marriage to the point that we are in counseling.—Jody

You and your partner are likely to turn to each other for support. But because no two parents cope alike, you are likely noticing the differences between you. Some differences are a natural result of cultural expectations and familial norms, some are due to the biological differences between fathers and mothers, and some are due to the dynamics of your relationship. Differing coping styles are also a result of differing temperaments, personal histories, and perspectives.

Unfortunately, differences can drive the two of you apart. Rather than focusing on your differences, notice the common ground. You are both engaged in the process of coping. If you are aware of your feelings and able to identify them, even if they don't make sense to you at times, you are coping. If you can be mindfully accepting of your feelings, observant as they ebb and flow, you are coping. If you are able to be present in the moment, rather than continually reliving the past or worrying about the future, you are coping. If you are *gradually* letting go of what might have been and adjusting to what is, you are coping. If you feel like you are learning and growing and reframing the situation in ways that give you hope even as you are grieving, you are coping.

Currently, my husband has a close relationship with our son and takes an active role in his care, but initially he was completely distanced. He wouldn't even visit me in the hospital right away because he was afraid of what could happen to our son. I still have occasional negativity toward him as a result.—Liza

My husband and I are very different in how we deal with things. Most of the time our styles complement each other. Under stress, it's more difficult. I tend to need to talk and express my feelings [and to] research and explore everything that's happening or may happen with our baby. He is optimistic she will be fine and tries to bury the fears. When I'm stressed about the whole situation, I cry and need to talk. When he's stressed about it, he gets irritable and withdrawn and needs to be left alone. If we're both upset at the same time, it's really, really hard because we need exactly opposite things.—Balbir

I would say that I tend to hold things in more, while my wife would want to talk about them right away. I feel like there are some things I can bring up and talk about but other things are too touchy and would cause a rift, however temporary.—Hugh

While talking and listening to each other can be challenging, doing so can build bridges, and you may both find it easier to cope as you reap the healing power of shared experience. As Jody says, "What helps most is learning to talk about what we are scared or afraid of, finding support groups, and talking to others who have been in our situation."

When you are listening, resist the urge to fix or judge. Simply affirm your compassion. If you need space or find solace in activity rather than talking, simply express your preference. If you want to talk more than your partner can handle, find additional support. Try to meet your partner in the middle.

It has put a lot of stress on our lives and our relationship, but we continue to keep the communication open and have become a stronger couple because of it. We have been through the best and been through the worst and I know we can get through anything as long as it's together and we continue to communicate.—Corin

I think we have a stronger bond now than before. We have been through hell and back together and know that each of us can do what needs to be done. But it took us awhile to get back to a good spot after the NICU.—Jody

My husband has been very supportive, and I do not know where I would be, emotionally, without knowing that I have his support.—Dina

My husband and I talked all the time. If I was getting too aggressive, he would pull me back a little bit; if he was getting too passive, I would poke him a little bit. And we know each other's capabilities. I'm more of the person to be there and hands on. And he felt that he needed to be home and help [our older son,] Cody stabilize, do the dad-son thing together, keep the home as mellow as possible, and let me deal with what's happening at the hospital. . . . Good balance and good communication.—Pam

Another good balance to strike is to have flexible roles, sharing involvement in the decisions and responsibilities that matter. When you each get some relief from carrying the burdens, you can both be more emotionally present and available.

Mat had a really hard time being in the NICU. It was very overwhelming to him. His focus in the early days was taking care of me, and I was totally focused on Lars. We were lucky to be surrounded by family, and I asked them to please take care of Mat. Also, having a special relationship with Lars's primary nurse made time at the hospital much easier for Mat. I dealt with all the insurance B.S. and learned everything I could about Lars's condition and care and supported Mat in caring for and about Lars when he was there. Mat did kangaroo care, bathed and diapered, and was amazing in the way he was able to go back and forth between work and the hospital, managing to be truly present in each place most of the time.—Kris

Supporting Your Other Children

It was very confusing for my five-year-old. Mommy was pregnant one day and not the next, but there was no baby when Mommy came home.—Cynthia

Cody (two years old) had been able to come up to the hospital before, but he was a little intimidated and overwhelmed by the whole experience. We took him into the family room, but still, the babies had wires and hooks and tubes. It was ugly to look at, and he was thinking, *My gosh, this isn't a baby, it's a machine.*—Pam

If you have other children, they can be deeply affected by the NICU journey. Younger children tend to be distressed by changes in you and your attentiveness; older children may have their own set of worries about their baby sibling's birth and hospitalization. Everyone may be disoriented by disrupted family routines.

We've got two other children. I wish that at the time we just would have been able to tell them that the baby was so sick, that we might lose him, and that Mommy and Daddy were very scared for the baby. But we didn't want to worry them. We were so scared we didn't even know what to tell them. We didn't know what to think ourselves. So at that point we hid the truth from them and just avoided talking about all those issues with them. We were gone all day and so nervous, and they didn't get a chance to know why. That was not fair to them.—Gallice

For most parents, as their children require more, they are only able to give less. Whether the NICU stay is long or short, you may feel terribly torn, guilty, and frustrated. How can you be a responsive parent when you are emotionally stressed and drained? How do you balance your newborn's need for you to be in the NICU with your other children's need for parenting at home?

Even though you can't be everywhere and everything to everybody, you can provide the kind of support that eases your children's coping and adjustment. Here are some tips. (See these and more at www.NICUparenting.org.)

On answering questions, offering reassurance, and visiting the NICU:

· When your children learn that "their baby" has to stay in the hospital, they may have lots of questions about why the baby can't come home. Because children are apt to imagine frightening scenarios when information is withheld from them, speak honestly and simply, in ways that quell their fears. For instance, you might tell them that this new baby was born too early or became sick and, for now, needs intensive care to grow and recover. Assure them that big, strong kids like them can handle being out in the world—and they won't ever need intensive care like the baby does.

· Show them photographs of the baby and the surrounding equipment. Use positive, reassuring language, such as, "This one helps the baby breathe," or, "When the baby is stronger, he won't need this tube anymore," or, "These wires are attached with tape that comes off easily and they don't hurt at all." Help them look beyond the machinery and see the baby.

· Your children can benefit from visiting the NICU so that they can see their new sibling for themselves and witness the necessity of intensive care. Visits can open opportunities for answering questions more thoroughly and offering tailored reassurances. Visits also reinforce family togetherness.

One thing my daughter is happy with is our weekly family visit to the hospital. We all go see the baby, then my husband goes to the family room and plays with or reads to her while I visit the baby. Then we swap places, and I spend time with her while he visits the baby. My daughter likes these visits a lot, and both our children get one-on-one time with us. —Balbir

Beth and Cassie, my daughters, were all grins when they finally got to see their brother. They really saw how small and fragile Geoffrey was firsthand. Finally, it was their opportunity to hold him on that visit, and they loved it. In fact, they did not want to leave, although the nurses were pushing us out. When we went back for another visit, there was the fight over who got to hold him first. I must admit to being very proud of both of them that day. —Shaw

- Prepare your kids for visits to the NICU so they'll know what to expect and how to behave. At home, practice the hand washing, gowning, and any other routines prescribed by the NICU. Explain that there are lots of sights and sounds in the NICU that may seem strange at first, but that it's the safest place for the baby to be. Also explain that the baby needs all her energy for growing so she sleeps a lot. Once you're in the NICU, remind them early and often that because the baby is tiny, he needs tiny touches and tiny whispers.

On providing emotional support and spreading calm:

- Remember that it's natural for your other children to be stressed by the NICU journey—and it's not your fault.

- When your children are acting out or in a funk, instead of trying to "fix" or make them happy again, empathize with them about how times are tough right now. Assure them that the whole family can prevail—and that all your children are important to you.

- When your children are showing signs of stress or problematic behaviors, listen for the concerns behind your children's words, questions, and behavior. Tell them you welcome their questions and want them to put their worries into words so you can offer the reassurance they need.

- Particularly if you observe troubling changes in your children, ask for a referral to a child life specialist. These professionals work with the siblings of hospitalized children, and many hospitals have such specialists on staff. Or ask your pediatrician to make a referral to a therapist who helps families weather this kind of crisis.

- Rely on familiar sources of support for your children. In addition to friends and family, recruit the support of your children's teachers and other caregivers by keeping them abreast of the situation.

- Know and honor your limitations—and remind yourself (and others) what your priorities are for now. Say no to everything else. It can wait.

- Hold onto the idea that, over time, the demands on you will ease and you'll have more resources to go around. This too shall pass.

- Boost your morale by pausing to appreciate the delight your other children can bring you. Set aside time for simply enjoying them.

- Remember that children need quantity time, not just quality time. More than anything, they need you to just be with them, hanging out, listening. And quality can be found in minimalism and effortlessness. Time spent playing cards, talking over breakfast, chatting in the car on errands, reading stories, or snuggling in bed can be far more comforting than a major outing or new trinket. Frequent little activities make the biggest impact.

· Maintain as many familiar routines as possible, as children will derive comfort from this. If you must institute some changes, establish new routines. Strive for simplicity and consistency.

My husband and I tried to keep things as normal as possible for my older child. I'm still home when she returns from school. Her dad takes her to school every morning, and she gets to visit her friend for playdates like she always did. . . . I asked my daughter how she was doing because I feared neglecting her needs in the midst of the chaos. She said, "I'm not worried because I know the baby's going to be fine." I said I wanted to know how she was doing, with me and dad being so busy. She said, "I know you love me and play with me and give me attention, so I'm fine." That's how I knew she was okay.—Balbir

On fostering relationships between siblings:

· To fold your baby into the family even during the NICU stay, make a baby book for your children, with photographs and keepsakes of their little sibling. They'll be able to turn to this special book when you're away at the hospital, and it can also be a catalyst for conversations and questions. Along a similar vein, work together to make a big sister or big brother book for your baby's incubator. Items such as these can help your other kids build a bond with their new little brother or sister.

· On the first NICU visit or on other special occasions, plan a gift exchange, where your other children bring small tokens to the baby and receive a small token "from" the baby. You can also have your children exchange photos, cards, and messages with the baby, with you acting as translator. These exchanges can build kinship bonds.

· As your children grow and mature, their perspectives will change—and new questions may crop up. In general, when you make your baby's special history or current needs a topic for continued open discussion, your children (and their peers) will likely have fewer unnecessary fears and faulty conclusions.

One day a neighbor boy came over and said that Mackenzie looked ugly with her oxygen on. That was it—all it took for me to get started. I then decided it was time for children around the boys to understand their plight and what was going on with Mackenzie. So I took Mackenzie in for show-and-tell at kindergarten for both boys. I showed them all about prematurity (on their level) and her feeding tube and oxygen. They soaked it in and began to love Mackenzie. (The teacher thought I was crazy!)—Dianne

Finally, keep in mind that children are resilient. Just as this family crisis is an opportunity for you to stretch and grow, it's an opportunity for them too. As you recover your parenting reserves, your renewed care and attention will add to their resilience and refill their reserves.

I realize now that kids understand lots of things, and they would've understood what they could. We should have faced the issue with them. Now they know that their baby was born early, too early, and he was very sick. They know that he almost died. They know they have to be very careful with germs, which I'm not proud about, but the word *germs* comes out of their mouths a lot. And they know that our baby is different. He needs more time to learn things. I think they need to know, maybe not everything, but they need to know part of it.—Gallice

Seeking Professional Counseling

The postpartum period is complex even under the most ideal circumstances, and getting help to untangle your feelings and identify your needs can make all the difference to your adjustment.

If I could relive that time, there are things I would do differently. Besides being more assertive with the hospital staff, I would have sought help for myself. I believe I could have served Molly better if I had had a grip on my feelings.—Renee

In addition to attending a parent support group, many parents profit from individual counseling as well. Individual counseling has the added benefit of letting you air your feelings at greater length and helping you work through other personal issues that may be affecting your adjustment. Just as you see a doctor when you suffer from physical distress, it makes sense to see a counselor when you suffer from emotional distress.

Some things are too big to work out on my own. . . . Is it uncommon to feel this way, to realize that years later, there's all this stuff that's still there, still unresolved? When does it end? . . . How many more layers of pain are there? Why is it that James has come out of this so much more whole than me? I'm sure that I was normal once. Now I wonder if I ever will be again.—Leanne

If you have overwhelming or persistent feelings of anxiety, fear, guilt, anger, numbness, or depression, professional counseling can give you the extra support you need and deserve. Counseling can get you back on track if you feel disconnected from your baby, are stuck in a rut of grief, seem to overreact easily, have trouble getting through the day, notice your relationships are deteriorating, or you simply think it might help. You may just want someone outside your circle of friends and family who can listen, understand, and support you. Family therapy can benefit your other children and your relationship with your partner. You may feel the need for counseling at any time, even years later, and at more than one point along your journey, particularly when you encounter situations that spark intense grief.

I guess until recently I had never really thought about the grief caused by the loss of rites we go through as our tiny babies are cared for by the medical system. I was too busy doing what needed to be done to get myself and my family through the whole ordeal of having Rowan so early.

Now it has hit with a vengeance. I find myself always on the defensive when it comes to general parenting and health issues. I am not as tolerant of well-meaning people and their advice as I was with my other two babies. I will often fly off the handle at simple things, like my father-in-law's commenting on how Rowan is holding his arms out to the side or the sterilizer still being used for bottles. I know that mostly the intentions are good and often it is just a way to find a topic of conversation meaningful to both of us, but I can't stop my defenses from stepping in and taking over in situations like this. My intellect goes onto the back burner.—Bess

Like many parents, you may have coping techniques that worked well enough in the past but are woefully inadequate now. And this crisis is too big for you to blunder, muscle, or sidestep your way through it. Your baby's hospitalization or condition can act as a catalyst for growth by compelling you to adopt healthier ways of dealing with crises and emotions. A skilled therapist can support you through this process of change and adaptation.

I do hope to have additional pregnancies. I thought I was ready, but when it became more of an imminent possibility, I realized that I am not prepared. I need to have some couples therapy with my husband so we don't repeat the same dynamic. It is possible that another child will end up in the NICU, and I need reassurance that he will not retreat into his own world and leave me to deal with our son and the new baby alone. I also need to process my experience with the NICU (using EMDR) and make it a memory rather than a recurring experience.—Liza

The stress of Lars's early birth and ongoing issues has brought new issues as well as preexisting things to the front. It's easy to blame problems on our situation, but recognizing that many of the things that are driving us crazy are old patterns has been very illuminating for us. And my husband, especially, is now dealing with issues like letting fear dominate his life, mild depression, and anger management that have been with him for a long time but that he has been able to deny in the past. I really feel that our relationship has been strengthened and deepened by our experiences with prematurity—not that I would recommend it.—Kris

Some people hesitate to enter counseling for fear they will never stop needing it. For many, getting into therapy implies weakness, mental illness, or character flaws. Actually, the reverse is true. Recognizing the need for counseling indicates personal strength, health, and courage—because being successful in therapy means facing your feelings and problems and boosting trust in yourself. Therapy also implies a commitment to your children and your partner, since those relationships will thrive as you become healthier emotionally. Therapy can help you to

- feel and express a wide range of emotions,

- understand your reactions,

- learn new ways of coping,

- acquire more skills for working through problems,

- feel nurtured and understood in a deep and complete way by a skilled listener, or

- feel better about yourself, more aware of your strengths, competence, flexibility, and resilience.

Ultimately, through the process of therapy you gain the ability to help yourself. When you stop going regularly, your counselor can remain available for occasional consultation if the need arises.

Even just a few visits with a counselor might give you reassurance and the boost you need. You might also want to explore other emotionally healing avenues, such as art therapy, yoga, meditation, journaling, acupuncture, homeopathy, naturopathy, and massage.

If you decide to try counseling, look for a licensed professional who understands your needs and the grief and trauma of having a newborn in the NICU. A reputable counselor can be a psychologist, a clinical social worker, a psychiatrist, a psychiatric nurse, or a member of the clergy. To locate specialists in your area, contact professional organizations or check local listings under Psychologist, Psychiatrist, Social Worker, Counselor, or Mental Health Services. Recommendations from people you know can be the most effective way to find a good therapist.

Looking back now, I didn't really cope; I just bottled those feelings inside, cried, and went back to the NICU. I got into counseling later. I work in a very high stress job and think that made me quickly see that I needed professional help.—Jody

I learned to recognize that when I was feeling particularly stressed that I probably needed help. I have sought the help of many therapists through the years for both the babies and me. I always tried to tell them my truth, and when I did, it almost always led to a breakthrough. When I go for help, I always wish I had done it sooner.—Susan B.

Remember, you're not the one who is flawed. It's the *situation* that is so aberrant. Most parents need some help adjusting.

Finding Solace in Your Beliefs

In Judaism, you are never supposed to pray *for* things; prayer is supposed to be about praise and gratitude. I never used to understand that philosophy until the time I spent in the hospital before my babies were born. I didn't even know what to pray for or how to pray. I bristled at first at the people telling me that they were praying for me and my babies. But at some point, I started to be in the moment. Almost every hour I would say to myself (or maybe to God, I'm not really sure), "Thank you for letting me get to this point." It wasn't anything radical, but it made sense to me at the time. On my good days, I still say it to myself.—Susan B.

Your beliefs may help you cope and adjust, or they may make you more confused or angry. Especially if you consider yourself devout, you may be surprised at your doubts. You may feel angry with God or disappointed in your religion. You may even reject some of the concepts you formerly embraced without hesitation. When life turns down any unexpected, challenging path, it is natural to question your assumptions. Whether you subscribe to a religious tradition or your own unique blend of philosophies about life, destiny, goodness, and higher powers, it is normal to reassess your beliefs and even to modify them based on the lessons you are learning.

Everybody's put here for a reason. There are a lot of times when I question my faith and I think that something like this shouldn't have happened, that I don't understand why, but I don't think it's for me to understand.—Betsy

Just having faith helps, I think. That there is a greater purpose out there. My beliefs have intensified in some ways.—Linda S.

I have struggled with faith and religion for some time. Our experiences changed our views on a lot of things. We still aren't really sure where we stand with religion.—Corin

If you have been taught that faith means unquestioning acceptance, you may worry that your current doubt and inquiry dooms your chances for righteousness or heavenly reward. You may wonder if your baby's condition and hospitalization is a test of faith and worry that you've failed that test. You may even fear that your lack of faith was lurking inside you all along and this crisis is your punishment.

If you are questioning your faith or feel guilty about your fears or doubts, here are a few ideas to ponder. As always, select the ones that feel right for you.

· Whether or not you consider yourself to be religious, you can adopt spiritual philosophies that give you answers and help you cope. Look for deeper meaning. Finding your spiritual path is its own journey.

· If being religious is important to you, your devotion is measured not by the blindness of your faith but by the honesty of your questions and the openness of your mind and heart toward different answers. It is far more meaningful to be a conscious follower than an obedient one.

· If you are struggling to understand what's happening to you within your religious framework, try finding a spiritual mentor who can help you make sense of your experiences.

· If your community of worship or your clergyperson cannot tolerate your questions or emotions, you are not getting the guidance and support you deserve. As you search for fellowship or direction on your spiritual quest, look for and associate with spiritual sources, including people, books and media, activities, and places. Open yourself to the possibilities.

· You can make choices. Even if your religious tradition emphasizes judgment, look for and trust the compassionate qualities of your God or higher power. Hold to the spiritual ideas that nurture, comfort, and empower you.

· If you feel tormented by your religion, explore other denominations or philosophies within it and even other belief systems. Learn about other values and ways of viewing life, purpose, and the big picture. Look for a spiritual path that feels right to you—not convenient, easy, or simple, but honest and heartfelt.

· You can choose to follow the teachings of those you would like to emulate in word *and* deed. The most respected, beloved, enduring religious leaders and teachers are those who not only encourage spiritual behavior but also lead by example.

· Don't use religion to hide from your grief or your imperfections. Religion cannot make up for the hidden parts of yourself or your life. Be your authentic self—and subscribe to a set of beliefs that celebrates that self.

Recognize that you can embrace a spiritual life without embracing religion. To be spiritual is to marvel at the wonder and mysteries of life (and death), to appreciate and respect the blessedness of nature and all living things, to ponder a greater power and knowledge, to seek, to question, to contemplate, to be willing to not understand. To be spiritual is to be conscious of the values you hold and to live your life consistent with those values. To be spiritual is to welcome the different beliefs of others because you know that each person's reality belongs to him or her, just as yours belongs to you. Of course, a religious person can be spiritual too, but there are plenty of people who profess religious belief without embracing much in the way of spirituality. You can strive to be spiritual whether or not you are religious.

Deciding to Move Forward

While Daphne was still at the hospital fighting for her life, one of the greatest gifts possible in helping me deal with Daphne's continuing challenges was the story likening having a child with special needs with a couple planning a trip to Italy but ending up in the Netherlands. Like that couple, I thought my pregnancy would lead somewhere completely different. I did not plan or intend to have a child with so many special needs. But I'm not about to simply give up on the trip, get depressed, or simply wish I could just go home. There are so many wonderful things to enjoy about my daughter, and I could never be disappointed in her. I have never denied my daughter's problems. There simply never was time. Circumstances required me to accept the fact that my daughter had CDH between when it was first detected and when she was delivered. The reality of my daughter's condition was only reinforced by meeting with various specialists, touring the NICU, and seeing what the doctors and NICU personnel did for her immediately after she was born. That said, while I accept the implications of my daughter's medical condition, I refuse to believe that I can do nothing to help my daughter try to overcome her various medical and developmental challenges. So long as we have the means, I will continue to seek out as much therapy as she needs. Every time I see Daphne make the most minute, noticeable progress in her development, I am filled with thanks, pride, and joy.—Dina

After a while, you can choose whether to accept your baby's special start and fold its consequences into your life or be defeated by them. You can move on with your present and into your future or remain stuck in your past. You needn't look too far into the future. Running a marathon is easier if you focus on each stride, not all the strides you have yet to take. Still, when there is movement, you know you're moving forward.

How did I cope? I have no idea. You just do. You just step up and do what you have to do to get through that day or even just that hour.—Jennifer E.

Many parents mention that eventually they reach a point where they stop wishing it hadn't happened and start learning to live with it. When you are ready, you can do that too.

I feel I got to the other side after that first birthday—that was the big step. . . . I still get emotional about it, but it's in the past now. We're over it, but it's still a big part of our lives and always will be. It's just not as devastating as it was. We've gotten past the pain, past the anger, and past the Why me?—Marcia

I think my key to surviving things with Sean is mainly the fact that he was such a little fighter himself. How could I sit there and wallow in my self-pity? If someone so tiny and helpless could fight so hard to survive, I had darn well better be fighting right along with him.—Ami

For me, I don't know that there was a key to integrating it (unless you count good old-fashioned bullheadedness). It was survived and integrated because there was no other option. It had to be.—Tracy

You've just got to move on and make it better for yourself and get stronger from the situation. . . . What doesn't kill you makes you stronger. That's our motto.—Betsy

Nod and accept it. What else could I do?—Jennifer E.

Looking for the Treasure in Adversity

As you move forward, you adjust to this experience and integrate it into your life. You claim it and own it as a part of what makes you *you*. You look back and say things like, "Before this happened, I was so shy. Now, I'll stand up to anybody to get what I need." Or, "I used to take so much for granted. Because of what we've been through, I can appreciate what is truly important." Or, "If I hadn't been through this, I wouldn't have the friendships, the job, the interests, the special joys that I so value now." By surviving this ordeal with your baby, you bear witness to your own resilience.

Now there are so many things every day that they do that make us laugh, and we just think, *Gosh, we're so lucky.* We've been just really lucky with them. . . . If you stay on the positive side of it, you don't get bogged down with the negative details.—Betsy

Three years later, I am less consumed, more able to concentrate, and once again an effective businessperson. But I will never be able to lose myself in my job, in my company, in my own life as completely as I once did. There is so much more in my life, so much more in my heart, so much more, both wonderful and painful, that none of it can ever be as important to me as it once was. I do my job well, but no business deal can ever mean as much now that I truly understand the blessings that we have and the risks that we face each day. I am better for my experiences. My priorities are based on what is truly significant, and I appreciate life's tenuous gifts so much more.—Susan C.

Finding the treasure in adversity is something you must do for yourself when you are ready. It can't be rushed—and try as they might, others cannot do it for you.

On a related note, many parents find it helps to make light of their predicaments whenever they're able and that doing so is a reassuring marker of their positive emotional progress. As you acclimate to each new situation, you'll be able to look more often on the brighter side, perhaps finding humor among the rubble. This will help you cope by lightening your load. Laughter—even chuckling with dark humor—is good medicine.

I want to tell parents at the beginning of their emotional journey not to forget to laugh at the little things. After Daphne was born and in the NICU, I decided to pump breast milk to keep my production at a level necessary for if/when Daphne would need it. I would keep a breast pump on a timer in my bedroom so that I could wake up and pump at regular intervals. One night early on, when the pump turned on, my husband shot out of bed looking for his pants and asking me how far apart my contractions were. It took a full minute for him to realize that Daphne was already born and that there was no emergency. After scratching his head and saying, "Oh yeah," Barry began to laugh hysterically at his mistake. I soon joined in, and we both felt much better having just laughed about a silly thing. In order to get through the emotional journey, you have to realize your life will keep on going even though your precious baby is still in the NICU.—Dina

For the longest time I was joking about being a part-time mother because the nurses were doing this and the nurses were doing that. I'd be able to come down for a couple of hours, but then I had to go home and do other stuff. . . . That is the way I deal with things. If I can't laugh about it, I can't deal with it. I had to look at the lighter side of it because if I looked at the more negative aspects of it, I would've just been useless. I would've gotten mired down in my own mind. So I would joke around about stuff like the insurance covering the time she was in the hospital. I'm like, "Man, I've got a full-time babysitter. I don't even need to pay for it. This is great."—Brooke

When he was doing so well—and I feel very bad about saying this, but—I even said, "Why are people pregnant for nine months if you can do it in six months?" Of course, I would not say that again now, after everything we've been through later. There is a reason for a nine-month pregnancy, for sure. But I was able to joke about it, which means I was able to feel better.—Gallice

Points to Remember

· *Trying to ignore, dismiss, or avoid your grief won't make it go away. Grief is patient—it will stay with you until you face it and let it flow.*

· *Grieving is not a sign of weakness. Rather, it is the healthy, smart, necessary, and brave thing to do.*

· *There are many effective ways to cope with grief. Whatever your preferred strategies, by facing your feelings and going with the ebb and flow, you enhance your ability to come to terms with your losses and move forward.*

· *By identifying emotions such as guilt, anger, and despair, you untangle them and make way for peace and healing.*

· *Reach for a sense of physical well-being. Practice relaxation techniques, eat healthy foods, and do some gentle, fun exercise to help you cope with fatigue, insomnia, and anxiety. Along with spending time with your newborn, if you accomplish anything else, you are overachieving.*

· *Getting close to your baby builds your confidence as a parent and moves you toward emotional healing.*

· *Try cognitive techniques such as reframing, mindful acceptance, going with the flow, focusing on the positive, and realistic expectations. These tactics can reduce your distress by restructuring your thoughts and perceptions.*

· *Tell your story: write in a journal or correspondence, talk to your friends and family, connect with other parents who've traveled this path. Rely on those people who can listen without trying to fix you.*

· *If you are feeling stuck or frequently distressed, you can benefit from counseling. Seeking professional help is a sign of your courage and willingness to face yourself. You needn't be incapacitated.*

· *Eventually you can find a balance between maintaining control over your life and accepting the limitations on your control. Focus on fixing the fixable.*

· *Let yourself take breaks from your grief and find respite in things you might enjoy.*

· *You will prevail.*

5:

Acclimating to the NICU

Finally, we got the call saying we could go up and see our son. I was put in a wheelchair, and we entered the NICU, the artificial womb that we all would live in for a while.—Laurie

When you first enter the NICU, you begin another chapter in your journey. You may feel besieged by the sights, sounds, smells, machinery, and activity. You may notice a palpable emotional intensity. Seeing all the worried parents and their struggling little babies, some of whom may die, can be very distressing.

The NICU was a bit overwhelming. There were a lot of very sick babies to walk by in order to get to Kitquin's bed. To my surprise, the NICU was actually pretty loud. It was filled with cries and pinging machines and whispering parents.—Jennifer E.

Even if you had a prenatal NICU tour, the emotional load is amplified now that *your* baby is here. As you approach your newborn, you can't help but notice that your baby is cradled by medical equipment and receiving technical care you cannot match. Diligent, authoritative nurses and doctors speak in alien terms, referring to anatomy, conditions, treatments, and gizmos you've never even heard of. When you meet with the neonatologists, every diagnosis sounds so frightening and so serious. You wonder how you'll ever understand your baby's medical status, master the language, and most of all, trust these strangers with your precious newborn.

He was so small. How could a person so small hold on to life? I remember wondering if he was in pain because of all the equipment he was hooked up to.—Cynthia

I wanted so badly to just hold and protect my child. The hardest thing in the world is to know that you cannot comfort or protect your child, to put your trust completely in the hands of others and simply stand back and watch. It felt so unnatural and broke my heart.—Corin

On my discharge day, it was so hard to leave. I was afraid to leave him. You've just started to bond, and with all your anxieties and fears, now you're going away from him. It really hurts because you don't trust anything at that point. You don't know he's in loving hands yet. You think you have to be there all the time to protect him.—Gallice

Our 100 days in the NICU were 100 days on another planet. My son's life depended on these people. My life depended on those people. Would they be kind to him, listen, respond, care, make good decisions?—Susan C.

Especially at first, when access to your baby may be most limited, it is natural to feel unsure about how and where you fit into the NICU. If your baby is unstable, ventilated, or recovering from surgery, medical staff may tell you to refrain from holding or even touching your newborn. Grateful that your baby is receiving skilled medical care, you may keep your distance for fear of causing your little one harm— and also deeply resent the fact that your baby has gatekeepers. You may not see these people as your allies, your teammates, and your advisors—yet.

Standing at this threshold, it's normal for you to feel hesitant. Give yourself the time you need to acclimate. Soon enough you'll become familiar with your baby's condition, knowledgeable about treatments, used to the equipment, fluent in the terminology, and friendly with the staff.

For the first two days I was able, I visited the nursery often, but only with my husband. I was still afraid to do much by myself. I was still overwhelmed by everything. Once I was released from the hospital, I quickly adjusted to visiting by myself. After my first solo visit, I began to relax and rely on the nurses for help when I didn't know what to do.—Kimberly

It took me a few days to be comfortable. It's hard to cope with. I didn't want to be there. In my mind, I was still pregnant, even though he wasn't in my tummy anymore . . . so it took me a couple of days to adjust. The third day was better. And then I wanted to be there most of the time.—Gallice

In the beginning I didn't even try to ask too many questions. I didn't try to learn the nurses' names. I wasn't there for social hour. I was pretty much just trying to sit at their bedsides and talk to them. Then the nurses taught me how to touch them—like, you're not supposed to stroke them but kind of cup them. When I was shown that, I was so grateful. Some of the nurses wouldn't let you even do that, but the ones who would, I was grateful.—Stephie

A question that kept running through my mind was *Why do they get to know more about my daughter than I do?* And at first the nurses and the neonatologists kind of intimidated me, but after I had a chance to get to know them, they were not so bad.—Stacy

The nurses were beyond amazing. They became my mothers, sisters, and best friends. They not only took care of my boys but also of me. During the boys' NICU stay, I lost both of my grandmothers; the boys were not stable enough for me to feel like I could travel away from them, and the nurses were there to give hugs and caring words. They are the most amazing people I have ever met.—Jody

And soon enough, you'll begin to find your place in the NICU, as your baby's parent. But at first, you cannot imagine how you'll fit in because all you may notice about Intensive Care is the "intensive." As you acclimate, you'll begin to see and appreciate the "care" and the many ways you can participate with your baby. You will shed the cloak of outsider and find yourself becoming an *engaged parent*. This transformation happens naturally, as

- your focus shifts from the NICU to your baby,
- your perception of *who your baby belongs to* shifts from "theirs" to "mine",
- your caregiving shifts from passive to active, and
- your voice shifts from tentative to advocating.

This chapter offers an orientation to the NICU that can help you acclimate and make this shift from outsider to engaged parent.

Modern NICU Practice

The current gold standard is gentle, responsive, and supportive care that embraces parent participation. But it wasn't always this way.

In the late 1960s and early 1970s, when neonatology was a brand-new specialty, it was standard to keep babies isolated, untouchable, and surrounded by technology under the assumption that this would speed their recovery. Unfortunately, as it turns out, many of these practices were detrimental to babies. Deprived of their parents' presence and touch, babies were stressed further. Bombarded by lights, noises, and medical procedures, their immature nervous systems were often overwhelmed. As a result, physical recovery, healthy development, and immune function were inhibited.

The technology-centered nature of early NICU policies also had a devastating effect on parents. Mothers and fathers were often treated like intruders, making it difficult for them to form close connections with their babies. Discouraged from asking questions, communicating their concerns, and participating in caregiving, parents felt powerless, alone, and incompetent.

As technology improved, survival rates climbed, as did the population of NICU babies—and the number of vocal parents who wanted and *needed* to be closer to their infants. These parents also pressed for certain issues to be addressed, such as a gentler, more nurturing environment for their babies; adequate pain control; parental decision-making power; and closer attention to long-range outcomes, not just survival statistics. Forward-thinking practitioners who observed the harsh conditions, poor outcomes, and professional burnout also sought change. So, in the 1980s and especially the 1990s, neonatology hit its stride. By that time, it could afford to turn its focus and research from the remarkable technology that was saving lives to the *quality* of those lives, both during hospitalization and after discharge. Research continues to show that parent participation is key to ensuring this quality, and state-of-the-art NICU care has shifted its focus from the infant to the infant-parent dyad.

In addition, to promote parent participation in the NICU and improve the infant's quality of life, two complementary approaches to care have been cultivated:

- Relationship-centered care
- Developmentally supportive care

Relationship-Centered Care

Relationship-centered care considers *relationships* to be the cornerstone of quality health care. After all, medical care is delivered to people, by people, and caring happens within the *relationship* between practitioner and patient. In the NICU, this means that each practitioner builds a relationship with your baby, seeing your baby as a unique and whole individual. This heartfelt connection results in medical care that is individualized, supportive, comprehensive, and compassionate.

Relationship-centered care also recognizes that quality medical care is delivered in the context of *collaborative relationships* on the care team. In the NICU, this means that all of your baby's doctors, nurses, and specialists consult respectfully and often with each other and with you.

Last but not least, it recognizes that patients benefit when *family relationships* are honored, supported, and incorporated into caregiving. In the NICU, this means *precious little should come between you and your newborn.*

In other words, parent involvement is considered central to your baby's best interests, and part of the NICU practitioner's job is to actively support your efforts to relate to your newborn. With tips and encouragement from your baby's doctors and nurses, you can get close to and nurture your little one. When care expands to address your needs, you can better cope with the situation, the uncertainties, and painful emotions, which in turn better enables you to nurture your growing infant. In short, your participation is not just important for your baby, it's important for *you.* Taking direct care of your baby and close contact with your little one whenever possible are what help you grow into your parenting role. Your participation happens in the context of your relationships with your baby's medical practitioners *and* your relationship with your baby.

The first time I held him was while the nurses did a bed change. I was so unsure of myself, and Gabe was still heavily sedated, but it still was an amazing feeling. The second time we were able to hold him was on New Year's Day. It was the first time his daddy was able to hold him, and I will never forget the happiness I saw in my husband's eyes. He finally felt like a daddy and was gleaming with pride.—Corin

Here are prime examples of relationship-centered care at work in the modern NICU:

- Parents are welcomed as *parents*, not visitors.

- Parents are recognized as having a critical role in their baby's recovery and development.

- Parents' presence, touch, and nurturing are encouraged and considered valuable.

- Mothers are encouraged to breast-feed or pump breast milk as they wish.

- Parents are encouraged to hold their baby skin to skin, as in kangaroo care.

- Parents are supported in becoming attuned to their babies.

- Parents are considered competent and able to carry out nontechnical caregiving.

- Parents are encouraged to ask questions, voice concerns, and share their observations.

- Parents are integrated into the care team.

As you can see, state-of-the-art neonatal intensive care encourages parents to get involved and close to their babies. Rikki recalls asking to see her twins a few hours after delivery, in the middle of the night: "I expected an argument but was given a wheelchair instead." Corin describes two very different NICUs, and you can imagine the effect on parents, babies, and their budding relationships.

The first NICU was crowded and unorganized. Babies were set up in rows next to each other with no space or privacy. It was loud and busy and uncomfortable.

The second NICU, where Gabe spent most of his life, was much quieter and more peaceful. It had private rooms and felt much more like a healing environment. They had a parents' area with showers, rooms with cots, a kitchenette area, waiting area with a computer and TV, and other accommodations for family. They allowed parents to sleep in the same room as the baby if they wanted and were very caring and tried to accommodate the family needs.—Corin

Even though your baby's hospitalization is still a painful life experience, you benefit enormously from the relationship-centered NICU. Your trauma can be ameliorated by the gratitude you feel for the therapeutic, collaborative relationships you form with the practitioners. Instead of feeling at odds with NICU practices, you feel included, involved, and intimately necessary to your baby's progress. In short, you can *feel like a parent.* (For lots more on this topic, see chapter 6; for more on kangaroo care and becoming attuned to your baby, see chapter 7; for more on breast-feeding and pumping, see chapter 8.)

I gained confidence in myself as a parent, especially because the NICU allowed us and taught us how to be active in our son's care (taking temps, swabbing his mouth, sponge bathing him, and so on). Being allowed to do these things brought home the fact that this was my living baby and I was a very active and good parent. Without realizing it, I became very comfortable with touching/handling my son and grew to love him very deeply.—Andrea

Relationship-centered care also incorporates *developmentally supportive care,* which also helps babies and parents thrive together.

Developmentally Supportive Care

Developmentally supportive care is individualized care that promotes, sustains, and enhances each baby's holistic health and development. More specifically, it seeks to accommodate the infant's immature physiology and nervous system by providing low lights, hushed sounds, warmth, swaddling, nesting, gentle touch, appropriate nutrition, and adequate palliative care (management of pain and discomfort). For example, proper body containment (swaddling, nesting) and careful positioning can improve posture and muscle tone development. Better oxygenation techniques and protection from constant or bright lights avoids damage to the eyes. Adequate palliative care lowers stress, protects the brain, and speeds recovery. Medical staff also tailor their handling to each baby's unique needs and sensitivities. Babies can grow faster and fight infection better when not taxed by unnecessary stimulation.

Developmentally supportive practices not only improve each baby's quality of life during the NICU stay but can also result in better long-term outcomes. It is certainly the most humane way to treat babies. It also aligns with the parents' own nurturing urges, helping them feel better about entrusting their baby to the NICU.

Because babies do better when their parents are involved, developmentally supportive care naturally includes parent participation, *which is developmentally supportive for the parents.* Your presence, caregiving, questions, and advocacy promote

- your developing identity as a parent,

- your developing confidence as you get to know your baby,

- your developing competence as you learn how to respond to your baby,

- your developing collaborative abilities with NICU staff, and

- your developing ability to cope with the emotional landscape.

For instance, at a time when your relationship with your baby is the most fragile, participating in his or her care helps you feel competent and connected to your newborn. As you become acquainted with your baby and practice being attuned and responsive to your little one, your confidence, your bond, and your parental identity grow. (See also chapters 6 and 7.)

NICU policies and practices are finally reflecting what parents have known all along: medical technology is important but so is holistic nurturing and a parent's touch.

What helped me feel like a parent? Being included as an active member of his [caregiving] team. The nurses would take the time to explain to me every little procedure that they were doing and talk to me about when he would go home, even when the prognosis didn't look good. They helped to remind me that he was still my son and hold on to the hope that one day I could be a normal mother to my son. Pumping also helped, as it was the one thing that only I could do for him.—Corin

The nurse who was his primary was on, and she put us right into that role of parent. She oriented us to the systems there and told us we had access to every scrap of information about him. She also helped us learn immediately how to touch him and what would be soothing to him. She got us in touch with him right away, and that helped a lot.—Laurie

I was able to touch my baby and hold him. It was wonderful to do the kangaroo care. It made such a difference to my bonding with him. The kangaroo care made a huge difference in terms of getting to know my baby and feeling connected. I also felt more connected when I gained confidence in feeding and changing him and felt more comfortable with the nurses in the NICU.—Liza

As you can see, there is much overlap between relationship-centered care and developmentally supportive care, and they dovetail beautifully and lovingly in the modern NICU.

Coping with the Technology-Centered NICU

I definitely felt supported by the staff but wasn't given enough information about how to bond with my baby. I was allowed to do kangaroo care, but I had to ask for it.—Liza

NICUs vary in how much they encourage mothers and fathers to take an active role in parenting their babies. In some units, care expands to provide tremendous support for parents and inclusion in caregiving and decision making. Other units hesitate to make room for parents on the care team or fail to provide adequate support for emotional and parenting issues. When a NICU is in the process of instituting a more relationship-centered, developmentally supportive approach, policies can be inconsistent, and sometimes the climate is determined by the staff on duty.

There was one nurse (isn't there always?) who seemed more concerned with being in charge than with being helpful. Other than that, I was so pleased with the way the NICU was handled.—Jill

I was grateful for anything that I could do that was somewhat of a normal experience because I knew [the babies] needed to be held and touched, and I felt so bad that I couldn't. If it were up to me, I would have taken them home and had private care so that I could have had some say in what was happening. The technology and stuff didn't scare me—it was the unlovingness of it that scared me. That they needed the nurturing and they weren't getting it, that's the part that bothered me. If anybody needed it, they needed it—more than any healthy baby did.—Stephie

I was his mother and that was it, although sometimes I had to remind the staff to let me know of things that were happening because sometimes they sort of forgot that the child had parents.—Pascale

Each twelve hours someone new took control of my child. Some were warm and inclusive and opened the door to me and my ability to begin to learn to be a mommy. Some were cold and controlling and kept me firmly on the fringes of my child's care. A few have become lifelong friends; a few have become enduring bad memories. Most fell somewhere in between. But when we were there, when I was waiting to see who would live, who would die, what would happen next, I was completely at their mercy.—Susan C.

I understood why the NICU was set up the way it was, and I understood the purpose for all the rules. However, I was also sometimes very frustrated by some of those rules. For example, as the weeks became months, Barry's and my presence in the NICU became more and more important because as Daphne required less and less critical care, the NICU nurses—who more often than not had to work in a triage fashion (focusing on the most critical patients before the less critical ones)—would leave her alone for longer periods of time. The problem was that we simply could not spend all our time at the hospital (as much as we wanted to). Although we had many friends and family members who wanted to be with Daphne whenever we could not, the NICU's strict visiting rules (requiring all nonparent visitors to be accompanied by a parent at all times) prevented this.—Dina

Even if a NICU is more technology centered, the staff may still welcome you and your parenting desires as much as they can given policies and layout of the unit. But if the staff is focused more on protocol than individualized care, you may struggle to feel accepted and appreciated in the NICU and feel thwarted in your attempts to be an active parent.

One of the doctors yelled across the room for me not to touch my child one morning. He said, "I just told you that he needs his sleep." Now, this doctor didn't know that I sat at the end of Casey's bed for sixteen hours a day and left his blanket over his bed so he could sleep. Part of our ritual was that first thing (when I was sure my hands were cleanest) I would reach in and touch him and say good morning. That day I had to leave feeling that he wasn't even my baby!—Kelly

I had to worry that he would desat while I was holding him. That used to piss me off, because the nurses could do all their stuff to him and do whatever they were going to do, and then you go to hold your baby and they think you've ruined him for the day. That used to make me mad!—Stephie

You have no control. I was like, "Could you please just listen to me? Maybe I know a little bit. Please, just listen to me. Just listen to me. How much can it hurt to *listen* to me? I'm not going to try to cause her any harm!"—Michelle

Asking for a more active role can make you an agent for change in your NICU.

We refused to leave during rounds. Our rationale was that it was our child and we were going to be involved in her care. We also spent long hours in the medical library and on the Internet looking for information. In fact, it got to such a stage that our neonatologist would ask us what our thoughts were during rounds. What really gave us confidence was the spirited debates that would be conducted by Ngioka's bedside during rounds. Our neonatologist, Scott, was willing to accept input from everyone—nurses, residents, and parents—everyone who had a stake in Ngioka. This made us feel that (a) her caregivers were willing to get the latest and best information available in relation to Ngioka's situation and (b) her neonatologist didn't have the "I am God and therefore my word is law" complex and was willing to accept input.

Later on, when she was in Bay 3, a couple of the nurses tried to enforce the no-parents-during-rounds rule. The neonatologists actually asked where we were and said we could be there for rounds. They also started to ask what we had been observing, and a parent sheet was placed by all babies' bedsides for the parents to write on. The rationale for this was that the parents were sitting by the baby's bedside watching. A nurse was responsible for two or three babies and therefore not in a position to notice everything.

While we were in a situation that made us feel hopeless, this small gesture from our neonatologist empowered us. In some very small way, he made us feel as if we were an integral part of Ngioka's care team.—Jo

If you ask for a more active role but are refused, you will grieve yet another loss. And you may wonder what impact these limitations have on your growing relationship with your baby. Try to remember that parents and babies are resilient and forming a relationship is a flexible process. You can still find meaningful ways to be with your baby and parent successfully. (For more on this topic, see chapters 6 and 7.)

Joining Your Baby's Care Team

I distinctly remember during Buddy's last week, a nurse asked me if I would like to help change his central line dressing. I remember this incredible excitement and anticipation as I put on a gown, a mask, and some gloves. All I really did was make sure that Buddy's arms didn't get in the way, but to me it represented a few things. First, I was able to help in the care of my son. I can't overstate the importance of that. Second, there was a sense that the staff saw me as competent because they had asked me to help, and in a way, I thought, *They wouldn't ask me to help unless they thought I was good enough and capable of doing it.* Third, I felt like I could—and would—do a better job than anyone else. I believed I could read my son's behavioral signs of discomfort or irritation and that I was uniquely qualified to do something about it. I could talk to him softly. I could gently move his arms. I could reposition him if it looked awkward. I wasn't real concerned about the central line site. I was concerned about how the patient, *my child*, was doing.—Ed

Part of acclimating to the NICU is becoming an integral part of your baby's care team. As you consider this, you may protest, "But I'm not a doctor, I'm just a parent." Especially if you tend to place medical professionals on a pedestal, you may feel inferior and believe they see you that way too. But you're not inferior; you're simply *different.* You bring a unique perspective, another orientation, and an extra level of dedication to the team. You also play an indispensable role in giving your baby extra nurturing and nonmedical care. Rest assured that practitioners know that you want and need to take care of your baby and that you care deeply. They *expect* you to ask questions and voice concerns. The relationship-centered practitioners want to draw you onto the care team as they respect your important contributions to the quality of your baby's care.

Still, you may envy the parent who happens to be a nurse or a physician, thinking they have it so much easier. But unless the medical parent's specialty is neonatology, he or she is most likely as uneducated as you are. Imagine feeling doubly incompetent, both as a parent and a professional. Gallice, a physician, explains:

People expect you to know about your baby, and they forget that you're a normal parent. It's really hard because you feel embarrassed to ask certain questions that a normal parent would be allowed to ask. They expect you to know things, or maybe they don't even think of telling you something. You may be a physician, but it's a completely different field.—Gallice

The situation is only further complicated if a medical professional parent's specialty happens to be neonatology. Imagine the profound disorientation of seeing your own baby in the NICU. Imagine the feelings of helplessness as you must step aside and simply watch. Imagine being in the position of vigilant parent but knowing your presence might be nerve-racking for the staff, as you are qualified to scrutinize every detail of their caregiving. Imagine trying to shake off your professional cloak, knowing that more than anything your baby needs you to be a *parent*.

I was lost. I didn't know who I was supposed to be when I stood by Mackenzie's bed. Part of the time I wanted to just be a parent and not know anything, but more often I reverted back to my neonatal nursing knowledge. . . . It was my safe zone, being a nurse, because being a parent was too painful. I often wanted to tell the nurses and docs how to do things, but I couldn't as I was afraid they would be mad at me and take it out on Mackenzie. Once I developed a rapport with some of her nurses, I could suggest things, but I had to be careful. . . . Over time and with the encouragement of doctors and nurses who were friends and could tell me to be a parent, I did learn to be more of a parent.—Dianne

In short, you *want* your baby's medical practitioners to assume you are an uninformed parent so they'll teach you everything they know, encourage you to get close to your baby, and expect you to immerse yourself in the role of devoted mother or father. Whether you work in a health profession or not, dive into your parenting role, ask questions, and let yourself be tutored and coached.

Getting to Know Your Baby's Medical Practitioners

Forming relationships with practitioners can be an intimidating task. You become acquainted under duress, and your postpartum hyper-vigilance can make you wary of their abilities and intentions.

I hated seeing him so lonely in his incubator and with his bandages and wires everywhere. I wished that the nurses would hold him more, especially when I was too sick to.—Ruby

I learned quickly in the NICU that nurses wield incredible power. My children were dependent on a nurse to recognize the symptoms that required a physician's intervention. Their attentiveness and reactions can literally have life-and-death implications for a critically ill child. And they set the tone for my life when I was there.—Susan C.

We didn't completely trust that everybody there was doing their best to take care of our kids. Even though they're professionals and are good at what they're doing, I guess I felt that nobody cared about my babies as much as I did. So I was very watchful of the nurses and quickly came to appreciate some nurses over others.—Debbie

You may also feel wary of the seemingly endless parade of new faces at your baby's bedside. Particularly if the NICU is in a teaching hospital, you may wonder how your baby can possibly receive consistent care and close monitoring.

The nursing staff is the key to your baby's care. Neonatal nurses are highly trained specialists. Many hospitals assign a primary nursing rotation for each baby so that twenty-four hours a day, seven days a week, one of your baby's primary nurses will be on duty. Your baby's nurses become familiar with you and devoted to understanding and meeting your baby's individual needs. Depending on the unit, your baby's primary nurses may be responsible for:

· assessing your baby's condition and progress,

· notifying the doctors of any changes,

· making recommendations to the doctors and other members of the medical team,

· carrying out doctors' orders,

· planning and implementing all nursing care, such as feeding, bathing, positioning, administering prescribed medicines, and managing IVs,

· educating you about the medical, technical aspects of caregiving,

· teaching and supporting you in carrying out the most nurturing aspects of caregiving, including feeding, bathing, soothing, interacting, touching, holding, and kangaroo care,

· supervising the care your baby receives from other specialists and assistants, and

· being involved in discharge planning.

The doctors are experts in neonatal medicine, but the primary nurses become experts on your baby's unique, broad, hour-to-hour profile. So if you have questions about how your baby is doing today, ask your baby's primary nurses. They can offer you valuable information on your baby's medical status as well as insights on temperament, behavior, sensitivities, communication, feedings, triumphs, and challenges.

As you collaborate in the care of your baby, you will likely form the closest relationships with your baby's primary nurses. They in particular can provide a holding environment that reassures and steadies you. As Michelle B. recalls, "The nurses were wonderful in calming me and explaining what was going on." Jody agrees, "The nurses basically told us everything on how to care for the babies and what was going on. They were our lifelines."

Some of the NICU nurses that we got to know in the sterile infant rooms were very supportive. They made us feel that Daphne was doing as well as expected at each stage of her recovery and were very receptive to our calling in for status reports whenever we could not be at the NICU.—Dina

The nurses became our family for the three months we were there. We shared our day-to-day lives with them. They knew our babies as well as, if not better than, we did! They were the people we entrusted with our babies' lives—the ones we left them with when we left the hospital. Had I not had the relationship I did with the nurses, I never could have left every day.—Sara

The NICU staff became an extension of our family. The nurses were Gabe's "aunts" as they knew him and loved him as well as we did. They laughed with us and cried with us, even calling or stopping by the hospital on their days off and checking up on him. Four and a half years later and I am still in contact with a few of the nurses and respiratory therapists. They will always be a part of my family now.—Corin

Of course, nurses work closely with doctors. Even though schedules for doctors tend to be less consistent than for nurses, at least one neonatologist is available in the hospital around the clock, every day of the year. *When your baby is unstable or needs critical medical attention, a neonatologist is called in.* The attending neonatologist may call in other physicians who specialize in cardiology (heart), neurology (nervous system), pulmonology (lungs), or other areas. Remember that everyone's number one priority in the NICU is uncovering and meeting babies' urgent medical needs.

In a teaching hospital, doctors have varying amounts of experience, depending on what year of training they're in. All doctors have graduated from medical school, but you may cringe at the thought of an intern (first year out) or a pediatric resident (second or third year out) taking care of your baby. Keep in mind that interns and residents work with your baby's highly trained neonatal nurses and are closely supervised by a team of neonatologists. Because there are so many people taking care of your baby, you may feel lost and unsure of how to work with them. Here are some guidelines:

- *Recognize that you are an integral member of the care team from the start.* Even when you still have so much to learn, your presence, input, and questions are critical to your baby's care. The doctors and nurses know that your involvement enables you to be a better advocate for your baby, and your advocacy helps them do their jobs well.

- *Identify your contacts.* Ask your baby's doctor whom you should contact when you want to check on your baby from home and whom you should talk to when you have questions or concerns. Write down the names, phone numbers, and pager numbers that you get from your baby's doctor and nurse, and carry this list with you at all times.

- *Welcome all support and guidance you are offered.* Many NICUs employ a variety of professionals to assist the doctors and nurses in providing psychosocial support to parents as a matter of course. If a social worker, a psychologist, a psychiatrist, or a member of the clergy approaches you, don't assume that the staff has reported you or that they believe you are not coping well. Instead, appreciate your NICU's devotion to parent care.

- *Speak up.* If you are uncomfortable with the care your baby is receiving, ask your baby's primary nurse to contact the attending neonatologist for a consultation—*immediately* if necessary—or make the contact yourself.

- *See your time in the NICU as training to become the leader of your baby's care team.* As you grow more confident and look toward discharge, your leadership role will expand because after your baby is discharged, you *are* the leader.

Valuing Your Own Contributions to Caregiving

With your baby safely in the hands of highly skilled doctors and nurses, you may wonder how you can possibly contribute to caregiving. But intensive medical care is only part of what your baby needs to thrive. Your baby also needs your nurturing and your presence. You have a special familiarity that your baby finds calming. Only you can provide your particular voice, your recognizable smell, and your attuned touch to your baby. No one else on the team can breast-feed or provide kangaroo care for your baby. No one else can cup or snuggle your baby for hours on end.

For hours at a time, you can also devote undivided attention. Your observations and input are important, even when your baby is being closely monitored by machines and practitioners. Monitors tell only part of your baby's story, and practitioners cannot continuously focus on your baby like you can. By keeping close watch over your baby, your eyes and ears and sixth sense will tell you more about your newborn than any machine can. And you will learn to discern the tiniest details. At times, your observations may be the most astute, and parental intuition is very powerful. Many parents can recall a time when they knew something was up before any monitor or medical practitioner detected it. Feel proud that you can play this attentive role in your baby's care.

I recognized trouble long before the professionals did. The nurses and residents just didn't share my concern. Finally, when Spencer's blood sats continued dropping without explanation, a very good nurse went over a resident's head and insisted on a visit from an attending physician. And knowing what I know now about NEC (things I didn't know then), I am at a loss to explain how those who should have seen the symptoms missed them.—Susan C.

They were considering amputating her left leg because it was not healing as quickly as they would have liked and it could threaten her life. I pleaded with them to wait, prayed a lot, and she did finally heal to their liking. It felt great to be right! It was a hard decision, but I knew it was the right one. I knew in my heart of hearts that she would heal up, and they were not going to ever again make up my mind on anything. I learned the hard way from the pregnancy itself that my instincts are usually right.—Janet

Overall, your most unique and vital contribution to the care team is your parental bond. Your love, devotion, and instincts are beyond compare. And unlike even the most devoted nurse, you as the parent envision a future with your baby.

Valuing the Staff's Contributions—and Knowing They Value Yours

To form effective partnerships, it is important for parents and practitioners to have a mutual understanding and appreciation for each other's roles and responsibilities.

For instance, it's easy to blame the practitioners for overlooked clues, belated or mistaken diagnoses, ineffective treatments, or a lack of definitive answers. Parents need to keep in mind that sometimes the diagnosis, the best treatment, or the outcome is not obvious, and it becomes the doctors' job to explore possibilities. Sometimes more tests have to be run or more treatments tried before the doctors can rule out possibilities and pinpoint the right diagnosis or the best care. Treatments may take longer than expected or be ineffective for your baby. Some babies defy logic or the odds. Often, only time will tell.

On the other side, it's easy to criticize parents for having unrealistic expectations, being emotional and hypervigilant, or asking too many questions. Practitioners need to keep in mind that it's your job to hold on to hope—to want your child to get better faster and to do normal baby things. You have a right to your intense emotions—the NICU is an intense place to be. And it's your job to watch over your infant and follow up on your concerns.

Not every parent will get along with every medical practitioner—it's simply human nature. The reasons are many: personality clash, emotional distress, bad timing, cultural differences, an unfortunate incident. Add the often arduous and dramatic backdrop of the NICU and it's a wonder there aren't more conflicts. On the flip side, most parents also form intense connections with certain practitioners to whom they look for comfort and advice. As a parent, it can help to rely on the practitioners who are supportive and forgive those who are less than helpful.

I tried to breast-feed, but Ricky was using more calories than he was taking in. One night I was particularly frustrated, and I remembered what one of the nurses had told me. "When you can't get him to eat, just hold him and let him know how much you love him. Both the food and the love make him grow and mature." So I was holding him and sobbing and talking to him when one rude nurse came over and told me that he had to be fed now and then returned to bed immediately, so as not to tire him out completely. I told her that I would like a few more minutes, just to hold him and love him. She said that I was too upset and should leave and come back another time to visit. I just looked at her and told her to butt out and leave us alone because Ricky was still my son and I was his mother and I should be able to hold and love my son. The overall feeling I got was that I was in the way. I will never forget the way I was degraded and belittled by that nurse.—Jenny

It's so important for parents and practitioners to remember that they share the same goal—that is, getting the baby as healthy as possible and homeward bound. Be mindful of the demands you place on each other and be fair in your assessments.

I understand now that medicine is at least equal parts art and science. I don't believe that anyone caring for my son intended any harm. I think that they most likely all did their best. I understand, though, that their best was highly dependent on individual levels of skill, experience, dedication, burnout, overwork, distraction, desire . . . They were people just like me, people with a little more knowledge, maybe, but no more power.—Susan C.

Being Informed

The attending neonatologist and the nurse both tried to orient us to the most important details about our baby's condition and about how long to expect he would be in the NICU—the standard "until his due date" warning. We were both so shell-shocked that not much sunk in. The only thing I think we both got was that we could come in any time and that we were in for a long haul.—Laurie

I felt constantly overwhelmed, not only with intense feelings but also with information. At times I felt as if I would never understand everything that was happening.—Claire

I could only deal with what was happening in the present. I didn't want to know what was happening tomorrow or in the future. I didn't want to know because I was so overloaded with what was happening right there.—Stephie

Information can be empowering but also overwhelming. You may want all the details right away or it may be a while before you are ready, as your mind is still reeling from the shock of your baby's early birth or newfound condition.

Sometimes parents are so dazed that they don't recall having a conversation about a particular issue. The exchange is documented in the chart, and the doctors are saying, "We discussed this yesterday," but you are convinced otherwise. It can take time and repeated exposure to absorb complex information, especially when you are emotionally distressed.

What would I do differently? I would have tape-recorded everything. I cannot remember most of what I was told for about three months. That is a frightening feeling.—Cindy

As you regain your footing, easy access to information is crucial. Being told by a nurse, "You'll have to talk to the doctor about that" in response to a request for even the most mundane information can be enormously aggravating. If practitioners deflect your questions or tell you, "Don't worry about that," you may begin to see acquiring information as a battle with desperate overtones. Withholding information only fans your feelings of incompetence, anxiety, and helplessness, and it can be difficult for you to trust the practitioners who aren't forthcoming. You may find yourself insisting on information that you don't really need or want—simply to establish your right to have it.

Some practitioners hesitate to reveal much about a baby's status because they don't want to overwhelm the parents or cause unnecessary anxiety. You may appreciate their caution, but if you are denied the information you request, you would likely feel barred from your role and excluded from your baby's care team.

I came to hate the word *stable*. As a mother, I wanted to know details, facts, incidents, things that happened—not just, "She's stable." That puts you out of the loop so fast. You feel, *Okay, they don't want to tell me anything. I have no part in this.*—Beth

In contrast, you will find it far easier to cope when

- you have full access to the information you want at the pace you set,

- you are told how the information applies to *your* baby,

- you are given information in caring ways that recognize how emotional and difficult it is for you to hear and absorb much of it,

- you are given information in a spirit of sharing, honesty, respect, and collaboration,

- you feel that the practitioners consider your questions important, not an imposition, and

- you are supported as you face reality rather than being shielded from it.

The doctor went through all of the problems. And he really prepared me, as opposed to making promises that he could not keep. And I preferred that. I'm more like, "Give it to me straight so that I know what I'm dealing with."—Vickie

Sometime during the afternoon I was in labor, the on-call neonatologist came down to talk to me. I remember sobbing, telling her that I was so scared that my babies would live short lives filled with pain. She held my hand, looked me in the eyes, and said: "When you were admitted ten days ago, your babies had virtually no chance of survival. We have bought them a week and a half, and now they have an 80 percent chance of survival. Better than survival. They have a good chance of leading wonderful lives. I can't promise you that everything will be okay, but I can promise that I will always tell you the truth." It was exactly what I needed to hear. And she did always tell me the truth.—Susan B.

By sharing their knowledge with you, practitioners are support-ing your efforts to step into your parenting role, and they are fostering a collaborative relationship that will enhance teamwork and caregiv-ing. For sure, the topics involved—complications of prematurity, birth defects, critical illness, and perhaps even disability or death—are dif-ficult topics to contemplate. Yet learning the details and filling in the blanks can help you come to terms with what's happening, establish a coherent picture of the situation, and participate fully in parenting your baby.

Additional benefits of being informed include:

· Replacing fear of the unknown with understanding the purpose of all the leads, lines, and machines, and seeing them as friendly beasts

· Feeling proficient and able to follow your baby's progress

· Being able to do your own research

· Being prepared to make important decisions and oversee the quality of your baby's care

· Easing the stress of facing uncertainties, as information sheds light on the possibilities and what can be known

· Feeling the comfort of teamwork and mutual effort to determine and carry out your baby's care

· Trusting the practitioner's decisions when you cannot or need not be consulted

· Building your competence and confidence to take over your baby's care upon discharge

About a week after the birth, the haze started to lift. I began to ask many questions. I was determined to be as involved in my son's medical care as possible. I got a book about premature babies so I would know what to expect.—Laura

Besides the NICU, I spent most of my time at the library trying to find information about prematurity. I believe the more you know about what you are facing, the better off you will be.—Kimberly

The NICU staff was great about letting me help out with T.J.'s care. Still, the major decisions about his health were in the hands of the doctors and nurses. In this instance, I was grateful to give them control because I felt very overwhelmed. I had faith in them.—Claire

On the second day, when another baby died in the NICU, that's when I realized I had to know and understand exactly what we were going to be going through in order for me to survive. I didn't want anything blind. So that's what made me start reading, asking questions, talking to people.—Vickie

According to the books, my girls had a slim chance of survival. Oddly enough, the information from those books gave me strength. I at least had some idea of what I was facing. It was overwhelming and very upsetting, but at least I *knew*.—Kimberly

Information-Gathering Tips

Here are some strategies for gathering the information you seek and staying informed:

- *Address feelings first.* Ideally practitioners can take the time to ask you how you're doing and give you the chance to air some feelings. If not, you can start the conversation by saying, "I think it might help me make the most of this meeting if I can first talk a little bit about what this is like for me." Be brief and succinct— this is not a therapy session, but brevity can still be therapeutic. Clearing your emotional decks even a little can make room for the medical information that's about to be imparted.

- *Take notes.* To help you absorb information, you might take notes during conversations and meetings so that you can refer to them later. Ask your baby's nurse or doctor to draw pictures and write out unfamiliar terms so that you know how to spell and pronounce them. This information will make it possible to ask others for information and do your own research.

- *Get online.* Ask your baby's medical practitioners to recommend websites.

- *Repeat the facts as you understand them.* By responding with, "So, what you're saying is . . . " or "Let me get this straight . . . ," you enable the practitioner to clarify as needed. Repetition can also help you absorb and remember the information.

· *Keep track of your questions.* Writing them down as they occur to you helps you make the most of your meetings and conversations.

· *Consider recording meetings.* Ask permission to audiotape discussions and care conferences, as this can help you absorb the vast quantities of information you're expected to digest. A recording lets you hear explanations more than once, and it's a useful tool for keeping other family members informed.

· *Ask how you might go about asking follow-up questions later.* Most parents cannot put all their questions into words on the spot. It's only natural to need extra time to absorb what you've been told and formulate additional questions.

· *Stay aware of your questions.* Let your questions—even the ones you're afraid to ask—guide you toward gathering the amount and kinds of information you need.

· *Let your hidden fears surface.* Then you can ask the questions that are tormenting you. You may hesitate, afraid that the doctors will tell you something you aren't ready to hear, but typically, imagination is more fearsome than reality.

· *Learn to read your baby's chart.* At first, it will be a challenge to decipher, but as you become fluent in the language and abbreviations it contains, this documentation can help you keep abreast of the situation. Chart reading can complement open communication with your baby's care providers. Consider the chart a tool for enhancing discussions with your baby's nurses and doctors, not replacing them.

· *Seek second opinions.* When a diagnosis, prognosis, or course of treatment is unclear, anyone on the team has the right to seek a second opinion. Responsible team members honor this right.

· *Accept that sometimes the answer to your question is "I don't know."* It is far better to get an honest admission of uncertainty than a groundless prediction.

Overcoming Communication Barriers

In spite of best efforts to stay informed, parents may encounter some communication barriers even after the fog of those early days has lifted. When the news is bad, parents can't always—and occasionally don't want to—hear what is being said to them. Stephie points out, "Being ignorant can sometimes be the best thing for getting through it." If you need to hold on to the hope that your baby's prognosis is good, or if you want to simply live in the present, you may resist the staff's efforts to inform you of a poor prognosis. If a certain practitioner tends to shed only pessimism, you may avoid those conversations. On the flip side, some practitioners are reluctant to be direct when the outlook is not good.

I did not care to read about Mikey's potential diagnosis because at this point I was very happy that Mikey was doing better, and I was beginning to hope that perhaps he would be okay. Even if it was Hirschsprung's, perhaps it was manageable and we could avoid surgery. The thought of surgery scared me.—Chip

The first doctor we had, I called him Dr. Gloom-and-Doom because everything that came out of his mouth was just horrible. I'm sure he probably had reason to be pessimistic, but maybe some doctors would have said it a little differently. Everything he said scared the hell out of me. If I didn't understand something, I might ask him, but I learned not to ask him for information because it was just too scary.—Stephie

It was hard to get information out of the doctors. I was often met with responses like, "Why would you want to worry yourself about that?" when I asked about the long-term outlook. Looking back now, I realize that the doctors didn't have much hope for my son. I, on the other hand, had nothing but hope.—Laura

Sometimes there is miscommunication due to the parent's frame of reference being different from that of seasoned practitioners. For example, you may take as gospel an offhand remark like, "This could be seizures" or "I've rarely seen such an infection" or "I'll be surprised if he responds to that treatment." The practitioner, meanwhile, may merely have been thinking out loud or expressing an incomplete thought. Unfortunately, before you have time to react, the practitioner may be gone, and there's no one to answer your questions. So, if you overhear something that bothers you, try to ask for clarification on the spot—for example, "What did you just say? I want to make sure I understand what you are thinking." Asking for clarification may not erase your fears, but it can give practitioners a chance to explain casual observations, retract guesses, cut out drama and exaggerations, or elaborate, as in, "I'll be surprised if he responds to that treatment . . . but babies never cease to surprise me!"

With Evan's blood fungus, the doctor literally said to me, "I wouldn't be surprised if he was dead in two days." He actually said "dead." Up until that time, everybody had used euphemisms, like "We'll have to wait and see" or "Let nature take its course." No one had said "die." When the doctor said that, of course, I sat there for the next forty-eight hours at my baby's bedside because if he was going to die, I wanted to be with him for the time I had left with him. And then forty-eight hours later, I'm sitting there at the bedside, and the doctor comes over and he says, "He looks great today, doesn't he?!" And I'm, "Huh?" And he says, "Oh yeah, his fungus is still there and stuff, but he's doing okay." And I'm like, "You mean he's not going to die?" And he shrugs it off, "What are you talking about?" And I'm like, "Hello??!!"—Stephie

Misunderstandings can also arise due to differing perspectives. For example, if a practitioner talks about your "sick" baby, you may wonder what is meant by *sick*. If your baby is premature, you may question, "Isn't she *supposed* to have trouble breathing or eating at this gestational age? That's not sick, that's normal under the circumstances!" If your baby is in for observation, needs a little a jump start, or had corrective surgery, you may wonder if there is more they aren't telling you. If you hear any term or reference you don't understand, simply ask for clarification.

You may also run into differing perspectives on medical events and NICU paraphernalia. The fact that your baby may have "lost a few grams" or be "a little jaundiced" or have "a few periods of apnea" may seem to the nurses like no big deal, just a "NICU thing." But for you, the news may seem ominous or be the straw that breaks the camel's back. Vents, shunts, needles, central lines, scalp IVs, cannulas, gavage feedings, and splint boards may be everyday sights to doctors, nurses, and therapists, but they may be horrifying to you.

Daniel started to do stuff that was scary. He got his first apnea attack and he stopped breathing and his oxygen level in the blood was not what it should have been and his heartbeats were inappropriate. We later found out that these little things were exceptionally routine and that these nurses do this day in and day out, but at the time I looked at it as this one nurse had basically just saved Daniel's life. I mean, he was going down, he'd stopped breathing. She bagged him and brought him back. So it was a very tense moment.—Mitch

I wished that the doctors and/or nurses had explained more about what feeding complications could arise so that when feeds were stopped or started, I felt like I understood more of what was going on. Once it was explained to me about such complications as NEC [bowel disorder], I dealt much better with the feedings being stopped because I understood that this was protecting her rather than hurting her. I think it's a parent's instinct to feed their child, but preemies aren't necessarily ready for actual food, and it needs to be introduced slowly. It was very frustrating for me when I didn't understand that.—Nola

To overcome these communication barriers and avoid misunderstandings:

- *Realize that practitioners cannot read your mind*—you must ask for the information or reassurance you need. Instead of assuming that practitioners are withholding the information from you, assume that it's an oversight, and ask them to tell you what you need to know.

- *Ask the questions that most trouble or embarrass you.* Doing so lets practitioners know what reassurance you need, and their responses can also help you trust their ability to take care of your newborn.

- *Know the difference between having worries and having questions.* When you feel anxious or desperate for reassurance, don't ask for more medical information—simply voice your concerns. For example, instead of "Please explain brain bleeds to me again," say, "I'm really worried about the condition of my baby's brain and what the future holds." Your goal is to try to understand the big picture and the range of possibilities, not to get information overload and *still* feel helpless to exert any control over the situation.

- *Consider yourself the most important person in your baby's life.* Looking at your role from that perspective should reduce feelings of suspicion, competitiveness, or timidity, and you'll be less likely to project unkind motives onto the practitioners.

I think that parents have to ask or tell somebody what they need—because, obviously, these doctors and nurses aren't mind readers, and everybody has got a different level of experience. Now, I went to the library and took out every book I could find, and I read everything, and I knew every term and understood every phrase that they were saying, and if I didn't, I would ask.—Pam

If you ever wonder whether you're being too inquisitive or vocal, consider this: Practitioners are far more apprehensive about overly optimistic or disengaged parents who do not ask questions or voice concerns. Some of those parents are not tuned in to their baby's needs and can miss signs of real trouble. Others are reluctant to engage with practitioners and are missing out on opportunities to receive important instruction and support. Many of these parents become extra-anxious or run into trouble after they take their baby home. They postpone all their learning to the time after discharge, making many frantic phone calls to the NICU and emergency room visits with a healthy baby. Being informed builds a parent's confidence and competence to handle caregiving, and practitioners vastly prefer discharging babies to confident, competent parents!

Advocating for Your Baby

I advocate strongly for my children because they don't have a voice, they can't talk for themselves. A lot of times people in the medical professions think they have a job to do, and they do it in any way they can, without considering that it's a baby with feelings. Even though babies can't talk, they still have all the feelings you would have if someone was sticking four needles into your head at one time.—Betsy

On the morning of day two, they did an X-ray and it showed Kit had some fuzzy lungs, which could be normal or could be infection, so they started her on some antibiotics. They called in the consulting doc from the Children's Hospital level three NICU, and we were told she should be okay. The consulting doc gave guidelines to the hospital staff on what her stats should be and when to call the level three NICU, if they got too low.

On the night of day three, Kit took a turn for the worse. My husband went in to look at her and noticed her stats were in the area where the consulting doc had said they needed to be called. He got in an argument with the nurse because she didn't feel the call needed to be made even though it was clear Kit was satting too low and she was clearly in the area where the consulting doc had requested a phone call. After the talk they had, she looked in Kit's chart and called the other NICU.

The doc came and agreed Kit needed to be moved. This hospital was just not equipped for her. The head nurse came back and apologized for the other nurse and told us that the ambulance was on the way, and they would be transporting Kitquin ASAP.—Jennifer E.

Being a good advocate for your child takes hard work and confidence.—Susan B.

As you acclimate to the NICU and take on your role as a parent, you will also ease into the role of your child's advocate. Your advocacy role requires you to understand the intricacies of your baby's condition, the pros and cons of each treatment, and your child's best interests. Along with becoming fully informed, it behooves you to share your observations and speak up whenever you notice a change, become concerned, or believe in taking a different tack.

It may take a little while to get up to speed as you integrate the medical information and become attuned to your baby. Like many parents, it may also take a while to realize that the doctors and nurses don't have ultimate authority over your baby—*you* do.

The true nature of the medical practitioner's authority is medical expertise. The doctors in particular are responsible for having the latest medical knowledge about neonatal conditions, complications, diagnostics, and treatments, including risks and benefits. They are also responsible for carefully and compassionately applying their knowledge and wisely advising parents. Doctors and nurses are not under any obligation to carry out aggressive intervention that is futile or to withhold treatment that is clearly beneficial just because a parent orders them to. But essentially, you are the one who has hired them. They are your valued consultants who treat your baby, share information, answer your questions, and help you navigate the NICU experience so that you can do your job as a devoted, loving, protective parent.

Because of a lot of things that happened in the NICU and after, I really realized that I had to be an advocate for my child because nobody else would. Just because a doctor says something, doctors are not God. It's an opinion; it's an idea. Doctors can have a bad day too. And they're not going to see everything a parent sees. Parents have to realize that their instincts are really good and to believe and trust those instincts. Not only trust those instincts, but then be an advocate for your child based on them.—Vickie

I broke all the hospital rules—I took one baby and then took the other and sat in a neutral spot with both of them together. Heck yeah, I did! And the hospital didn't like it, but they lived with it. Because, I thought, these babies had been inside me, together, for as long as they were, and I'm sure, when they were born and separated, they were like, "What happened, and why am I here, and where is my counterpart?" You know? And that's probably what I felt worst about: having to have them separated and not be together and have that bonding thing. I was worried about that for a long time.—Pam

Many parents find it difficult to trust their observations, but you can very quickly develop a keen eye for how your baby is faring. Other parents find it difficult to muster the courage to speak up. If you feel hesitant, seek out the caregivers you feel most comfortable with. Like so much else about parenting in the NICU, becoming your baby's advocate is a process of adjustment, and it coincides with gaining confidence in your parenting role. (For more on this, see "Building Confidence" in chapter 6.) Also keep in mind that most practitioners value your input as it serves doing what's best for your baby.

If you have twins, triplets, or more in the NICU, you bear a multiplied obligation to stay informed and advocate for your babies. This can be very challenging because all of your babies will seldom be experiencing the same thing at the same time. You may have many conditions, complications, and treatments to learn about in order to stay on top of their situations. (For more on this and coping strategies, see "Multiple Realities—Multiple Roller Coasters" in chapter 9.)

Being able to stay on top can pay off. Sometimes, although very rarely, orders get mixed up, particularly with multiples. For instance, Pam's baby girl, Riley, got abdominal X-rays, but her baby boy, Banning, was the one with a bowel disorder. Banning's medication levels were checked, but Riley was the one who was receiving the drug for apnea. So Riley was exposed unnecessarily to radiation, and Banning received an unnecessary blood draw. Pam talks about taking charge:

At that point I said, "*Nobody* does *anything* to either one of these children without prior consent, no ifs, no ands, no buts. If it's an emergency and if it's life-threatening, then sustain life and *then* call me. But nothing is to be done." And I hated to be such a jerk about it, but I had to be. These babies couldn't speak for themselves, so they needed somebody to do it, and I thought that was my job, you know?—Pam

Being There for Medical Procedures

As your baby's advocate and wanting to keep an eye on your baby's care, you might feel strongly about being present for certain medical procedures. Hospitals and practitioners vary on how comfortable they are with parent presence at these times. But it is your right to be with your baby, as long as you can conduct yourself responsibly, cooperatively, calmly, and quietly, and you do not interfere with the procedure being carried out, the staff's ability to do its job well, or a sterile environment (which is why you can't be present during surgery).

On the other hand, it can be very difficult for most parents to be present for certain procedures. Your deep empathy with your baby can cause you great pain, and the resulting queasiness (or your general tendency toward queasiness) can get in the way of your being able to handle yourself properly. So remember, you don't *have* to be at your baby's bedside during every procedure. It is better—for yourself and your baby—to leave rather than force yourself to stay when you're feeling squeamish or distressed. If you're having difficulty soothing yourself, you won't be able to soothe your infant. Instead, from a safe and calming distance, you can send your positive thoughts toward your baby and then comfort your little one when the procedure is over.

Making Medical Decisions

When the benefits of a medical treatment clearly outweigh the risks, parents want to (and are expected to) agree to it because it's in their baby's best interests. But when the best interests of the child are unclear, parents need to be included in the decision making. For example, when there is more than one treatment option, and it's not clear which one is the way to go, you may be consulted as to which intervention you think is best for your child. If a treatment is experimental or of questionable effectiveness for your baby, you must decide whether to consent to its implementation.

In fact, your informed consent is required for all experimental procedures, as well as all major treatments aside from life-threatening emergency care. You can also request that even the simplest changes in routine care be run past you before they are carried out. As an emotionally invested parent and as a member of the care team, part of your job is to study your baby's care and watch over it.

I was worried about the effect that [the medication] would have on him long term. When I was pregnant, I don't think I took regular-strength Tylenol more than five times, and here they were pumping all this stuff into him.—Micki

They had a lot of X-rays. I didn't like that. My mom never wanted us to even get dental X-rays. So here were my babies, who weren't even supposed to be born yet, getting X-rays every day. I was not very happy about that. But it couldn't be helped. It had to be done.—Debbie

Of course, you make these decisions in collaboration with your baby's doctors, who provide information, statistics, and their opinions. You bring your values, preferences, points of view, priorities, and hunches to the process. You also bring your heartfelt hopes and fears for your baby's future and your parental devotion to do what is in your baby's best interests.

When giving informed consent for a treatment or procedure, there is so much to scrutinize. In fact, you may feel overly informed because the hospital has a legal obligation to disclose every possible risk, no matter how unlikely. Reading the long list of dangers, you may feel reluctant to grant permission. Ask about the likelihood of a particular danger befalling your baby and how the risk relates to the potential benefits. Also ask what is likely to happen if you refuse consent. For instance, transfusions pose potential risks, but if your baby will die without one, then the scale would clearly tip in favor of the transfusion. If your baby will probably do okay without the transfusion, then you might safely opt to refuse permission.

On the flip side, sometimes the benefits of a treatment are overblown. Perhaps you're wondering about the true necessity of a particularly invasive procedure or a certain aspect of your baby's care. Perhaps your baby's condition doesn't appear to be that serious to you, or you see improvement, which makes you reconsider. It's difficult to question a plan when the practitioners are recommending it. But in the face of an unclear diagnosis, questionable benefits, possible side effects, or an uncertain outcome, it is important for you to weigh in. Voice your concerns and observations, gather more information, make inquiries about other options, and get second opinions.

I would say, don't feel compelled to do what everyone says is the best. Follow your heart and do what you would want done to yourself. Make sure it's really necessary. Take him home and see how he does without the treatment. The doctors paint this picture of resolution and closure when it's possibly just a mirage.—Chip

If I could go back in time, I'd tell myself, "Don't let anyone railroad you. *You are his mother.*"—Linda S.

Dealing with differing medical opinions is particularly trying. It is common for different doctors to have not only different ideas about your child's condition, but different approaches to diagnosis and treatment. Some tend to wait and see; others do every test available to them. One doctor may be very aggressive about intervening; another might suggest trying the least invasive treatment first—and then going from there. Of course, you may be more in tune with one approach than the other. If you're lucky, you'll have a doctor whose philosophies match your own. In any case, if you have questions or concerns about how a doctor is planning your baby's care, you can seek another opinion. You may want to contact either your baby's primary doctor or the specialist you trust for consistency and guidance. And if you're given contradictory opinions, you have to put your parental intuition to work—and trust what your gut and heart are telling you.

They kept telling me, "He's going to need surgery still, any day." And I kept telling them, "No, he's not. They told me at Children's Hospital that he's not." And then they thought I was being this really rude parent and not believing them, like I was in denial or something. It was awful. This is not something you want to mess with. But he was sent over to Children's for a second opinion because they were the experts, which I kind of did intuitively believe.—Stephie

Your advocacy and assertiveness are essential to your baby's care, but you may wonder if being assertive will cause you to be labeled difficult—and, as a result, cause your baby to receive inferior care. But babies are not held responsible for their parents' behavior—and medical professionals don't perform less competently or lower their standards to get even. Babies are *never* denied the best care possible, no matter how assertive, emotive, questioning, demanding, or challenging their parents are perceived to be. In fact, *constructive* assertiveness can benefit your collaborative relationships with practitioners, and advocacy can improve the care your baby receives.

I think that I had a pretty good relationship with the doctors and the nurses because I was there and I was on them, in their faces, all the time, asking "Why? Fine, you're going to do this blood test. What is the blood test? What is it going to show you? What are you going to determine by the results of this blood test?" I was constant, on them, on them, on them. I mean, I would find the doctor, hunt down the doctor, grab him, and say, "In the child's chart it says _____. . . . Explain that to me." And he's like, "Well, that's the nurse's writing." And I would say, "I don't care whose writing it is. You're the doctor, you tell me why!" I wasn't afraid to do that. I wasn't one of the people who wouldn't look at the chart because that's a private thing. I don't care. If it's there, I'm the mother, I'm gonna read it, you know? So I was on them constantly, and I wanted them to know that I was there, and I wanted them to know that I wanted to know and I wasn't going to take no for an answer. I think they gave me, I don't mean to say preferential treatment, but maybe people thought of me as someone to contend with and to be slightly leery of and *If we don't do everything right, we're going to hear about it.* And I'm not a nasty person, but I had to do what I had to do for the sake of the kids.—Pam

This mom was very assertive, and her style may be different from yours. You can advocate effectively in your own way, as long as you are constructive, by

- not attacking the doctors and nurses personally,
- sticking to "I feel *this* about *that situation*" statements,
- identifying what's in your baby's best interests,
- assuming that the medical staff has your baby's best interests at heart, and
- approaching in a spirit of collaboration, not conflict.

For instance, to begin a dialogue instead of a war, instead of, "Why did you do that? I want to talk to your supervisor!" try, "I'm really scared about my baby's setback. Can you please help me understand what's going on?"

Remember, as your baby's advocate, it is your goal to be informed, vigilant, and protective so that your baby receives care that you understand and approve. You are expected to ask questions like: What are the side effects and risks of this test or treatment? Will this hurt—can you give my baby something for pain? When can my baby medically tolerate kangaroo care? Practitioners understand that you have a right to answers and you have a right to object or disagree with care plans that may be risky or unnecessary. You have a responsibility to question any plan that ignores the big picture or overlooks your baby's comfort or developmental needs. When, in your opinion, something is not clearly in the best interests of your child, you can propose another path.

We were a pain, but we felt that was our right, our kids' right. I think they knew that we weren't going to go away, that they had to deal with us—and that if we weren't satisfied with what was going on, we would seriously question it, and we'd call a meeting to figure out a solution or to have them make us understand exactly why they were doing it. They understood that.—Betsy

Such decisions are not easy. Look at what the expected outcomes are of doing something now or waiting and doing it at another time. Talk over the options with others to get important feedback that might otherwise be obscured by the information overload you feel when trying to absorb everything in an attempt to understand it all. Do your best to balance your feelings and preferences with those of your [partner] and family. Be more cautious when your feelings or preferences are in opposition to the others that are part of the decision-making process. Once a decision is made, accept that you did the best you could.—Chip

For information and support around life-and-death decision making, turn to "Making Medical Decisions in the Gray Zone" in chapter 9.

Dealing with Regrets

If I had to do it over again, I'd write down my demands to feed the baby and be called when he was awake. They encouraged breast-feeding, but some nurses were very impatient.—Linda S.

Looking back, many parents wish that they could have been more constructively assertive during their baby's NICU stay. Some parents don't have enough time or experience to muster the necessary fortitude or skills. Others just need to survive the NICU experience and get out; only in hindsight do they wish they could've been stronger advocates. Still others are too stressed to have the energy to communicate judiciously. Whatever your style or timetable, remember that you were who you were, and embrace the growth that has come from this experience. Also remember that it is much easier to be an effective advocate when you are working with practitioners who understand and respect your advocacy. Although second-guessing yourself is a normal part of parenting in the NICU, give yourself credit for doing your best at the time under difficult circumstances.

My deepest regret is that I let them perform surgery that may not have been necessary and that may adversely affect him in the future due to side effects as a result of the surgery. I have the same regret with regard to the circumcision.

I can rationalize the decisions I made because many or most parents would make the same decisions. I'm also comforted by the fact that in every way our beautiful, fun, active boy is having a completely normal life in every way, and so far there is no evidence of any adverse effects.—Chip

Children's Hospital has a team that runs the ambulance. They look like a NASA flight crew. They rolled Kitquin into my hospital room so I could say good-bye to her. To my shock, Kitquin was awake and pretty alert. They had put a pacifier in an oxygen mask and she had that over her face. The increased oxygen was obviously doing her well. To my shock, they asked if we wanted to tell her good-bye and even touch her! We couldn't pat her, but we could hold her foot for a few seconds if we wanted to. It was amazing. I knew then that this was the best thing that could be done for her, and I wished we had just been moved there from the start.—Jennifer E.

You may wonder if better observations or assertive demands from you would have made a difference for your child. It is more likely that your baby's outcome, under the highly skilled, attentive care of your NICU's medical staff, would have been the same, even if you had behaved differently. After homecoming, as you deal with pediatricians and perhaps therapists and more treatments, you can continue to practice a more assertive approach.

Stay strong and listen to your instincts. Mothers instinctively know what is best for their babies. Remember that this is *your* child, and you have every right to be a part of his/her care.—Corin

Your evolution as a parent is ongoing, and you will continue to learn about your child, become increasingly skilled at caregiving, and develop as an advocate. Parenting in the NICU is but your first step in mastering this aspect of your journey.

Points to Remember

· *By understanding modern NICU practice and the overall intentions of your baby's medical practitioners, you'll be able to appreciate and embrace your critical role in your baby's care.*

· *Give yourself time to get used to the NICU. Very soon, you will learn your way around and come to trust the nurses and doctors who are caring for your precious baby.*

· *In the relationship-centered, developmentally supportive NICU, parents are involved and encouraged to get close to their babies. Medical technology is important for babies, but so is nurturing and the parents' touch.*

· *In the relationship-centered, developmentally supportive NICU, each practitioner builds a relationship with your newborn, learning about your baby's sensitivities and preferences, strengths and weaknesses, and tailoring care to be responsive, individualized, holistic, and compassionate.*

· *As you regain your footing and spend more and more time with your baby, you'll be able to absorb and integrate the necessary medical information.*

· *When you start to understand what is going on with and around your little one, you can begin to find your place as your baby's parent—and a full-fledged member of the care team.*

· *To keep the lines of communication open with your baby's care team, approach them in the spirit of collaboration and request the kinds of information and support you need.*

· *As a parent, it is your job to ask questions, learn, make mistakes, have intense feelings, be informed, and advocate for your baby.*

· *Overall, your most unique and vital contribution to the care team is your parental bond. Your love, devotion, and instincts are beyond compare.*

· *You are your baby's best advocate.*

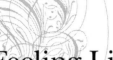

6:

Feeling Like a Parent

Suddenly I was no longer pregnant, and yet I was far from being a mother. At night I'd dream that I was still pregnant and wake up full of hope—and then remember that I wasn't. I'd lie in bed at night and wonder if my baby was peaceful, if he was calm. Was he agitated, did he need his mummy? And instead of peeping in his bassinet, I'd have to phone a nurse and ask. I wasn't a mother.—Leanne

For a while, Katie wasn't our baby. She was the NICU's baby. We were in this odd state of limbo.—Mark

Feeling like a parent in the NICU presents many challenges. You can be well aware that your baby was born and is in fact lying right here in front of you, but emotionally you may not have signed in yet as *the parent*. Especially if your baby was born prematurely, you may resist the idea outright.

It seemed so surreal. Nothing was happening the way it was supposed to. At first, I couldn't believe that I was pregnant. Then right around the time I started believing I was pregnant, I had her. So I didn't feel like a mother right away. I came in when she'd been in the NICU for two or three days, and the nurse says to her, "Oh look, Mommy's here!" And I'm like, "Whoa! Stop that. I'm not a mother." And they're like, "Yeah, you are." And I'm like, "Well, yes, I am, but don't call me that because I'm not quite ready to accept that yet."—Brooke

No matter that you delivered your baby, your mind is still pregnant. It took me a long time to adjust to that, to not feel pregnant, to see a pregnant woman on the street and not think, *That's what I am*. Because your mind is scheduled for a nine-month pregnancy. You want to be pregnant. And you don't want to face the preemie thing.—Gallice

I think the worst part was trying to make myself believe that I did give birth to a baby, he didn't die, and I could take care of this child when he came home.—Ami

It is also difficult to act and feel like a real parent when

- your baby is a full-time resident of the NICU and you aren't,
- your baby needs a different kind of care than you alone can provide,
- your baby's medical condition keeps you at bay,
- medical technology covers and surrounds your baby,
- your baby's condition, treatments, or simple immaturity keep your baby from responding to you, or
- your baby's medical practitioners are hovering, if not over your baby, then nearby, ready to swoop in whenever necessary.

Overall, it can be hard to believe that you are a mother or a father when so much separates you from your newborn. It can be hard to *feel* like a parent when there is such a wide chasm between your vision of parenting and what your baby needs from you.

I had no idea what I expected to feel or what kind of parent I thought I would be, but I do know that dealing with this threw everything completely out of whack. It was really hard for me to feel like a real parent to Nicholas for the first few weeks. After all, I was not his primary caregiver, and that felt just plain wrong to me.—Sterling

I wanted to touch him, to stroke his face and skin, but that felt unsafe. He seemed so fragile. I felt distanced because of the tubes and wires. I was afraid of pulling something out. I felt I had to wait for instructions from the nurse. That wasn't what I was expecting when I first met my baby.—Laurie

Even seasoned parents can be set back on their heels. Deprived of close contact with your newborn, you may continue to feel out of sync and out of touch, even as you spend time in the NICU. In addition, your infant may not look or respond like a typical newborn. How can you fill your intended role when your baby isn't playing the expected part or occupying the expected mark? This is not the duet you'd practiced in your mind. You want so much to do all the nurturing and cuddling that is supposed to be good for babies, but your baby may not tolerate the kind of caregiving you have to offer. You may feel frustrated and dejected.

The way you think about being a mother is, *I'm a mother. I'm sitting here. I've got my baby.* But of course, for me, it never happened like that because she was in the hospital for so long. So I had problems believing I was a mother.—Brooke

I felt like I was just tossed aside. "Okay, your job is done, you didn't do a great job at it, but you did it. So thank you and we'll see you later." I didn't feel like a parent at all. Even touching her that one time, I don't think I comprehended that [not feeling like a parent] was what was inside of me.—Michelle

It seemed so wrong to give birth to this baby and then leave him for someone else to take care of. I was supposed to do it. I'm his mommy. Not these nurses. Not the doctors. Me. So it should be me taking care of him. It wasn't fair. That's all I could think. It just wasn't fair.—Ami

It hurt having to go see Alison in the hospital and watch others taking care of her. That was supposed to be my job. I almost felt as if she were not even my baby—as if I was just her babysitter, going in to hold her every once in a while.—Stacy

In fact, your baby's needs may be so far beyond routine newborn parenting that you feel hesitant and clumsy, unqualified to even touch or hold your tiny baby. You want to get close, but you don't want to do anything wrong. Unsure of your role and fearful of being an agent of harm, you may feel helpless to mobilize yourself as a new parent.

I couldn't touch them. I couldn't hold them. I couldn't feed them. I felt totally useless as a mom, and often felt in the way of their "real" caregivers. This was almost entirely on me, because 99 percent of the time, the staff was welcoming and encouraging.—Susan B.

I didn't get to hold her for eight days after surgery, and then when I could, I didn't want to do it. I was afraid to do it. They said, "Do you want to hold her?" and I said no. I was scared that I would hold her and she'd have another setback, and it would be twelve days before I could hold her again. Or weeks—and I'd never get to hold her and she'd die. I'd do something wrong: knock the ventilator by mistake, or kill her.—Beth

The thing I remember most was the fact that I couldn't get close to him. I felt as if I had hurt him so badly and that I could never make it up to him. I also remember feeling helpless and extremely useless.—Jenny

It took me quite a few hours before I'd go back in to see Sean. I was scared, I guess. I didn't know what to do with him.—Ami

When your baby has such urgent medical needs and is so inaccessible to you, you may believe you have no place in this baby's life. Wanting to feel like a parent, you may struggle to

· claim your parental identity,

· close the gap between you and your baby,

· get privacy with your baby,

· manage your fears,

· get past the medical barriers,

· build confidence in your caregiving abilities,

· trust that your baby benefits from your presence, or

· make the most of the time you're in the NICU.

At first, these struggles may seem insurmountable. But as you acclimate to the NICU and get your bearings, you will prevail as a parent too. With practice, you will become competent at meeting your baby's unique needs. Over time, you will build confidence in your abilities and instincts. With experience, you can feel like a real mother or father in the NICU. This chapter offers encouragement and practical suggestions to clear these common hurdles and come into your own as a parent to your little one.

Developing Your Parental Identity

I expected Katie to do the roller coaster thing, but my emotions were even more out of whack. I wanted to hold her and love her. I wanted to be that strong parent—and found myself in tears a lot of the time.—Angel

Becoming a parent is an emotional business for anyone. Intensity and turmoil are normal during the last trimester of pregnancy and the weeks after delivery. This upheaval is considered adaptive because it mobilizes the mother's and father's emotional energy toward adjusting to parenting and forming a relationship with their baby.

In the NICU, this emotional upheaval is particularly intense and consists of both heartwarming *and* heart-wrenching moments. But your turmoil is adaptive too. Although often uncomfortable and overwhelming, it mobilizes your emotional investment in your baby.

The first time I really held Ricky was when he was almost a week old. I felt as if I was holding him away from me, so I wouldn't hurt him anymore. I thought that this was all my fault, and I couldn't bear to hurt him anymore. He felt heavy, not like a burden but like a weight around my heart, pulling and pulling me toward him. I wanted to hold him forever. I looked up and saw that I was not the only one crying. The nurses who took care of Ricky knew my pain; they had seen it before. I just held him and looked into his eyes and begged him to forgive me for failing him so miserably. He didn't open his eyes, but he did yawn and wriggle. I held him that way for about five minutes, and then the nurse told me I had to put him back. I was so happy that I had finally gotten to hold him, but I was hurt deeply at having to leave him there. I went home and laughed and cried and fell into an exhausted heap at my husband's feet.—Jenny

Derek's and David's eyes were still fused shut, and they were covered in fine hair. You could literally see their veins, as they were almost translucent. A nurse told me I could touch David. I was so scared thinking I would hurt him because he was so small. I held his tiny hand and just cried.—Jody

It is natural for you to hang back at first. Approaching your baby tentatively, staying for short periods, and touching with just fingertips, you may wonder about your hesitance and caution. But your subdued interactions are appropriate and not necessarily a sign of detachment. In fact, parents of term newborns instinctively imitate their babies' level of responsiveness to avoid overwhelming the infant. Parents of hospitalized babies have this same instinctive reaction. When your baby is inactive and unresponsive, it is only natural for you to tune into and respect those signals. Keeping some distance can show your connection and empathy with your little one. (See also "Becoming Attuned to Your Baby" in chapter 7.)

They were on warming tables in the NICU. There were tubes and wires everywhere. I was afraid to touch them, but I asked the nurse if I could, and she said it was okay. I stroked their feet. It seemed like the only safe place to touch them.—Lorraine

If you are concerned about any feelings of hesitation, detachment, or ambivalence or are simply searching for ways to develop your parental identity even when your baby is inaccessible to you, try the following suggestions.

- Forgive yourself and your baby for not being the way that you had imagined. Let yourself get to know this baby rather than waiting until he or she seems more like the baby you had envisioned.

- Remind yourself that feeling detached isn't a sign that you don't or cannot care about your baby. It could be an expected after-effect of trauma, the result of separation, or due to postpartum adjustment. As the circumstances (or your hormones) stabilize, so will you. Seek out the support and counsel you need to move beyond feelings of detachment.

- Accept that you may have mixed feelings about seeing or being with your baby. It is normal to feel reluctant, especially at first. Many parents need to warm up to their baby—and the NICU. (See also "Bonding Occurs Over Time" in chapter 7.)

- Remind yourself that even your painful emotions reflect your parental connection to your baby. If you didn't have this connection, you wouldn't be so emotional.

- Spend time in the NICU. The more you stay and the more you learn, the more familiar this place will become—and then you can make strides in getting to know your baby. As your baby becomes a part of your everyday existence, you'll feel more and more like a parent.

What helped me feel like a mom was just living it—accepting it—because it was something I had to do day by day by day. Also, seeing her react to me.—Brooke

- If you're the mother and you are able, pump breast milk. (For more on pumping and breast-feeding, see chapter 8.)

Each day, I felt more like a parent, but I often felt completely helpless and useless. Pumping made me feel like it was the only thing I could do for them and that I was the only one who could do it. Maybe all mothers feel that way, but it's more pronounced in the NICU.—Susan B.

- If this is your first baby, recognize that perhaps part of what's holding you back is that you've never been a parent before. All new parents feel incompetent, overwhelmed, and anxious at times. Having a baby in the NICU magnifies the intensity of these feelings, of course, but hesitancy is a natural part of being inexperienced with this new role.

- If you have older children, recognize that this baby may challenge your self-image as an experienced parent. It's difficult to go from feeling confident to feeling unsure. It's natural to feel like a novice as you learn how to meet *this* baby's needs.

- Remember to identify your painful feelings and their sources, so you don't displace emotions like anger and disappointment onto your baby. Dealing with your emotional pain can free up your energy to invest in your little one.

- Let yourself cry when you feel like it. You may find yourself moved to tears while you pump or while you hold your baby skin to skin. Tears of joy and sadness can mix together, and floods of emotion are natural. Your tears won't harm your baby. Shedding them can help you move through your grief and mobilize yourself as a parent. (See also "The Emotions of Kangarooing" in chapter 7.)

- If you feel anxious about being around your baby, talk about your feelings with someone you trust. If you are worried that your presence might harm your baby, keep in mind that your worries are likely based on your intense wish to protect and nurture your infant—even if you conclude that doing so requires you to keep your distance. Inkan confesses: "I was very afraid about giving him any infection. It felt more secure to stay away from touching him." This sentiment—to shield your infant from harm—is profoundly parental.

- Talk about your emerging parental identity with a trusted friend or with other parents of NICU babies. Seek out reassurance and support for doing the things you want to do with your baby in the NICU. There are many good books that support parents' desires and needs to be close to their babies. (For a list of resources, go to www.NICUparenting.org.)

- Refer to your little one as "my baby" and "my daughter" or "my son." Even if awkward at first, practice using the phrase in your mind, on paper, and verbally.

The birth certificate lady asked, "What did you have?" "A boy." "What's your son's name?" I said, "Oh, my son." I hadn't said "my son"—those words—[before]. I hadn't thought of him as my son. I loved saying those words after she said them.—Nettie

- Refer to yourself as your baby's "mother" or "father." Although you may not yet feel competent in the role of mother or father, you are still your baby's parent. Even when you have so much to learn, you have a unique relationship and connection with your little one.

There's so little you can do. I remember them coming in soon after he was born, and I asked them, "What can I do? Does he need my kidney? He can have it. Anything that he needs, he can have." And there wasn't anything I could do, except give him breast milk. So that's what I did. And be there for him. I did those things with everything I had.—Marcia

I would just stay by his side whenever I could, especially when he was awake and tell him how much I loved him. I would stare into his eyes, and I felt like he knew me and loved me too.—Corin

- Keep in mind that you can create your own firsts—the first bath you give, the first diaper you change. You or your partner will also be the first to breast-feed, the first to give kangaroo care, and the first to take your baby home. No one else can do those parenting tasks.

- Decorate your baby's temporary home. Ask the medical staff where you can place family photos, small toys, and special name tags or signs. Bring a baby blanket from home to drape over the incubator. Bring clothes for your baby to wear. These activities indicate that this baby is yours and an important member of your family. (For more ideas on this subject, see "Making the Most of Your Absences" later in this chapter.)

Here's one more tip that also offers reassurance: whether your baby was born prematurely or not, view your baby's hospitalization as the last trimester. While not what you'd envisioned, this time can be seen as the continued gestation of your baby and the continued incubation of yourself as a parent. This perspective has the added benefit of seeing the NICU days as an intrusion into the pregnancy rather than as a thief of the newborn period. Indeed, the newborn period you get to experience at home is also known as the fourth trimester, in recognition of every parent's continuing development of identity as a mother or a father.

Many of the actual newborn experiences still happened once they came home. Even though they were five months old, their corrected age was about one month old, and developmentally they mostly behaved like newborns. In fact, the newborn stage lasted much longer with them than with typically developing infants, since they grew slowly and reached their milestones much later. It didn't exactly make up for what we missed, but we tried to relish their babyhood.—Susan B.

Closing the Gap

Each evening I'd blow my child a kiss through his plastic walls and walk away, every nerve ending screaming that this was wrong, every fiber of my being wanting to hold that child close and never let go, and yet night after night I left. How could I do this one more day?—Leanne

To cope with separation from your baby, there are many activities and thoughts that can close the gap between you—even when your baby is inaccessible or you are away from the NICU. Closing the gap also helps you grow into your parenting role. Try any of the following ideas that feel right to you:

· Acknowledge your baby's birth in ways that comfort you. It may help to decorate the nursery; shop for baby clothes, toys, or supplies; or start a photo album or baby book.

· Send out birth announcements. Notify people of your baby's birth, sharing the details that let them know that this is neither easy nor routine for you. Creating this announcement also gives you a chance to welcome and show your love for your newborn.

· Write down your observations about your baby: preferences, features, resemblances, expressions. Keep a journal or record milestones in a baby book.

· Learn more about your baby's birth. Talk with your partner. Ask the attending nurses and doctors about the details. It may also help to ask why things were done the way they were. This information helps you reclaim memories, satisfies your need to know, and fills in the gaps of your story.

· Share your story with anyone who wants to listen. Telling your story over and over can be tremendously therapeutic. You can also write your story in a keepsake journal or baby book.

· Trust that your baby knows who you are and that you are someone special to him or her. Follow your intuition about this connection. You don't need concrete evidence. Just sense and feel the connection—and build on it. (See also "Recognizing the Importance of Your Presence" later in this chapter.)

· Place breast pads or a cotton shirt you've slept in for several nights in your baby's incubator. To your baby, your scent may be a comforting reminder of your presence.

- Ask the nurse if you can have something with your baby's scent on it to take home with you. Smelling this item can help you feel close to your baby.

- Record yourself talking, singing, or reading a story and leave the recording in the NICU with your baby so it can be played at low volume when your baby is fussy or alert.

- Spend as much time as you can or want with your baby. Don't cave into others' urging you to take breaks or to get away when you truly want to stay. Also, don't listen to criticism for taking time away. Trust your instincts.

- Take photographs of your baby and look at them regularly. It is especially important to keep updating the photos as your baby's appearance and condition change.

- Write notes to your baby about your thoughts, wishes, and devotion.

- Write notes "from" your baby to post at the bedside to remind practitioners about special needs, sensitivities, preferences, or requests.

- Post notes at your baby's bedside to remind practitioners to wait for you to arrive if you plan to be there for feedings, caregiving, or tests.

- Ask your baby's primary nurse to write short notes to you "from" your baby reporting on his or her condition and new developments from your baby's perspective. (There is more on baby diaries, later in this chapter.)

- Don't underestimate the power of breast milk. If you can do it, breast-feeding and/or pumping feels like you are doing something motherly. Even if your baby isn't ready for breast milk yet, pumping and storing the milk is a way to bank on the future.

- Buy a special piece of jewelry or other commemorative object to represent your baby's presence in your family.

- Turn to religious or spiritual rituals and symbols to mark the birth of your baby. Welcome and shelter your little one in ways that feel meaningful to you and your family and community.

I always made sure that Dominique had a little something—a charm—to help keep her safe while I was away.—Rosa

As your baby's condition improves, some barriers will disappear, and you'll be more confident about negotiating the remaining ones—and the gap between you and your baby will become narrower. In the meantime, when you can't have your baby in your arms, let your voice, your touch, and your presence hold your little one.

I just sat there beside him, talking to him. We tried massaging him, but he couldn't take the stimulation until much later in his hospital stay. So we settled for just hanging out.—Sterling

I discovered that they all loved to be read to. I would sit there and read to them, go from station to station. So I knew I could do something to make them happy. So even when I couldn't hold them, I could still care for them.—Julie

Finding Privacy

Being a first-time mom, I was already nervous that I would do something wrong. Having to be a mom to a NICU baby, I felt like I was constantly on display and was afraid to touch of talk to him in fear that I would do something that I wasn't supposed to.—Corin

I was taken to see my girls on the third day of their life. It was not a pleasant experience. The nursery was crowded and noisy. My husband was constantly trying to explain what all the machines were doing for them. At that point, I really wasn't interested in listening. I just wanted to pick both of the girls up and go to a quiet place and hold them.—Kimberly

Forging a parental connection with your baby is an intimate, heartfelt activity. But there are many eyes and ears in the NICU. Surrounded by medical staff and other parents, you may feel exposed and self-conscious. You yourself may watch or listen to other parents out of curiosity or a desire to learn.

As you become used to the NICU, you may be able to tune out others, or you may simply not be bothered anymore. Also, you may develop territorial feelings about "your" space and naturally feel more comfortable in it. But if a lack of privacy ever bothers you, ask your nurses to help you get the privacy you need. Screens are available in some units. As your baby's condition improves, you may be able to take him or her to a more private space in the unit. But for most parents, getting enough privacy remains a challenge until discharge. There's no place like home.

The NICU is, of necessity, a very cold, loud, and sterile place with very little privacy. Because of the NICU's heavy caseload, it was not easy blocking off times to use a family room to be able to hold Daphne against my chest, skin to skin, for so many hours. More often than not, I had to use a surgical curtain so that I could do kangaroo care; however, there were a number of other NICU patients in the room too, and I had to deal with the constant noise of various life-support machines and alarms as well as interruptions whenever another NICU patient had an emergency.—Dina

The best of times were at the end of the NICU stay, when we could go to a private room and nurse lying on a bed, all alone. I used to sing soft lullabies to him and dim the light. In the NICU, there were so many other people all the time, and it was hard to relax in the same way.—Inkan

I wanted to hold him and mother him, in my own home and on my own terms.—Claire

Dealing with Fears

My babies did not look like babies. They were so small. I knew I was supposed to feel an overwhelming love for these children, but all I could feel was fear. I was scared to get any more emotionally involved because I knew the chances of their survival were very slim. I was scared to touch them.—Kimberly

Becoming a parent in the NICU involves dealing with fear. Seeing your baby, perhaps way before the due date, inundated with sterile, humming, blinking medical intervention, you may feel paralyzed with trepidation. Your imagination can run wild with frightful scenarios.

Deep down I felt completely out of control. I would lie awake at night in a panic imagining her living with awful handicaps. How would we be able to take care of her? What if she was a vegetable? What if she lived for three or four months and then died?—Karen

At the beginning, I was most afraid of my daughter dying. Later on, after she made tremendous progress and I could hold her, I was most afraid that my efforts to get her to bond and orally feed would not be successful.—Dina

The thing I was most afraid of was that she would die. The very close runner up to that was that she would be severely disabled. I was picturing basically a vegetable. There, breathing, but gone.—Brooke

Especially early on, your anxieties may mount each time you see your baby: Has my baby's condition changed? How can I risk getting close when my baby looks so sick? What can I possibly offer as a parent? What if my baby dies? In the dark recesses of your mind, you know that not every NICU baby goes home. Every time your phone rings, is the hospital calling to report a turn for the worse? Fear can be paralyzing.

Throughout this time we worried quietly to ourselves, never voicing our concerns. I am usually very expressive about my emotions, but I was too afraid to say anything, certain that my biggest fears would come true if I gave them a voice. I also was in denial that anything was really wrong. Still, I would dread going to the hospital in fear that there would be bad news and that I would have to face it alone. Sometimes there was. Other times I would have my husband call ahead to get a report before I went to the hospital.—Laura

Strange, but I can't remember [holding him for the first time] very clearly. I was still so afraid I was going to lose him. I do remember that I was afraid that I would give him germs. Seven weeks with PROM [premature rupture of the membranes] had made me very frightened of germs.—Inkan

It was like the whole thing was a dream. It didn't feel like I was looking at my child. [I was] afraid that if I got attached to him, I would only end up getting hurt, because I didn't see how such a little person so sick would ever survive.—Susan C.

I tried not to let myself think that they are going to die, but each moment was so scary—like, *What does that machine mean?* In the beginning, I had to wonder, *When that beeps, is my baby dead?*—Stephie

I didn't read any books for a good four months, and I listened to the radio because I didn't want to be in the middle of a good book or listening to one of my tapes that I really like when I got the phone call that she had died. . . . I didn't want to taint it. So I did crossword puzzles because I figured, *I hate crossword puzzles. If she dies, it's okay because I [already] hate crossword puzzles.*—Brooke

I don't know how I managed the fears. I certainly didn't acknowledge them at the time. When Sarah was born, I didn't allow myself to really consider her death. I knew it was a possibility but never once spoke of it aloud. I approached any physical or mental impairment the same way. It was never spoken of. . . . What was I most afraid of? Going down to the unit and not finding the baby where she was supposed to be.—Cindy

It is normal to have fears about what's going on, what's next, and what the future might bring. It can be scary to admit your fears, but doing so will not make them materialize. Rather, by facing your fears squarely, you can overcome them. For example, by facing your fear that your baby may die, you might become aware that you are keeping physical or emotional distance to protect yourself from getting too close to your little one. With this kind of awareness, instead of your fears creating another barrier between you and your baby, they become something you deal with and put aside, allowing you to stay mobilized and involved with your baby. Instead of being paralyzed by what *might* happen, you become engaged with what is happening *now*.

Even though contemplating disabilities or death is especially frightening, bringing these fears into the light lets you move past them. Ask your questions, gather information, get support, and know the options. (See also "Balancing Hopes and Fears" in chapter 9.)

It was an awful time. . . . I wanted to be sure that if Shayna were to die, I would have no regrets about how everything was handled. So I planned for the worst. I made my sister-in-law pick out a family plot and talk to the funeral director about different options. (I couldn't bring myself to go there; my husband wanted nothing to do with this.) I know this must sound terribly morbid, but it gave me a sense of control. I needed to be ready for anything.—Karen

In the beginning, David was very sick and the outcome was not good. I was scared to get to know him because we might lose him. A nurse told me not to be afraid and to let him know I am there because even if he does pass, he needs his mom.—Jody

You might also find it helpful to focus on what the medical team *does* know, rather than what is unknown. And remember, if a fear becomes a reality, you can cope, adjust, find meaning, and prevail over that too.

Negotiating Medical Barriers

You can't just hold a NICU baby. You hold a NICU baby and their stuff.—Jennifer E.

Particularly when your baby is in critical condition, there are many medical obstacles between you and your little one. It's hard to get past the tubes, wires, tape, eye masks, earmuffs, machines, and the plastic walls of the incubator. Sometimes, your baby may be too sick, overwhelmed, or tired to be responsive or held without compromising vital signs.

Kitquin was much more fragile than I expected. The oxygen tent was at a max and her stats were not getting better. We were told that we cannot touch her, talk to her, move too much around her or her stats would crash. Her oxygen would go down and her heart rate would go up. There was nothing I could do. I couldn't sing to her, talk to her, hold her toe, or even hover over her. I had to stand a foot away and just look.—Jennifer E.

When he was very sick, he was on paralytics. Without movement or being awake, it felt like he wasn't completely there and I couldn't connect to him.—Corin

Daphne was sedated and on the high-frequency oscillating ventilator taped to her mouth. There were tubes, wires, and machines everywhere. She had earmuffs on to prevent the noise of the NICU from disturbing her, and at this point we were not allowed to hold her or even stroke her in any way because of the risk of complications if she had a reflex action.

I felt completely helpless. There was little I could do. For the first week, we couldn't touch her, so I spent much of my time in the NICU just sitting next to Daphne and reading or singing to her. My visits were always interrupted because of some crisis requiring a team of doctors and nurses to make adjustments, during which time I had to leave the room she was in.—Dina

As a parent, you want more than anything to be able to *do* something, to get involved, to *nurture* your little one, yet you do not want to interfere with your baby's care or hurt your fragile infant. You know that these technological obstacles are necessary for your baby's survival, and yet they are so *in the way*.

I had been carrying him around for seven months, and I could not get used to the idea that I had to look at him in an open warmer with tubes in him. We couldn't hold him because he was on an oxygen hood, so all I could do was lay my hand on him and cry uncontrollably.—Jenny

I wanted so badly to pick him up. To hold him close to me. To rock him and sing to him and feed him. But all I could do was reach in and touch his tiny hand. I couldn't even stroke him. Any more stimulation than just a touch would be too much for his little system to handle just yet. I was crushed. This was not how it was supposed to be. I should have had my boy in my arms—not in this bed. I went back to my room and cried—again.—Ami

I can remember that right after the surgery I could not touch her. At all. Period. If I touched her, she had a tachycardia. She would [set off] her alarms. And the nurse said, "I have to tell you not to touch her because you're disturbing her and stopping her from healing." And I just sat and cried and cried. It kills you. . . . Going through that was the worst thing that's ever happened to me in my life. The absolute worst.—Beth

Here are some suggestions for getting past medical barriers:

· See your frustration as a sign of connection. When you feel impatient with the barriers between you and your baby or feel envious that other parents are able to be closer to their babies, consider these feelings as signs of your growing courage and involvement with your newborn.

They were each about three weeks old when I finally got to hold them. I was thrilled, but it wasn't at all like holding my full-term babies. In fact, I was barely holding them at all. Two nurses worked to move the baby from his or her isolette, managing the ET tube and the IVs and monitors. I held each baby on a pillow on my lap, while the nurses hovered, monitoring their temperature and oxygen sats and holding up the hoses and wires. Still, I remember feeling completely overjoyed.—Susan B.

· Focus on your baby, not the medical equipment. Ignore the stuff, and see the little person behind it all. If you tend to watch the monitors, try watching your baby instead. To gauge your baby's condition and progress, even medical practitioners rely largely on their observations rather than on monitors and measures.

I had a tendency . . . I never looked at her, I was always watching the monitors. And then one day this one nurse came in and said, "All right, we're going to fix this," and she took a blanket and just threw it over the monitor. And I was [gasp], and the nurse said, "If it alarms, we'll know it, but you can't sit there and just keep staring at the monitor." Because every time her heart rate would go 160, 140, 150, I was panicking. So [covering the monitors] helped a lot.—Suzanne

- Ask the nurses to show you their tricks of the trade. For example, you might ask how they handle your baby without disturbing the wires and tubes. Ask about what kinds of handling your baby can benefit from and how to get your baby out of the incubator and into your arms. Model their behavior, and soon you'll easily work around the lines and equipment.

After a while, I had gotten to know the NICU routine, watched numerous times how the NICU nurses changed Daphne's diapers and applied moisturizer to her skin and, after I asked, was allowed to assist with those tasks under supervision. I also learned how I could "hold" Daphne by placing my hands firmly on the top of her head and on the bottom of her feet (no stroking), which calmed her when she became agitated with her restraints and tubes.—Dina

- Try any avenue you can to relate to your baby. You may find yourself doing "strange" things in an effort to feel close to or get to know your baby. Remind yourself that you are facing unique challenges in parenting and in forming a relationship with your little one. Unique challenges often call for unique behavior.

The first time Josh got off the ventilator, we kind of tortured him, as only a parent of a preemie could do, but we wanted to hear his voice. He liked the pacifier by then, and we kept pulling it out just so we could hear him cry—because it was so magical to hear any kind of voice. We would put it back in and pull it out just so we could hear him complain. It was so amazing to us to hear that. Some of the stuff we did, it just wasn't normal. But it was all we knew.—Stephie

As you adjust to the NICU and your baby, you will be able to negotiate the medical barriers with ease. In the meantime, remind yourself that you are doing the best you can in a difficult situation. Rest assured that over time your best will become even better.

Building Confidence

When they're in the hospital, it's not your baby; it's their baby. You have to ask to do everything. Or you feel like you have to ask to do everything. Even though you probably don't, you feel like you do.—Beth

Having to ask to touch/hold your baby—you feel like you are not really the mom. And it didn't help when newer nurses to our boys treated us like we had no clue what we were doing even though we had been there the longest.—Jody

It was not me taking care of my babies, it was the doctors and the nurses. And I hated that, and I was resentful of the fact that they were the ones who were taking care of our children instead of me. But I'm not a doctor, and the doctors and nurses were giving the babies the life-sustaining whatever they had to have, but they weren't nurturing them the way a parent would. I mean, the nurses were very wonderful. I would see the nurses in there holding babies just because they wanted to. But you're a nurse, you're not me. You know?

At home is where I actually feel like their mother. In the NICU, I was their supplier of food and that was about it. I bathed them, I changed their diapers, and I did what I could do. I held them, I rocked them while I was there. But it's like babysitting. You give them back. They couldn't come home.—Pam

It is normal to feel displaced by the medical practitioners, especially when you cannot get close to your baby. This sense of displacement only compounds the feeling that your baby isn't quite yours. You may view the nurses and doctors as so much more important than you are. After all, they are *saving a life*. All you can do is hold a tiny hand and whisper endearments.

Feelings of displacement can give rise to envy, frustration, and resentment, especially when you see how adept the nurses are at holding and taking care of your baby. You want more than anything to know what they know and to know it *now* so you can participate in your baby's care with confidence. You appreciate their ability and expertise, but you may feel twinges of irritation. Knowing that you alone can't meet your baby's needs only intensifies any feelings of helplessness and parental incompetence.

When I had to return to work, the long hours away were torture. I counted every minute until I could bolt to my car, wolf down the portable food I kept there, and race across town to the hospital. I ran breathless up the stairs, sprinted to the NICU, and looked eagerly for a task I could participate in to remind me that I was a mommy. I will forever carry the rage, the wounding I felt when I faced nurses who backed me down, forced me to the sidelines, and asserted their authority at the cost of my parenting.—Susan C.

I always had to ask permission to touch her or hold her. Much later on, she was almost off the vent, and I was more comfortable picking her up while she was on the ventilator. I did it by myself without asking, and I thought that was a really big deal. It seemed like I was always asking permission. I wasn't encouraged a whole lot to do things for her.—Suzanne

After a few days, I became possessive. I wanted to change his diaper, take his temperature, feed him. One day, I was running a little late, and I had called to say I was going to be in at this time and I want to do everything, and his nurse said okay. Well, she went on break, and the nurse who took over went ahead and fed him. I was so upset because I felt like they were doing my job. They get to do all the medical things that I can't do, and so the few things I get to do, I want to do them to feel like I'm a part of this baby. . . . And I remember I was really down in the dumps that day because I didn't get to do my job.—Vickie

While I was thrilled that Josie was doing so well and was at a good hospital, I couldn't help but feel that her nurses were far more competent than I was. They were so confident holding her and changing her diaper. I was a nervous wreck just picking her up. It took me twice as long to change her diaper, and I actually dreaded bathing her, even though the nurses highly recommended it. I wondered why she would need a bath when she wasn't out playing in a sandbox or making mud pies, but I felt too intimidated by these skilled nurses to question them.—Rebekah

You may feel frustrated, thinking that if only the practitioners would step aside, you could really be with your baby, yet at the same time you may dread being given that chance because you feel so inadequate and unsure of how to handle your infant. You don't want to fail your little one. This fear of failure can make you back off even more, and being so removed can make you feel like even more of a failure. This vicious cycle can deepen feelings of detachment.

Probably one of the rougher aspects was saying, "No, I'm the mother, I'm supposed to be the one to do this. You're not supposed to be doing this. This is supposed to be my job." But I was so scared of her. I didn't want to touch her because I was afraid that, like, her arm would fall off, which of course is a completely irrational fear but one that was very real in my mind at that point in time. It was like a double-edged sword. On the one hand, I was really happy that other people were doing [the caretaking] because I didn't feel quite ready to, and on the other hand it was, "Wait a minute here!"—Brooke

I remember one time when my husband was pushing me to change her diaper, and he was saying, "C'mon, Michelle, they have to watch you do it. They need to know you can do this." And I was like, "Why? They do it all the time. Let them do it. I'm too afraid to touch her. She's too tiny." I felt like, *You know more about it, you just do it.*—Michelle

One of the things that got frustrating was that some nurses would let me go in and change a diaper or hand me [one of] the babies and walk away, and other nurses wouldn't let me touch them. Or they would say things like, "Your baby is so over-stimulated today," or "Your baby doesn't like to be touched." Excuse me? I know my baby. You never even had my baby before today. But I couldn't defy them and put my hand in there and touch. Since [these babies] were my first, I didn't really know. If that happened today, I'd say, "Sorry, I'm touching my baby. Go get the doctor if you want to kick me out of here. If my baby starts desatting, I'll take my hand away." But back then, it was, "Okay, this nurse says no," so I didn't do it. There's a sense of powerlessness.—Stephie

My lack of knowledge made me feel completely powerless. I visited her in the NICU but did not know what to say or do. I felt useless and conspicuous standing beside her bed. To make matters worse, days later I still felt no connection to her.—Renee

Even as your baby's condition improves, your feelings of helplessness and detachment may persist. You may find it hard to believe that you can do much of anything and decide that it's better to leave your tiny baby in the care of the people who "really" know how to do things for him or her. You may wonder if your baby even knows who you are.

Tips for Building Confidence

The antidote to feeling displaced and unconfident is getting more involved in your baby's care. As your baby's care becomes less intensive, you will gain more access and practice. With the encouragement from your baby's nurses, your growing comfort and competence in caregiving will translate to growing confidence and feeling more like your baby's parent.

Your confidence will also simply grow over time as you adjust to the NICU and your baby. The unfamiliar becomes familiar, your distress lightens, and you can tolerate more, absorb more, and accomplish more.

At first, I was scared to touch T.J. He was so fragile. Also, I was overwhelmed by all of the machines and the information that I had been given. I didn't feel as if I was really his mother because I had so little control over what was happening to him. Gradually, I became more confident.—Claire

Here are some more pointers:

- Consider that one of your responsibilities as a caring parent is entrusting your little one to the skilled care of others when that is necessary. Lean on their expertise. Chip attests to this delicate balance when he reports, "We are spending a lot of time at the hospital, holding Mikey and doing whatever we can to help or stay out of the way."

- Recognize that your parental devotion is apparent in your desire to nurture your baby. Your feelings of limitation or inadequacy reflect your baby's medical condition and hospitalization, not your competence as a parent.

- Get more involved by asking your baby's nurses to explain what they are doing and to show you how to do the tasks you want to carry out.

- Ask the nurses to show you how to read your newborn's responses and point to the evidence that your baby knows you and is comforted by you.

Initially the nurses were saying, "He knows who you are." And I said, "Oh, come on. I believe that when a baby is eight or nine months old, it knows who its mother is, but I don't think when babies are this premature they know." And they kept saying, "Yes, he does." So by the second day, when I was saying I just don't believe it, they said, "Come in and don't say a word. Look at the monitors. Then touch him and watch what happens." His respirations got more stable, his heart rate got more stable, and he always responded. I put my finger into his hand and he rolled his fingers around my finger, so I said, "Reflexes." The nurse said, "You want me to do it?" So the nurse did it, and there was nothing. So I put my finger near his toes, and he rolled his toes around my finger. When the nurse did it, nothing. So I said, "Yoni, I guess you know who I am."—Micki

- Take the time you need to regain trust in yourself. By participating in your baby's care, you will see that you are an agent of comfort and affection.

There were all those damn machines and people and procedures and tests. I never really felt like Sarah was in my control until she was moved from the critical area. Once she was in a regular bed like a full-term baby, swaddled for all she was worth, I began to feel more like a parent. That's when I started becoming less frightened and more protective—because I could protect her. I knew (or thought I knew) what she needed to feel secure and loved.—Cindy

- Go easy on yourself when you feel awkward or unsure. Nobody expects you to be comfortable with your tiny baby right away. When you're feeling incompetent, remind yourself that nobody is more protective of or cares more about your baby than you do. If you had the power to make everything better, you'd do it.

- Break the fear cycle. If you are afraid to fail, to make mistakes, or to show your inexperience, your fear may keep you from relating to your baby. A way to break this cycle is to confront your fears, which will empower you to tap your courage, take risks, and step up to the plate. Try telling your baby's most supportive nurses that you're unsure of yourself. Coaching and practice can boost your confidence.

- Spend blocks of time caring for your baby. Practicing skills across the span of many hours helps you get the knack of it faster, which helps build your confidence. If you live far from the NICU, ask the hospital if there are nearby accommodations for parents.

- Be persistent in your requests to be involved. If you ask for a more active parenting role or want to hold your baby more often and for longer periods but are refused, continue to bring the subject up with your baby's doctors and nurses. Encourage them to review the research for themselves. Give them a copy of "Modern NICU Practice" from chapter 5, the section on kangaroo care in chapter 7, or share other resources with them.

- Practice speaking your mind as you begin to feel more sure of yourself. If you have a question or an opinion, voice it to a practitioner with whom you feel a connection. Over time, you will develop the confidence to speak directly with others on the care team.

- Recognize that the actions and attitudes of individual practitioners can affect your degree of involvement. Some may welcome your presence and participation, teaching you in a way that nurtures your parenting spirit. Others may feel uncomfortable handing over caregiving tasks. Embrace the welcoming messages and ignore the negative ones.

- Recognize your essential role as nurturer. You, the devoted parent, are responsible for and the one most able to provide the nurturing your baby needs and to make sure that he or she feels loved.

When I finally got to hold Sean for the first time, he was three weeks old. I finally held that tiny child and cried at how beautiful he was and how much of a precious miracle he was. I realized then that this little boy needed me as much as he needed the doctors and nurses that were caring for him. —Ami

· Do the kind of parenting you want to do. As you get to know your baby, you'll increasingly be able to read your baby's cues and respond appropriately. You'll learn what soothes him or her and be able to identify when there is a problem. As you note that "Hey, I was right," you'll begin to trust your instincts about your baby. (See also chapter 7.)

As he grew, I could hold him to my breast, and even though he wasn't supposed to be able to nurse, he could rest and be comfortable there.—Inkan

· Recognize what constitutes parenting. Your prenatal care, your dreams for this child, your loving thoughts, your quest for information, your advocacy, your simple presence, and your attempts to do practical caregiving all count as parenting.

I never felt like I wasn't a parent to my baby. I just felt like a parent who wasn't in control of what was happening to my baby. In my opinion, a parent is one who does her best to make sure each of her children grow up to be the best person they can be. Using that definition, I felt like I was able to act like a parent from the moment I discovered I was expecting Daphne. I took care of myself during pregnancy and did everything I could to keep her inside me maturing for as long as possible. I got to the right kind of hospital in time and made sure all of the doctors and other professionals in the delivery room knew what was wrong with my daughter and they were prepared to receive her. And I kept trying for a vaginal delivery, which would help Daphne's lungs develop and give her a better chance of surviving. When she was finally in the hands of doctors who could stabilize and work on making her better, I knew that it was my efforts as a parent that got her there.—Dina

Parenting from a Distance

Perhaps the biggest barrier to feeling like a parent is physical distance. Even if your home is around the corner from the hospital, your baby is not there. You cannot see and hold your baby whenever you want. Even when you can spend a lot of time in the NICU, there is still a sense of distance between you and your baby.

I hated being a mother during the time the girls were in the hospital. I was a new mother, and yet I had no baby to show off. It was strange.—Rosa

Most parents struggle to fit a NICU caregiving schedule into complicated lives. Other obligations and limitations make it impossible for you to be with your baby as much as you'd like. If you have other children to care for, your heart and your time are pulled in opposite directions. You may feel as if you are never in the right place.

Even if the hospital isn't far, you must set aside extra amounts of time, energy, and money to be with your little one. If you live close to the hospital or can stay nearby, you may feel even more pressure to spend lots of time there, neglecting your other responsibilities. And if you live far from the hospital, you may have mixed feelings, at times wishing you lived closer so you could go more easily, other times feeling relieved that the miles give you an excuse for taking a break.

Regardless, you may feel guilty whenever you're not there. You may feel selfish for needing a break, wanting more time for other responsibilities, and resenting the constant trips to the NICU. When you think about your baby struggling, you may feel embarrassed for complaining.

To reduce your angst, simply find the balance that works best for you each day. Stay flexible, recalibrating the balance as your baby's condition changes or as other factors weigh in. After homecoming, you'll have a whole new balancing act to manage!

Of course, one disadvantage to living far from the hospital is that your options aren't very flexible. Parents who live close by can stop in just because they want to or as time becomes available. But if you live farther away, spending time with your baby takes more effort and planning. Even a half hour's commute each way can be time consuming and draining when done regularly. When you live some distance from the hospital, you may also feel scared and especially unsettled that your baby is so far away from you.

Making the Most of Your Presence

To make the most of your time spent in the NICU, figure out what you need from each stay. Is it meeting with the doctors face-to-face? Talking with your baby's nurses? Watching your baby, even as she or he sleeps? Holding him or her? Taking photographs? Fussing over the toys and homey touches in your baby's incubator? Learning caregiving tasks, such as bathing, changing, and feeding? Watching how different your baby's reactions are to you than to the nurses?

As you read all the ideas in this book, you may feel that you must concentrate lots of parenting into very small segments. But don't expect each precious stay to be perfectly satisfying. Each time will be what it is—a typical slice of your newborn's day. Expect variety in what happens as well as in how you feel. You can also adopt Janet's perspective: "There was no 'most meaningful' way. Every minute we got to spend with her was meaningful." You might also figure out the best time of day or days of the week to be there, as Susan B. did:

We discovered that visiting in the middle of the night was a good time. That's when the babies were weighed and bathed. There were fewer docs around, and almost no procedures were done. Silly things go on among people who work midnights. The nurses would dress up our babies in Cabbage Patch doll clothes and take pictures for us. We found we had more access to them on midnights.—Susan B.

Many parents—even the ones who go to the NICU daily—don't feel much like parents until their baby comes home. You might feel restless and dissatisfied even if you could spend all day, every day at the hospital. It might always be less time than what you wish for.

Making the Most of Your Absences

Making the most of your absences means discarding the idea that when you and your baby are apart, you are disconnected. Your absences are inevitable, even necessary, but you can still maintain contact in ways that have meaning for you. Call often. Try to telephone at a scheduled time when your favorite primary nurse can speak with you at length to give you a full report. Many NICUs try to accommodate the needs of parents by connecting through the Internet. As computer technology continues to advance, parents can see digital photographs or even videos of their baby and communicate online with hospital staff, including video conferencing.

Also remember that physical distance need not equal emotional distance. If it helps to write to your baby, talk about your baby, or just think about your baby, do it. When you can't be at the bedside, let your heartfelt thoughts connect you. And each time you go to the NICU, you can pick up where you left off. (If you are concerned about bonding, see chapter 7.)

Having two other kids at home and trying to finish up some of my work, I was not the most present. Some parents stay night and day. I wanted to be there a lot, especially when he was awake, but if he was sleeping, it was okay for me to leave him asleep—since that's what he had to do a lot. We gave him some animals and a blanket to feel at home. I was there mentally even if I wasn't there physically. He was in my thoughts constantly.—Gallice

I encouraged Andrew to leave my side and go meet our daughter. I'm not sure what was going on in my mind at the time. I don't remember wondering when my turn would come to meet her. I have reflected over and over to myself, wondering why I didn't scream out for her, why I didn't have the sense of urgency to be with her. Why I didn't demand to hold my little girl, the way any new mother should be able to. If I'm honest, I think I had a strange sense of peace that had washed over me, an acceptance of our reality. I felt a strong connection to my baby and it was as though I knew that I didn't need her in my physical proximity to know and feel that she was mine.—Angie

I was very glad I made the choices I did. For example, pumping breast milk from the beginning made sure that I had enough available when Daphne made surprising progress and we ended up needing it sooner than expected. I'm even glad that I began scrapbooking the whole experience to feel like I was doing something to chronicle Daphne's life, no matter how it turned out.—Dina

Making the most of your absences also means tending to yourself and your other business when you're away from your baby's bedside. By keeping your home life running as smoothly as possible, maintaining healthy habits, and doing what nurtures you and gives you respite, you can really attend to your little one when you *are* there. You can be more nurturing and soothing when the rest of your life isn't pure chaos. In this way, your absences benefit both you and your baby.

For a little while, our son was very fragile. We could go there and hang out, but we couldn't even open the incubator, so we didn't go as much or for as long. How were we helping our child? We were doing normal activities, seeing friends, getting support, sleep, food, time together, downtime. We were healing ourselves too!—Maren

Baby Diaries

Baby diaries are notes written by the NICU nurses "from" the baby to the parents. This idea, which originated at Simpson Maternity Hospital in Edinburgh, Scotland, grew out of the messages and notes the nurses would leave for their replacements coming on shift. The nurses began sharing these diary entries with the babies' parents, who were delighted and comforted by these little notes from their babies. Here is an example, the first note Susanne and her husband received, followed by this mother's recollections of how the note affected her:

Good morning, Mummy and Daddy,

I just woke up from a lovely long sleep, and I have been a very good boy. My special breathing machine is making breathing a bit easier for me: small boys like me need some help. I have a cozy wee house a bit like a greenhouse but more comfortable. I have some lovely blue stripy socks on, and I think I look very handsome. There are lots of funnily dressed people here to keep an eye on me, and I have worked out how to make them come and visit me by making my bells ring!!! Hope you had a long sleep, Mummy, and that you can come and see me today if you feel better. Daddy said you will have to get rid of your drips [IVs]. I need mine for a wee while longer till I grow a bit bigger. Phew, I must stop now because I am tired with all this typing. It is hard work when your fingers are only small. Bye Bye. Love, Connor XXXXX

Well, you can imagine I was both delighted and overwhelmed with emotion. It was very powerful and comforting, and after having never seen this baby they all told me I had, all of a sudden I really felt as if I did have a baby after all. It also prepared me for how Connor would look, to an extent, in a lighthearted way. Over the next few months when they had a minute or two, the nurses would add to Connor's diary, and when we would arrive, a little note was taped to the end of his incubator. And even though we knew it was done by the nurses, we would laugh and say, "If he could talk, these are the things he would say." Good days and bad, when he put weight on or when he had to be reintubated, he sent us a lighthearted note, which gave us a relationship with him and made things easier. It helped us immensely. I can never stress to anyone enough how much this meant to us.—Susanne

Even if your NICU doesn't provide baby notes, you can write them yourself if the idea appeals to you. Share the notes with your partner as a way of conveying information about your baby and your solitary treks to the NICU. Writing notes from a lighthearted point of view can help to ease the trauma of your baby's hospitalization and help you see your baby as a real individual and a member of your family.

Recognizing the Importance of Your Presence

As you begin to feel more like a parent, you'll learn to recognize the importance of your simple presence in the NICU and your participation in your baby's care. At first, your attempts to hold your baby's hand or cup your baby's head can seem so small next to the life-sustaining medical intervention he or she is receiving. But, in fact, many experts believe your touch can make a significant difference in promoting weight gain, how soon your baby gets off the ventilator, how well she or he continues to breathe without it, and reducing the length of hospitalization. Your baby benefits greatly from your nurturing. As you get to know your baby, you will observe how she or he is soothed by your comforting presence.

He would calm down if I stroked his head in the incubator. My husband noticed that his vital signs would change when I spoke near his incubator or when I would stroke him. I never noticed that because I didn't look at the monitors much, but they were somehow comforting to my husband.—Laurie

I always felt that he knew me, even from the beginning. I spent every day by his bed talking to him and making sure he knew that we loved him. He always was very calm when I was with him—very rarely did he have any bad times when I was by his bedside. If he was upset, I could open the porthole and put my finger in his palm, and he would settle down.—Kelly

A nursing student was holding my son, and he was crying inconsolably. I took him from her, and he stopped crying instantly. My presence helped them thrive. They loved being touched and held and cuddled.—Erica

Even when her eyes were still fused shut, Emma would acknowledge our visits. Her little eyebrows would raise up and down.—Diane

I was pretty sure he knew me after a few days. I know he could recognize me by smelling me. He wouldn't do it every time, but I got the feeling of him turning toward me or moving when I got there, or when he was sleeping, he would start to do little imperceptible movements when he was perfectly quiet before, but he could feel that I was there. And against me, he was just breathing, not getting agitated but just breathing quietly against me, and I'm sure he knew it was me.—Gallice

When you start to see that you are not simply another set of hands to your baby, you can begin to embrace your parenting role. Realizing that you're special and important to your infant can be very comforting. Of course, with this realization comes the belief that you should be even more available to your baby. Discovering the powerful effect of your presence makes being away that much harder.

But your baby does not need you at the bedside constantly. Your infant can benefit from long stretches of uninterrupted sleep. Your baby also needs you to be healthy and resilient, so you taking time to rest, run errands, or catch up with a friend is time well spent. Put aside your guilt. You do not need to remain hospitalized with your baby.

Finally, keep in mind that staying informed, advocating, and making the most of both your presence and your absence are all ways of staying meaningfully connected to your child. Recognizing the importance of your presence doesn't refer only to your presence at your baby's bedside but also to your ongoing presence in your baby's life.

It's painful to be separated from your baby when he or she needs you, but be reassured that the time you spend with your baby really matters, and the benefits don't disappear when you leave. Your nurturing presence builds your baby's capacity to endure your absences. Have faith in your baby's ability to manage when you're away.

Spreading Yourself among Multiple Babies

When they were first born, Evan was so much smaller and so much sicker that we were just really concentrating on him. If we had to sit by somebody's bedside, we'd sit by Evan's bedside. I would go and look at Josh and make sure he was okay, and I would talk to him, but we concentrated on Evan. And then a couple of days later, they did the brain ultrasounds, and we found out that Josh had a grade III brain bleed. And that's when the thought of having twins that are so sick just really got to me. How can I do this? How can I sit by two babies who need me so much? [tears] Josh really needs me, he's got this brain bleed, and Evan is so little and so sick. How can I do it? I just didn't know how.—Stephie

I was so wrapped up in Jacob, I wasn't thinking that I had other children. Then I realized that I had better start paying attention to all of them. It wasn't just Jacob who was critically ill, Claire and Emily could have problems. I guess I was feeling like a pretty lousy mother.

I wish I could have cloned myself and stuck one of me next to each of them. I felt pretty inadequate—like I didn't have enough of me, I didn't have enough to give.—Julie

If you have more than one baby in the NICU, it's only natural to feel torn. The best you can possibly do is to put your energy and resources where you think they are needed the most. You can't do any better than that. Trust yourself to give each infant what he or she needs on any given day—or even hour by hour.

Also remember that it isn't so much the amount of time but the quality of your focus that's important. For instance, Pam discovered that when her twins were in different sections of the hospital, both babies benefited from her being able to devote her full attention and energy to each, one at a time. To her, spending half the time truly present with each one was better than spending all the time ricocheting between the two.

On certain days, if you feel especially drawn to one of your babies, spend more time with that one and perhaps encourage your partner to focus on the other(s). Have confidence that your babies will do just fine even if your attention is split at times.

Also appreciate and rely on the attention your babies' nurses give them. The nurses are there to help you care for your little ones. Finally, remember to give yourself credit for being your babies' round-the-clock advocate.

When you have three babies in the NICU and you're going from one to another to another, dealing with what each one of them has, you just have to know that they're in the best place that they can possibly be and that they're going to be taken care of. And that there's nothing you can do to make them better but advocate for them.—Betsy

Becoming a self-assured parent of multiple newborns challenges all parents. Give yourself the time and space to become a parent to each child individually and to become adept at meeting their inevitably various needs.

Managing Your Regrets

I would have touched him more, been more active in his care, and read to him. I was so afraid that I left everything up to the doctors and nurses. Even when they suggested that I do a diaper change or rub lotion on him, I was often too afraid to do so. There are so many things I would have done but wasn't sure if I should or even was allowed to. I would have asked more questions, done more research, and been an active part of his treatment and care rather than just stand by and watch silently.—Corin

I wished I'd taken more control right away. By the first week's end, I was just going in and picking her up, but those first few days, I'd wait to be offered, as if she belonged to these strangers and not me. I would touch her through her little incubator, apologizing still.—Linda

The very nature of parenting in the NICU can give rise to feelings of inadequacy and regret. Even if you are in the most relationship-centered NICU on the planet, you can still feel out of place at times and unable to nurture your baby in the way you want.

Some parents fault themselves for not being the "perfect," sacrificing mother or father during their baby's hospitalization. You may regret not spending more hours in the nursery, or you may feel burdened by your constant vigil, believing that all the hours you do spend are still not enough.

If constant attendance in the NICU is wearing you down, remember that although being with your baby because you *want to* can be good for both of you, it's not necessarily beneficial to be with your baby because you feel you *should* or you *must* to quell your anxiety or grief. It can do you far more good to take some time and energy to work through these feelings of obligation, worry, and grief by journaling, going to counseling, attending a support group, talking with a supportive friend, or engaging in meaningful activity. This emotional clearing can keep you from emotional and physical exhaustion. Plus, you can enhance your ability to be truly present with your little one by setting aside regular times every week to write, think, share, talk, create, and play. Also try viewing all that you are doing for your baby as if in hindsight. When you can look objectively at all you are juggling and accomplishing, you can give yourself the credit *and* the breaks you deserve.

I drove myself into the ground trying to watch over Vincent while he was in the NICU, and it left me very fragile.—Anne

I probably should not have acted so much like a martyr by spending so much of my time at the NICU when there was nothing I could do but worry.—Dina

If I had to do this again, I wouldn't beat myself up so much. I'd take a day off when I needed it without feeling guilty. In the months my kiddos were in the NICU, I was there all day, every day but one. I was so exhausted that day that I broke down in tears at the thought of [finally] driving in at 9:30 at night to see my babies. I look back now and can't believe I pushed myself so hard and didn't totally fall apart mentally and physically.—Julie

If you are looking back now with regrets, be compassionate with yourself. Remember how flooded with feelings and fears you were. You were not the same recharged, adjusted, confident parent you are currently. Recall your baby's condition and all the medical obstacles in your way.

I can think of all sorts of things I wish had been different, but mostly I realize that none of them were possible because I couldn't figure out a way to [deal with] my own anxiety, fear, frustration, anger, sadness, and, on some levels, resentment. . . . I believe the bottom line is that I wish I could have felt more a part of the whole situation rather than like a spectator at a horrific accident.—Sheila

Also recognize that most of the limitations you have to work within—such as your baby's medical status, your own physical and emotional conditions, having more than one baby in the NICU, your other family obligations, the distance between your home and the hospital, the NICU policies—are largely out of your control. Instead, commend yourself for the ways you work within or overcome these limitations. Also remember that there's no such thing as a perfect parent. Reaching for being the best that you can be every day is a worthy goal, but on the days you feel as if you're falling short, reassure yourself that it's okay to be "good enough."

Feeling More Like a Parent

One long night, a midnight shift nurse told me that I was perfectly capable of performing some of the tasks involved in caring for my son. She recognized my motherhood—and stunned me, honored me, by helping me do the same.—Susan C.

Over the course of your baby's hospitalization, as your baby increasingly responds to your voice, your touch, and your scent, you'll feel more confident in the critical role you play in your baby's care and recovery. Your tentative touch will gradually develop into a more confident, protective hold. Your hesitant requests will become more assertive and your convictions more firm. Only your baby's own growth will rival your development as an involved parent.

There are so many things I learned about myself, walking in there. I'm a very confident person anyway, but to realize that there's a certain amount of confidence you need to be able to go in there and do what the nurses do. You know, they're flipping these babies around, and they're not afraid of this stuff. As the days go by, you start learning, okay, I can have the confidence to hold this baby, to know which cord is for what, and when to be alarmed and when not to.—Vickie

We set up vigil at his bedside and reminded the occasional hurried medical student to wash his hands between beds, asked janitors to avoid clanging trash cans near his bedside, argued with doctors about placing infected babies adjacent with single nursing care when beds got scarce.—Susan C.

As you get more confident and involved in your baby's care, you may notice an emotional shift. You can begin to let go of some of your sadness and guilt. You develop ways of relating to your baby that go beyond grief and shock. Most significantly, in bits and spurts you have moments of feeling parental. You feel bolstered by the simplest incidents—noticing that your baby responds uniquely to you, being asked to consult on a medical test, soothing your baby during a procedure, or even noticing a family resemblance. The more you behave like a parent, the more you can feel like one.

You can also see that your baby doesn't depend entirely on technology and skilled care. Your baby also depends on you. Gradually, you gain assurance that you can know what your baby needs and that your presence can calm and comfort. You begin to feel more in sync with your baby. As that rhythm develops, you realize that you are connected and important to your baby. This realization is both reassuring and a bit anxiety provoking. After all, your last big job as a parent was to complete a pregnancy or bear a healthy baby. But no matter why your baby is in the NICU, your ability to parent this child remains intact.

During his first week, he was so critically ill that he did not respond to anyone. When he was more stable, he began to respond to my voice by trying to open his eyes. At around the same age, he began to show high sats and fewer bradycardia episodes when one of my breast pads was laid next to him within sniffing range. Once I was able to hold him, he began gaining weight at a more accelerated rate than when I was not allowed to hold him. The first time I held him for an hour, he gained seventy grams that night.—Jayna

In fact, as you become accustomed to the monitor beeps and more comfortable with the tubes and wires (or as they disappear), you can reclaim the simple, basic caregiving you had hoped to do with your newborn. Holding, cooing, singing, rocking, reading to your baby, even just sitting nearby—when done with care, all of these activities foster increased intimacy and connection. As your baby grows, you'll be able to do more feeding, bathing, dressing, and interacting. The more you are able to meet your baby's needs, the more confident and parental you'll feel.

As Nicholas grew and I got more comfortable with him, we got to know one another. I guess we all end up adapting to the NICU environment in our own time. But pretty soon, I was doing almost everything for him—so, in a sense at least, maybe he saw me as one of his primary caregivers and hopefully the one that wasn't causing him any pain.—Sterling

No matter where your baby sleeps, you are still the parent. No matter how much skilled care your infant requires, you are ultimately the one in charge of your little one's welfare. Even a shaky start doesn't doom your ability to feel like a parent. As you blossom into an effective parent, you'll look back and wish you had been able to imagine your future success. Dare to imagine it now.

Points to Remember

· *Feeling like a parent in the NICU presents many challenges.*

· *You are likely to be flooded with confusing and overwhelming feelings as you try to ease your way into your parenting role. The intensity of your feelings mobilizes your development as a parent.*

· *When your baby is inactive and unresponsive, it is only natural for you to hold back. In fact, your hesitance can be a sign of your attunement and empathy toward your child.*

· *Recognize that many parents need a certain amount of privacy to forge a close connection to their infant. As you adjust to the NICU, you'll be able to carve out quiet, private moments.*

· *No matter how your baby is doing in the NICU, it is normal to have fears about what's next and what the future will bring. Facing your fears can decrease their power to disturb you and bar them from intruding on your relationship with your baby.*

- *Parenting in the NICU demands that you build confidence in the face of some unusual obstacles. Spending time with your baby and increasingly participating in caregiving can help you become the confident parent you had imagined being.*

- *No matter how much technical care your baby needs, your presence is extremely important to your baby's healing. As you get to know your baby, you will observe how she or he is soothed by your comforting presence.*

- *Your caregiving schedule will depend on many factors in your life. If you can't go to the NICU as often as you'd like, find other ways to feel close to your baby.*

- *Parenting multiples in the NICU challenges your view of yourself as a good enough parent. It's normal to worry that there isn't enough of you to go around, but your babies don't need all of you all the time. They can thrive on your focused attention for part of your stay.*

- *At some point in the future, perhaps as you hold your little one close to your heart, you may wonder how you could ever have doubted your ability to feel like a parent to this baby.*

Relating to Your Baby

I remember devouring the sight of his face—trying to see the person inside. I remember his hands flailing and having a sense that he was afraid. I wanted to soothe him but wasn't sure what I could do.—Laurie

I had read about how important it was to hold a baby skin to skin as soon after birth as possible. I couldn't help thinking about the possible harm being caused by every day that I couldn't actually hold her, especially seeing her in such discomfort at times.—Dina

Like many parents in the NICU, you may wonder how to relate to your baby and develop that special, loving connection. Central to forging a meaningful, two-way relationship are bonding, feeding, and becoming attuned. But how can you bond when you struggle with feelings of detachment and lack easy access to your baby? How can you feed a baby who cannot suck or swallow, be held, or digest normally? How can you become attuned to a baby who is unresponsive or so easily overwhelmed?

I was very sick and was kept about a week in the hospital to recuperate. I remember that I did not feel connected to the baby and was disappointed that I didn't learn to recognize his cry right away (never did, really) and, embarrassingly, could not even recognize him visually. . . . I worried that someone was going to realize that I couldn't recognize my own baby.—Shaina

Because of her very ill health, I couldn't even touch Daphne for the first week of her life. And until her ventilator and her chest/drainage tube were removed (when she was almost a whole month old), I couldn't really hold or caress my baby the way a mother ordinarily should be able to. Emotionally, this was very hard for me. What mother doesn't want to hold her suffering baby?—Dina

He really didn't respond to anything. This really was hard. You always hear how a newborn knows his mother's voice, and I wondered if he had had enough time in the womb to know mine. Would we have the bond mothers and babies have? Does he know I'm his mommy?—Cynthia

My son was so inactive that it was hard to believe he was even alive sometimes.—Terri

It is important to remember that becoming acquainted with and attuned to any newborn is a learning process. Just as you're meeting the NICU challenges of getting close, getting involved, and feeling like a parent to your baby, you can meet the challenges of interacting and building a relationship. This chapter covers bonding, kangaroo care, infant massage, co-bedding multiples, and attunement; the next chapter focuses on feeding your baby. Both chapters provide information, tips, and support for connecting with your baby in ways that you'll both find rewarding.

Bonding

I remember that he seemed to weigh nothing. I kept trying to orient his weight to know how to hold him. He was so bundled that it all felt awkward and unreal. I couldn't get any sense of connection because I couldn't feel him at all. I felt like I held an empty blanket.—Laurie

Bonding refers to the connection, devotion, or emotional investment that parents feel toward their baby. But when your baby is admitted to the NICU, instead of feeling completely connected and devoted to your infant, you may feel worlds apart.

A nurse brought me pictures of her, and I studied them very closely. Was this really my baby? She looked so strange and unfamiliar. Why don't I immediately feel close to her? Shouldn't I immediately feel close? We didn't have that initial bonding that so many books advocate. Does that mean we'll forever feel distant from each other?—Rebekah

The first time I held her, I didn't really feel much emotion. It sounds bad to say that. I was happy, but at the same time I was just really numb. I don't remember feeling *Yes, I feel this wonderful outpouring of emotion*, because it wasn't really like that. I was just there, and she was just there, and there wasn't really any connection.—Beth

Bonding was by no means an immediate occurrence for me. For a long time I looked at those babies and thought, *They're cute, but are they really mine?* I wondered if I would ever bond with them. I knew I should love them, bond with them, be a mother to them, but I didn't feel anything! I felt numb. I didn't cry—and I feel I should have. Why didn't I? It wasn't until a month after they were born that I cried.—Sara

I wish I could say here that I soon bonded with my daughter. I'm not at all sure I ever did while in the NICU. It was weeks before I felt she was mine. Perhaps my heart was afraid to get too close to an infant who could die at any moment. I was becoming increasingly depressed for perhaps the first time in my life. I was concerned about my lack of emotional closeness to the baby. I felt that I should feel more for this baby, that I should love her more than I did. My feelings of failure over her birth were multiplied by my guilt over not feeling loving toward her.—Renee

As discussed in chapter 2, most parents struggle with feelings of detachment in the face of separation and the barriers created by your baby's need for intensive care. You may worry about the impact of missing out on early opportunities for closeness, such as being able to hold your slippery little newborn against your body, spending the first few days together in peace, or freely snuggling and nursing your baby.

It is natural for you to grieve deeply over missing these bonding opportunities, but in the long run these activities are not critical to becoming emotionally invested in your infant. That's because bonding is a *process* that

- occurs over time,

- has peak moments,

- is flexible, and

- is resilient.

As you read the following sections, you can be reassured by how close to the mark you are with your baby.

Bonding Occurs Over Time

When parents think about bonding, they often imagine instantaneous rapture upon their baby's delivery. Although this emotional spike may happen for some, it doesn't happen for everybody. For many parents, falling in love with their baby is a slow warm-up, not an explosion. And even for parents who do experience love at first sight, bonding remains an ongoing process of emotionally investing in their baby as their face-to-face relationship develops.

In fact, for many parents, the bonding process starts even before conception, as they imagine welcoming and raising future babies. These dreams for the future continue throughout pregnancy and persist after birth—throughout the life span, really. When a baby is born early or with serious problems, these dreams are momentarily derailed, but the bonding process isn't. It just continues on a different track, and parents dream new dreams.

I loved Alex before he was born. I felt very connected with him when I carried him inside. . . . When he was born, he was whisked out of the room, and I had to ask if he was a boy and was alive. But I felt so close to him, it was like we shared memories. When I entered the NICU for the first time, it was like I saw it from his perspective and from my own.—Allison

While you can probably identify the bonding you've done before and during the pregnancy, your baby's need for intensive care can complicate your developing bond. But as discussed in chapter 6, just as you feel more and more like a parent as you become acquainted with your baby, establish your role, and gain confidence, your bond will follow a parallel course, continuing to strengthen as you feel more knowledgeable, more in sync, and more in charge.

I felt terribly lonely and cheated when T.J. was whisked away to the NICU. I wanted desperately to hold him and to marvel with my husband at the little miracle we had created. I felt I had been robbed of the initial closeness to my child. I just wish I could have held him right after I had him. However, now, I feel as if we bonded just as well afterward.—Claire

Over time, you'll experience many opportunities to feel close to and connected with your baby. Although not anticipated, these opportunities can be just as precious, extraordinary, and meaningful, if not more so because you have to wait for them. For example, as your baby stabilizes and matures, you'll eagerly await and appreciate eye contact or the turn toward your voice that much more. Touching or holding your little one can be such a tender and endearing experience, a highlight that is special every time. Homecoming may mark another turning point, when you finally begin to feel the intense bond you've been wishing for.

I bonded with him the first time I put cream on his leg—because that was all we could do. Every day, he was like a little white ball of cream because that was all we could do.—Nettie

For me, the realization that he was mine was when the nurse wrapped him up and handed him to me and I was able to hold him. I was looking at him, and I couldn't believe how a baby could be so small. I mean, I know they're that small when they're inside of your stomach, but how could this baby be so small and be alive? . . . And he just looked at me, and he probably couldn't see past his eyelashes, just staring right at me, and I just remember crying and thinking, *This is my baby. How wonderful. How wonderful.*—Vickie

Bonding Has Peak Moments

Bonding between parent and child has many peak moments: receiving a positive pregnancy test result, seeing the baby's image on an ultrasound screen, feeling the baby move for the first time, meeting the baby after birth, when watching the baby sleeping peacefully. As mentioned in chapter 2, the father experiences his own special peak called *engrossment*—gazing in wonder at his newborn after birth, as if the rest of the world no longer matters. In general, peak moments are when parents feel a heightened level of commitment and devotion. Experiencing and remembering these precious moments reinforces the parents' bond with their little one.

You've already been through the peaks of pregnancy test results and perhaps ultrasounds and feeling the baby quicken. But once your baby is born, it's hard to imagine when you'll be able to experience another peak moment. You may feel surrounded by valleys instead. But although the peaks may be brief, bittersweet, or few and far between, you *will* experience significant bonding moments. You may find them when and where you least expect them.

Fabian didn't need to be intubated on the spot. He was breathing and he cried, and so I even got the chance, which I never even imagined could be possible, but they put him on my breast for a few seconds. . . . It makes me cry. . . . That was one of the most beautiful gifts on earth, to be able to have him on me. It was really good. Because at that point, you're so scared you don't know what's going to come out of you. And I could see, of course, he was really tiny, but still he was a baby and doing well and to just have him on me, that was really wonderful.—Gallice

I held my son the night he was born. I had to beg them to let me hold him. When they put James in my arms, I started to cry. But it was the most wonderful feeling in the world, holding my son. I could only hold him for a few minutes, and I didn't want to let go. When I held him, I felt that everything would be all right.—Jennifer A.

They came up with a picture, a Polaroid picture—oh, that's him. It didn't seem real to me at that point. But when I could hold him, I can't even describe it. I was just trying to hold him as close as I could—I guess trying to put him back [into my womb]. . . . It was a big moment.—Marcia

The baby I held first was Jacob, but that's only because the nurse bent the rules. He was twenty-eight days old, and they were getting him ready for the first of his surgeries . . . and one of the nurses said, "Why don't you hold him while I get the bed ready? What if I pull up a rocking chair and you can sit down and hold him?" I'll never forget. It was at that point in time I knew everything was going to be okay.—Julie

Words cannot adequately express what holding my baby after so long meant to me. It felt like a victory of sorts. Finally, after all we had been through, Daphne was in my arms where she belonged.—Dina

Some parents are too dazed or scared to appreciate the peak bonding moments when they occur. It can be difficult to feel warm and fuzzy when your baby is in peril. Nevertheless, in spite of your worries and hesitation, when you feel so thankful that your baby is alive, when you touch, hold, or feed your little one for the first time, when you start making discharge plans, or simply when you savor thoughts of how precious this new life is, you are experiencing a peak moment. Sometimes the feeling may seem closer to terror than to love, but it is still a peak moment.

I remember that I started to cry before we even entered the room the babies were in. It felt as though my heart was attempting to get out of my chest, and I was shaking.—Michele

About a couple of weeks after my son's birth, a nurse practitioner called me with some results of a brain scan and described a small bleed to me over the phone. We had been told he hadn't had any bleeds they could find, so this was quite a shock. . . . I spoke to the neonatologist that night, and he explained the brain scans. The news wasn't nearly as bad as I had thought, and the bleed was so minor they didn't even classify it as a grade I, but I was hysterical. This was the first time it really hit me that this is a real baby—and he was mine to protect and raise.—Andrea

The first time I really felt close to my son was when Sean was three weeks old, the day I finally got to hold him. It was only for ten or fifteen minutes, but I got to hold him. I sat in the NICU rocking chair, looking down at my tiny infant son. The realization suddenly hit me for the first time that rather than wasting all this time and energy feeling sorry for myself, I should be giving him love and encouragement. At that moment, as I looked at this miniature baby bundled in his blankies, cuddled up in my arms with all his wires and tubes and such, I was suddenly hit with an overwhelming feeling of love and pride for this little boy. He had fought so hard, come so far already. He amazed me. He was my miracle. . . . I was going to take care of this baby the best that I could. I would give him everything I had. This little boy was going to live. It didn't matter anymore what I had to do to make that happen.—Ami

I didn't get to see my son for five days after his birth because I was very sick also. I had expected to see a big, bubbling baby, and instead there was this little tiny thing lying there, and I was afraid to touch him. He had all these tubes and pipes coming from everywhere. The nurse was very friendly and helpful, and she finally got me to touch his hand—and it was the most electrifying experience. I've been holding that hand for three years now.—Jonette

Bonding Is Flexible

The bonding process is flexible—flexible enough to overcome obstacles such as anxiety, illness, the NICU, and separation. For example, parents needn't go through a term pregnancy, much less see their newborn upon delivery, to develop a bond. Just ask any adoptive parent. Even if you haven't yet been able to nest or nuzzle, you are bonding with your baby simply by wanting what's best for him or her. Whether you're able to look past your baby's medical fragility and necessary treatments or you agonize over them, your reaction is a measure of your intense devotion—and your bond.

I looked at them, and it was the standard, classic, overwhelming feeling of total and complete love for these babies. . . . From the moment I found out I was pregnant with them, I was in love with these babies. And then, looking at them, I could see beyond the wires and these monitors, these little teeny tiny humans that were my children, that will someday run and play and have a good time. I wasn't focused on the situation. I could see beyond that and see these tiny babies with their teeny tiny hands, and I saw a term baby in there. I loved these little babies, regardless of how different they looked.—Pam

No way could I look past their prematurity. It was like a knife in my heart. My most fervent wish on bed rest was that they would be boring [need few interventions] to neonatologists. As it turned out, they weren't boring. I was tortured by their fragility because it meant that they needed things that I couldn't give them. . . . I desperately wanted to be able to give them everything they needed and everything I had.—Rikki

You and your partner may differ in how you show your devotion. One parent may learn every medical term and pore over the chart; the other may want time spent with the baby to be jargon free. One parent may spend hours over the incubator, while the other may work overtime to pay the mounting bills. One may search medical libraries, and the other may want only to count toes and sing silly songs. All of this is bonding. And if, for whatever reason, you can't be with your baby, taking comfort in your partner's presence at your baby's bedside is another expression of your bond.

When she was first born, I was already thinking that whatever it took to keep this child alive, if I had to go into debt and live in a shoe box, I would live in a shoe box to keep this girl with us for the rest of our lives. . . . I would make sure this girl would be happy.—Charlie

Bonding Is Resilient
If you had a very high-risk pregnancy, you may have tried not to become invested in your baby. If your baby was unlikely to survive, you may have refused to see your little one at first. Even if you find yourself falling in love right away, you may fight the feeling, hesitant to invest

emotionally in an infant who looks too frail to survive. But in spite of these barriers, you can still feel a bond.

It's really weird, but I kind of felt bonded to her and detached at the same time. It was like I was bonded to her, but I didn't want to be because I didn't know how she would turn out. I didn't want to get too attached if she was just going to die on me. I didn't let myself feel like a mom until I didn't have to worry so much about losing her.—Brooke

She was extremely tiny—transparent skin, I could visualize her every vein. She was beautiful. Such a sweet, innocent, frail little baby. My baby. And I fell deeply in love with her from the moment I laid my eyes on her, even though I tried so hard not to love her because I was so afraid of losing her.—Jillian

Even if you remain reluctant to get close to your baby, you are still gradually adjusting to the reality that this baby has arrived—and is possibly here to stay. Even if you try to stay detached, your love remains, just waiting for an opportunity to bloom. As your baby's condition improves and you are finally able to get closer, you can feel more emotionally calm and open to bonding. When your baby finally squeezes your hand or when you hold your baby in your arms, you can feel more mobilized and nurturing. As you do more caregiving, your love and investment in your little one naturally grows.

I watched as she was wrapped in warm sheets and handed to me. I think that was when I realized she was a real baby. I could hold her and kiss her just like a full-term baby. It was a moment in my life that I will never forget. Until this point, I was unconsciously holding myself back from loving this child. That ended when I held her. She was so small and innocent, I could not help but feel an overwhelming surge of love for her.—Kimberly

The first time I saw Liam was beautiful. Here was this little baby I was so scared to get attached to but couldn't help it. Here was the baby I kept thinking I was miscarrying. Here he was. And once I saw that face, I immediately started crying. I had tried so hard not to love him when I was pregnant for fear of getting hurt . . . but it turns out that I did love him all along. I kissed his head and took in his smell. I will never forget those first few minutes.—Kimi

I was afraid to really let myself believe that he was real and was mine. But when he was a little more stable and I had a little more say as to how he was cared for, then I began to look at him as my baby. But it really wasn't until I had some semblance of control over the situation that I could allow myself to feel that.—Sterling

For me, that bond wasn't really there [in the NICU]. Yeah, she's my baby, but until we really got her home, it wasn't as significant. As she got healthier and bigger, it was definitely easier. The bond was there. But in the first month and a half or so, it was hard.—Sandi

Bonding during Crisis

As your emotions rise, keep in mind that bonding in the NICU (and beyond) involves more than just positive feelings such as love and joy. There is also a dark side to feeling invested in your baby. You may worry about the terrible things that might happen. It will hurt you to see your baby struggle. You may struggle as well. You may feel rejected when your baby can't tolerate handling. It can be tiresome and depressing to pump breast milk when you'd rather just put your baby to the breast. It can be overwhelming to seek out and absorb medical information. It's anxiety provoking when your baby continues to be medically or developmentally challenged. Setbacks are devastating, and you may be filled with feelings of anger and dread. But these emotions are signs that you *care.*

It's different. It has to be so different. Especially with the firstborn [who was full-term and healthy], I was just amazed when I came home and this child was lying in a bed next to my bed, and I'm thinking, *This is mine now, and no one's going to come and take it away. This human being, this beautiful creature I was given as a gift.* With Erin [the preemie], there was so much in your head, going around, there just wasn't any peace—from *Is she going to have problems when she's older?* to *Are the oxygen sats levels at 100 all day?* There was no time for me to think about the beautiful things. It was just more of the awful things. I kept thinking of all the things that had to be done. . . . And you get to the NICU for the day, and they explain what's going on—and just trying to remember all the medical stuff. There just wasn't that much time to lean over and look in the incubator. The love was the same, but the worry was higher.—Charlie

Your bond to your baby includes all the joy that comes with childbirth *and* all the agony that comes with crisis. While "typical" newborn parenting includes occasional feelings of distress and being overwhelmed, NICU parenting includes these feelings in spades. But this only makes your parenting journey more intense, not wrong.

So rather than getting bound up trying to follow a script that doesn't fit, turn toward your baby and accept the emotional terrain that comes with NICU bonding. Acceptance can free you to behave more naturally and spontaneously with your baby and strengthens your growing connection to your little one.

I did everything I could to get to know her and, more importantly, for her to get to know me. During Daphne's first week in the NICU, I tried to spend as much time as possible sitting near her reading or singing so that she could hear my voice. During Daphne's second week, I asked and was permitted by the NICU personnel to assist in changing her diapers and apply moisturizers. I also took every opportunity to have physical contact with her by placing my hands firmly on the top of her head and on the bottom of her feet, which calmed her. And after I was finally able to really hold Daphne, I worked long and hard to get her to adjust to being held, to actually bond with me, and to even breast-feed.—Dina

Certainly, as discussed in chapter 4, seek help from a qualified counselor for unflagging distress or for persistent depression or anxiety. In some cases, medication is indicated to treat the biological components of your symptoms. Even if you simply have some nagging concerns about your parental feelings, you can benefit from additional help and support. You and your baby deserve to experience all the complexity and richness of your budding relationship.

I didn't see my son for a week after he was born. Those days were horrible. I went into a deep depression. When I finally got to see my son, he was off the oxygen and breathing on his own, and I got to hold him the first time I saw him. That was when it was all worth it—it didn't seem real until then.—Cyd

Also keep in mind that because your bond grows in spite of your attempts to protect yourself, if your baby were to die, you would be devastated no matter how much you tried to harden your heart. If you avoid the NICU and then your baby dies, you will always wonder what small but powerful knowledge of your child you might have gained had you been there. And if your baby ends up with long-term challenges, you will grieve over them and for your child whether you are in the NICU for fifteen minutes or fifteen hours a day. So you might as well reap the benefits of involvement. Dare to get close to your baby. Dare to bond like a parent. The road can be challenging, but the rewards of loving devotion are immeasurable.

In some ways, we are even more bonded. We know what it's like to almost lose them—to be faced with that. Maybe we're even more appreciative of just having them.—Debbie

To make a long story short, I overcame my fears of my child and of the NICU. I could not love my daughter any more than I do now. The special circumstances of her birth just required some adjustments in my thinking!—Kimberly

Enjoying Your Baby

You may hear from your family and your baby's practitioners, "Just enjoy your baby." This suggestion can be confusing or irritating. You may wonder, *Enjoy? Really? Does anyone enjoy the terror of watching their newborn struggle or tiptoeing around a fragile, unresponsive infant in this public setting?*

Naturally, enjoying your baby means something different in the NICU. It means learning to pay attention to those little moments when your infant grips your finger or turns to your voice. It means appreciating each moment you can touch your newborn and every time you can be together. It means being genuine and heartfelt with your baby. As your terror and anxiety subside, enjoyment will come more easily. But even in the midst of your worries, your anger, and your regrets, you can stop and smell the tiny roses.

Kangaroo Care

Kangaroo care is the practice of holding your unclothed, diapered baby on your bare chest (between your breasts, if you're a mom), blanket draped over your baby's back. Both you and your baby can benefit greatly from this skin-to-skin contact. After the trauma of crisis and the barriers between you and your baby, the sensation of having nothing between you acts as a balm to heal the wounds of your separation. Being so close to your baby feels so right, so good, and so natural, at last. Holding your baby close can transport you to a different world.

When I was allowed to hold Alycia, I kangarooed her and loved every minute of it. The warmth of her skin against mine was a feeling that I cannot describe! I felt like a mom for the very first time! And each time I held my babies, I felt a bond that no one will ever be able to take away. The hardest days were the ones on which I wasn't able to hold them.—Michele

Of course we were excited about the prospect [of kangaroo care]. The doctors finally relented and allowed us to hold Sarah after she weighed enough. Sarah handled kangarooing so well, the doctors were amazed. And I felt alive finally—at least for those few, short minutes each day.—Cindy

I remember the feeling of pure joy. I don't think I had ever been that happy before. I could see the relaxation in Glen's face. I could tell it was so much more comfortable for him than lying in the warmer.—Sharon

As appealing as the idea of kangaroo care is for many parents, you might feel reluctant to hold your tiny baby, especially at first. If your baby is premature or otherwise fragile looking, the natural fear of hurting your baby may stand in the way of your enthusiasm. If you feel at all responsible for your baby's plight, the opportunity to hold your baby so close to your body might feel both exhilarating and frightening—after all, you may not yet have banished the feeling that you and your body are agents of harm. Rest assured that your scent, your touch, and the rhythms of your speech and breathing are beneficial to your baby. Your little one needs you, and you need your little baby.

Frankly, I was terrified of picking her up—she was so tiny and weak. I was actually somewhat relieved that the doctors didn't want me to hold her at first. In just two days, though, the nurses told my husband and me about kangaroo care. I held her frail body against my bare skin and slowly started to feel like, yes, this was my child.—Rebekah

The first time I held Zane, our smallest triplet, it was by kangaroo care. He weighed just over three pounds at birth. I was so surprised and comforted when I held him and found that he felt just like a baby. He looked so tiny and fragile that I think I assumed he would be like china, but he was soft and warm and cuddly. . . . We calmed and comforted each other. I could feel myself relax as I held Zane, and I could see from his monitors that he was relaxing too.—Jill

Kangarooing is so natural that, with encouragement, most mothers and fathers seize the opportunity. After a gentle initiation, even the most hesitant parents can become ardent kangarooers.

They put her on me kangaroo-style. She felt like a wet dishcloth. That's what went through my mind. They placed her on me, us both unclothed, right between my breasts. I have never felt more content in my life.—Timmesa

The Benefits of Kangarooing

The physical and emotional benefits of kangaroo care are many. Research (most of it with preterm infants but similar results are found in term infants) indicates that after just a few minutes of kangarooing, marked results are observed in babies and their parents. In recent years, research has uncovered the additional benefits of implementing kangaroo care earlier, more often, and for longer periods in the NICU, further demonstrating the value of this simple yet profound intervention.

Compared to being in the incubator, kangaroo care may help your infant

· maintain body warmth more easily,

· achieve more stable heart and breathing rates,

· spend more time in the restful, deep sleep that promotes recovery,

· spend more time in a quiet alert state and less time crying,

· gain weight more quickly,

· be more successful at breast-feeding,

· tolerate better and recover faster from painful procedures, and

· achieve faster neurobehavioral maturation.

Kangaroo care is good for parents too. It can help you

· feel like a parent,

· grow more confident about your parenting ability,

· be more eager and able to take your baby home,

· feel closer, more bonded, to your baby,

· be more sensitive and attuned to your baby, and

· feel less stressed and more relaxed.

Kangaroo care can help the mother

· have more success with breast-feeding and a better milk supply, and

· be less at risk for postpartum depression.

If you have twins, triplets, or more, you and your babies can benefit from shared kangaroo care, where all of you snuggle together.

Why is kangaroo care so beneficial? Skin-to-skin contact releases the hormone oxytocin in the brain. This hormone's influences in the brain result in most of the growth, calming, physiologic improvement, analgesic effect, and recovery-enhancement observed. This hormone also plays a critical role in promoting human bonding and attachment and is primarily responsible for your observation that skin-to-skin contact simply *feels so good*.

Overall, kangaroo care enhances rest, recuperation, and healing by making intensive care less taxing and less disruptive to the infant.

The Emotions of Kangarooing

For parents, the emotional and psychological benefits of kangaroo care are important. Instead of watching your baby through plastic or holding what essentially feels like just a blanket, you can finally snuggle up, smell that sweet baby smell, and touch soft skin. Knowing that your infant is responding well to kangaroo care strengthens your recognition that you can actually *do something* to help your baby recover and grow. When that *something* is so natural, significant, and nurturing for your baby, it can boost your confidence and morale. It's as if you've regained control over the situation, and you can finally claim and protect your infant. Nurses and doctors, for all their skill, do not do kangaroo care with the babies in the NICU. Only parents hold their baby with such intimacy.

While he was in the hospital, I felt he needed to be held—[he] couldn't just be in the incubator all day, only held when the nurses needed to feed him. He needed that interaction. That was pretty much why we were there.—Richard

The kangaroo care for sure helps so much. You've got your baby on your skin, and he's yours and you feel him and he's living and he's breathing, he's warm and he's a real human being. Everything else in the world disappears. There's nothing else but your child. You feel him and he's just . . . you forget all about the whole situation, the fears, that you're scared for his life. You forget everything, and he's just on you. It was just so relaxing. At the same time, you remember that that's still where he's supposed to be, so he should be there. It's the best thing to have in the world. You forget all about time. You'll never forget that feeling, it's so special.—Gallice

Especially the first time, it can be an intense emotional experience and perhaps a potent catalyst for releasing pent-up emotions. Most parents believe that their baby reaps emotional benefits as well.

This dear nurse asked if I wanted to hold him. She got him out, and we were able to kangaroo for almost an hour. It was the first time I had cried since the whole emergency began. It was so wonderful. He spent only a little time looking at me or awake, but it didn't matter.—Trish

Thaddeus cuddled right down when I would hold him against my heart. I had the feeling that that was familiar to him. He was quite peaceful that way right from the start, and that told me he felt safe there.—Laurie

If you feel like crying during kangaroo care, your tears may have many sources. As you feel your tiny baby curled up on your chest, calm and content in your protective embrace, you can rejoice at your closeness and at the same time grieve for your cruel separation. Kangaroo care can also build your hopes: you may start to feel confident that your baby will survive and that you can have a close relationship with this child. As you hold your baby, you may feel more certain that you can monitor your little one's health and safety, and you can feel more positive and patient with the NICU experience. If you've been feeling displaced or inadequate, the way your baby sinks into your bare chest can make you feel valuable and capable. If you are struggling with guilt, you may sense that this child forgives you for all that you imagine to be your fault. You may even begin to forgive yourself.

Your tears will not hurt your baby, who may be in a deep sleep and undisturbed by your crying. If you'd rather not cry in the NICU, you might try to visualize kangarooing your infant and having a good cry before you go in.

Some nursing staff may be uncomfortable with your tears and try to take your baby away. One mom bitterly recalled, "A nurse ripped my baby away from me when I cried. Told me it was bad for the baby." But as long as your infant is resting comfortably, there's no evidence that your tears are bad for him or her. You can be assertive and advocate even through your tears: make it clear that as long as your baby is content and comfy, you're going to continue kangarooing.

When your kangaroo session is over, your baby may protest being removed from you. This won't undo the benefits of kangaroo care. Your baby was able to have a valuable rest. Research also shows that right after kangaroo care, babies sleep better. For that reason, you might consider kangarooing in the evening so that the benefits to your baby continue into the night. You want to encourage your baby to sleep well at night, partly because of the NICU routine (in units that practice developmentally supportive care, nighttime may provide more opportunity for uninterrupted sleep) and partly in anticipation of discharge, to encourage a day-night cycle that matches your family's.

Arranging to Kangaroo Your Baby

If your hospital's NICU is hesitant about kangaroo care and you feel up to it, you can be an agent for change. Many books and articles touting the incredible benefits of skin-to-skin contact have been written in recent years. Go to www.NICUparenting.org for a list of resources and consider sharing them with medical staff.

In some NICUs, infants are kangarooed only when they are medically stable and in good condition, but research identifies the benefits of kangaroo care for younger and sicker babies as well. Some hospitals use kangaroo care from birth onward, as well as during simple, routine but painful procedures such as heel sticks. This makes sense because babies may need kangaroo care the most when they are struggling or in pain, which is usually when the doctors and nurses want to surround them with machines instead of their parents' arms and skin. It is often logistically possible to kangaroo a wired, intubated, hooked-up baby, machines, practitioners, and parents working together. This kind of kangaroo care has been tried with great success in many NICUs.

If you feel strongly about wanting to try kangaroo care to help your tiny baby recuperate, become stable, or weather painful procedures, talk to your baby's doctors and nurses. Encourage them to review the research for themselves.

If your baby is very sick and the doctors tell you there's not much more they can do, *you can do kangaroo care*. If they believe your baby is dying, there is absolutely nothing to lose. Kangaroo care probably won't save your baby's life, but it will improve your baby's comfort and give you a chance to be intimately nurturing at this important time. Kangaroo care always provides precious moments to cherish.

If you are never allowed to kangaroo your baby or if you must wait for weeks and weeks to do so, know that you can still form a strong bond with your baby. Kangaroo care is simply one of many ways in which parents and their babies can be close.

If you and your baby happen to be at home now, the two of you can still enjoy the many benefits of skin-to-skin contact. Kangarooing at home can help heal your disappointment over not having a "normal" birth, one where your naked baby is placed on your bare skin. It offers a chance to reclaim the intimate holding and snuggling that you missed in the early days or weeks of your baby's life. Your baby's health and growth can profit from kangarooing at home, helping your baby fall asleep more easily, calming both of you after a fretful period, and even reducing, interrupting, or preventing crying spells or fussiness. A sick baby may recover faster if he or she spends time sleeping on you, even when you are both fully clothed. Consider holding and lying down with your baby to be the best way to invest your time. Enjoy the respite, relaxation, and connectedness for yourself too. You will cherish these sweet times and the treasured memories they make.

Infant Massage

The greatest happiness we had together when he was a baby was when I massaged him. I tended to get lost in the beauty of his little body, and our interaction seemed much more instinctive and comforting to us both.—Anne

Offering the same skin-to-skin benefits as kangaroo care, infant massage can also benefit your baby. According to the research, your touch can calm your baby and promote healing and weight gain. The first step is simply to contain your baby by cupping one hand around his or her head and the other hand around your baby's feet. You can also cup by placing your hand on your baby's chest or by holding your baby's arms and legs in a flexed position. Cupping can be especially soothing to a baby who cannot tolerate stroking. As you become accustomed to cupping, experiment with different kinds of touch and pay attention to what your baby seems to enjoy. Most babies prefer small amounts of firm, gentle stroking. Avoid anything that seems to irritate, startle, or overwhelm your baby. You can also try using nonirritating natural oils or a gentle unscented lotion that your baby's doctor recommends. Your NICU may have a nurse or therapist who can teach you more about infant massage, or you can find information in books or online or consult with a certified massage therapist.

Okay, so you can't hold the baby—the baby's in the incubator. And I'm asking the nurse, "Can I touch the baby, can I put cream on the baby?" It's that skin touch that gives you that connection. There's not much to touch, but just being able to make a connection skin to skin, that was so important. And I know it's important to the babies. It's got to be. Because being in an incubator or a warmer is not the same as being in a mom. . . . It was a few days before we could hold Peter, and I knew that I just had to have my hands in there to just touch him—to touch his toes if that was the only thing I could get to, or a hand. That's what I did.—Vickie

Co-bedding for Multiples

In many hospitals, babies from a multiple gestation are placed together in the same bed in a practice called co-bedding. Like shared kangaroo care, co-bedding is a natural source of cuddling and touch for twins and triplets and so forth. In fact, if your babies are kept in separate beds, you may be sensitive to the fact that they cannot snuggle together. Besides missing your womb, they might be missing each other.

Multiples can benefit from co-bedding because they are comforted by the familiar touch and boundaries the others provide. As their sleep-wake cycles become synchronized, they cuddle with, suck on, and provide mutual warmth for each other, and they support each other's ability to stay calm and adapt to life outside the womb. There are case studies of putting twins together when one twin is struggling to stabilize, sleep, stay calm, or eat and gain weight. Within minutes, the struggling twin calms and starts to improve. Just as kangaroo care mimics the comfort of the womb, co-bedding mimics cohabiting with one's womb mates.

Parents of co-bedding multiples take comfort in the thought that their babies are together in the NICU. They perceive the NICU to be a gentler place, and, perhaps most important, parents can practice and gain confidence in taking care of all their babies together, instead of alternating between or among stations. Finally, parents report that their babies' synchronized sleep-wake cycles make it easier to take care of them in the NICU and especially after discharge.

Overall, co-bedding of multiples can reduce stress in parents *and* their infants. And once again, research confirms what parents already intuit about the value of a natural and nurturing practice.

In the final weeks before my twins came home, my son was doing fabulously. But before we could take him home, he had to have some surgery. They did four surgeries at once, which included bowel resection, hernia repair, circumcision, and ROP Stage III laser surgery. Well, after this surgery he was a mess. He stopped eating and took about five giant leaps backward. My once fairly docile son would not stop screaming. It was like all the pain he had suffered bubbled to the surface. No one or no amount of fentanyl could calm him. One day, one of the nurses decided to sneak my daughter into his incubator to see if maybe that would help. Well, lo and behold, the minute she was laid near him, he took one look at her, reached for her hand and held it, and fell quietly asleep—and calmness had returned. It was one of the most miraculous things I had ever experienced. The entire nursery was silenced by the beauty of this. I get teary just remembering. That night, he started eating again, and his fentanyl was discontinued.

After they connected like this, I insisted that I wanted to start kangarooing them together—so they let me when the docs weren't around. I had always felt that my kids had been cheated out of the twin bonding by being born prematurely, so I think co-bedding and co-kangarooing is an absolutely wonderful idea.—Becky

If your NICU doesn't already practice co-bedding and you would like your infants to try it, your practitioners may be open to the idea, particularly if your babies are breathing room air, stable, and without infection. If there is concern over confusing the babies, everything can be color coded, including lines, monitors, charts, supplies, medications, and wrist and ankle bands. As some of the parents in this book can testify, twins can get mixed up even when they *aren't* in the same bed. And in fact, it may well be easier to keep them straight when they *are* together.

Co-bedding can also be a workable option after discharge. Whether or not your babies had the opportunity to share a bed in the hospital, you can try co-bedding them at home.

Becoming Attuned to Your Baby

Becoming attuned is more than just getting to know your baby. Over time and with trial and error, you will come to understand your baby's temperament, preferences, and cues and learn how to respond in ways that both you and your baby enjoy.

When your baby is in the NICU, becoming attuned is challenging, partly because your access is limited but also because your baby may not show much interest in the world. Extremely premature babies don't interact much for a few weeks or even months after birth. The same is true of very sick babies, who need all their energy to recuperate. But with growth and recovery, your baby's awareness and responsiveness will increase, and you will be able to interact more. With practice, you'll learn how to encourage your baby's interest in the surroundings—and in you.

Becoming attuned to your baby is another cornerstone of nurturing your baby. The following sections explain how to decipher your baby's behaviors so that you can confidently respond and build a rewarding relationship.

Honoring Your Baby's Uniqueness

Like everyone, your newborn has a unique temperament, as well as particular sensitivities and thresholds for stimulation of the senses. Babies who are premature or have a long recovery tend to have especially immature nervous systems, which can result in even more extreme sensitivities and thresholds. For example, some infants have strong aversions to certain sights, sounds, touch, or movement. One baby may have trouble tolerating noise and also have difficulty noticing soft voices, leaving a very narrow range of sound that is just right. Another baby may have trouble tolerating movement and also have difficulty detecting slow rocking, leaving a very narrow range of movement that is just right. Escape from overstimulation and a lack of responsiveness are two reasons newborns spend a fair amount of time in a state of drowsiness or sleep. Newborns who have trouble regulating themselves may disintegrate into fussiness when under- or overstimulated, as they cannot stay calm when they're unable to tune out or tune in.

Fortunately, parents can discover their baby's sensitivities and thresholds by interpreting their infant's behaviors. You can learn what bothers your baby, what keeps your baby soothed or attentive, and what restores calm. You can also use your baby's many cues to read her or him and recognize readiness for different kinds of interaction with you.

Reading Your Baby

Much of your interaction with your baby will be instinctive. When your baby is sleeping quietly, you'll feel compelled to leave her alone. When your baby is bright-eyed, you'll feel like getting his attention. When your baby cries, you'll try to satisfy the expressed need. But sometimes your baby's cues will be more subtle than a silent snooze, rapt attention, or a lusty yowl. Read the descriptions below to decipher your infant's level of sleepiness, alertness, or fussiness.

- *Deep sleep.* Your baby is fast asleep, breathing regularly, eyes closed and motionless, with no bodily movements except the occasional involuntary twitch. In this state your baby is difficult to awaken, will not respond to your voice or touch, and cannot effectively eat from breast or bottle.

- *Light sleep.* This sleep state is associated with dreaming. Breathing is irregular, eyes are closed but moving beneath the lids, and your little one may move, suck, or fuss although still asleep. Your baby can be awakened enough to feed but probably not enough to play.

- *Drowsy.* Your baby is in the transition zone between wakefulness and sleep. The eyes may open and shut, the arms may move voluntarily, and breathing may become more rapid and shallow. Babies who have been awake are ready for a nap when they become drowsy; those who have been asleep may be ready to wake up and enter the quiet alert state.

- *Quiet alert.* Your baby has a bright, wide-awake look and can focus and attend to the surroundings. Because your baby is so focused, he or she may not move much or make much noise. This is the best state for playing with your baby because your little one is calm and attentive.

- *Active alert.* Your baby is awake and slightly agitated. Breathing is irregular. Your baby may move and startle more easily in response to sights, sounds, and touch and may be fussy. Your little one cannot tolerate much more stimulation without dissolving into crying or drowsiness. Try lowering your voice, stilling your touch, or averting your gaze (or all three, depending on your baby's sensitivities and thresholds) to see if he or she can return to the quiet alert state or take a needed nap.

· *Crying.* Your baby is awake and agitated. Breathing is irregular, shallow, and rapid. Your infant can no longer tolerate or attend to playful interaction or feeding or cope with any stimulus that isn't calming.

As you can see, deciphering your baby's behavior lets you know when it will be easiest to encourage sleep, coax a feeding, or enjoy some play.

There are additional observable physical signs—called physiologic cues—that suggest how your baby is perceiving and coping with the surroundings. For instance, look at your baby's color, breathing (respirations), movements, and eyes. Under each bullet in the list below, the first description indicates calm; the second, in italics, indicates stress:

· Is your baby's skin tone healthy, even, glowing, pinkish under-tones—or *relatively pale, mottled, gray, or bluish?*

· Are your baby's respirations stable—or *uneven?*

· Are your infant's limb movements smooth—or *jerky?*

· Are your baby's eyes bright—or *glassy, squinting, frozen, or looking away?*

· Is your baby leaning into your touch and settling into your hold—or *startling easily, arching his or her back, or squirming?*

· Are your baby's muscles toned—or *limp or rigid?*

When your baby is calm, he or she is better able to attend to and tolerate what's happening—and is open to its continuation. When your baby begins to show signs of stress, she or he is telling you that it's too boring, too unpleasant, or too much—and time for a change, a break, or a nap.

Engaging Your Baby

To effectively engage your baby, you need to support his or her growing ability to stay interested in the surroundings and calm and attentive during interaction. Some newborns can regulate themselves by sucking on their own hands, looking away, or falling asleep when they need a break or some soothing. But their repertoire of regulating actions is quite limited. Tiny babies can't cover their ears when it's too noisy, walk away when they're tired of visiting with somebody, or find something else to do when they're bored or overwhelmed. They haven't yet figured out how to change the channel. And so, all newborns rely heavily on the responsiveness and protectiveness of their caregivers.

In this light, you can try the following strategies to bolster your baby's growing ability to engage with you:

- Follow your baby's lead.
- Honor your baby's attempts to moderate stimulation.
- Protect your baby from what's overwhelming or unpleasant.
- Provide what soothes your baby and sustains interest.

You probably know these strategies instinctively, but when confronted with a challenging baby in the chaos of the NICU, you may be afraid to trust your instincts. The next time you are with your baby, notice how easy it is to take these approaches and how right you feel doing them.

Follow Your Baby's Lead

Many parents become more actively engaging when they are eager to attract and hold their baby's attention. Unfortunately, this approach can overwhelm premature or recovering babies, causing them to disengage their attention. Instead, it's important to tone it down and imitate your baby's actions and level of interest. When your baby averts her gaze to rest, you can rest too. When she is ready to reengage, she'll look at you, and you can respond by smiling and looking back. This intimate dance shows your baby that you are responsive to her pace. By imitating her and following her lead, you encourage her attentiveness.

Honor Your Baby's Attempts to Moderate Stimulation

Touching or making eye contact with your baby can be very rewarding, but it's important to remain responsive to your baby's ability to notice and handle your advances. As you get to know your baby's signals of distress, you can adjust your interaction. If your baby arches her back, change your touch or stop completely. If she averts her gaze, let her go and wait until she is ready to come back for more—which may not be until after a good nap. If she tries to reengage, try changing your interaction. In a similar vein, let her sleep when she is tired and feed when she is hungry.

When your baby gets overwhelmed, she may recover if you back off—or she may quickly pass the point of no return. Recognize that your baby's inability to recover is not an indication of your parenting abilities but a measure of your baby's fatigue, gestational age, unique temperament, and immature ability to stay calm (to *self-regulate*).

As you learn more about your baby, you'll become more sensitive and skilled at reading cues. As you become more experienced and your baby becomes more mature, the two of you will be better able to regulate the amount of stimulation and extend fun playtimes.

Protect Your Baby from What's Overwhelming or Unpleasant
If you notice that your baby is particularly sensitive to light, sound, or touch, you can take steps to protect him or her. Ask that the overhead lights be dimmed, request that the monitors be turned down, and do what you can to reduce the kinds of touch your baby finds irritating. Put a sign in your little one's incubator to remind everyone on the care team to take these sensitivities into consideration. Ask that your baby be given eyeshades and earmuffs for sleep. Unfortunately, in the NICU, as in life, you cannot always protect your baby from unpleasant or overwhelming stimuli. To compensate, you can soothe and nurture whenever you're there.

Provide What Soothes and Sustains Interest
Your baby will respond uniquely to various sights, sounds, touches, tastes, smells, and movements. Like all parents, you will figure out through trial and error what your baby finds tolerable and interesting. By reading your baby's physiologic cues, you and your infant work together to figure out what's calming and what's interesting but not overwhelming.

For example, how does your baby react to a noisy environment? Does your baby drift off to sleep, stay awake but unfazed, remain alert and interested, or startle easily and become fussy? What kind of voice does your baby turn to? Experiment with a high pitch and then a low pitch; then try a soothing voice, a singing voice, and finally an animated voice. Which objects (or which parts of you) does your baby like to suck on? Does your baby respond best to your face when you smile gently and silently or when your smile is lively and you're talkative? What kinds of touch does your baby lean into? Some babies like to be swaddled (wrapped in a blanket or other covering); others like to hang loose. Some babies like to be held firmly; others just want to be cupped with the hands.

Also note that some babies are flexible and easygoing, while others are more discriminating and less adaptable. To encourage growing flexibility, provide the kinds of stimulation and interaction that interest and soothe your baby. By accommodating and working with (rather than against) your baby, you are helping your baby stay calm and attentive to the surrounding world. That the world (including *you*) is intriguing, fun, and safe is a significant lesson for your baby to learn. Your emerging ability to provide a calming attitude, a soothing touch, and an interesting distraction is a skill that you can use effectively throughout your baby's childhood.

The nurses said that she was more calm when we were there from very early on. In the first few days, we could cup our hands around her feet or lay our hands on top of her to give her boundaries, and she responded well to this. It was so important because this was the first direct thing we could do to help.—Mary

My son opened his eyes a little and watched us, but mostly he slept. He rarely cried when we held him but watched us very closely when he was awake. We talked to him very quietly when he was awake, and he seemed to respond very well to our voices by having really good readings on his sats and no apneas or bradycardias.—Andrea

There will be plenty of times, especially early on, when your baby won't engage with you. Instead of feeling rejected, remember that your baby's ability to fall asleep or to turn away from you is a sign of his or her ability to control the amount of stimulation being taken in and an attempt to avoid becoming overwhelmed. This reaction is much like they way you behave at your favorite museum: even though you're fascinated, after a while you simply need to take a break from the exhibits. When your baby tries to find a balance between paying attention to what's interesting and becoming overwhelmed, this is evidence of growing adaptation to the outside world.

As you become more responsive to your baby, your baby can become more responsive to you. Your infant's growing attentiveness and your emerging ability to engage and sustain that attention are reassuring signs that you are building a rewarding relationship.

If you have more than one baby in the NICU, it's challenging to get to know and connect with each one separately. It takes time to discover each baby's preferences and sensitivities. It takes energy to engage each baby and to decipher each unique set of cues. It takes practice to become responsive and to build a rapport that suits each baby's special style. Give yourself the time you need to get to know each of your precious babies.

Points to Remember

· *Parental bonding is a wonderfully powerful, resilient, and flexible process. You can bond during the most anxiety-filled pregnancy and infancy. Your bond can thrive in spite of your baby's hospitalization.*

· *Many parents develop the full depth and joy of parental love over the course of many months and especially after discharge from the NICU.*

· *Kangaroo care is an important way of feeling close to—and providing respite for—your baby. Other beneficial forms of touch are massage and, for multiples, co-bedding.*

· *When your baby is very young, unstable, or struggling, you may feel frustrated by his or her lack of attentiveness to you. Rest assured that your baby will be able to show interest in you and the surroundings as he or she heals and matures.*

· *As you get to know your baby, you will learn how to read your baby's behaviors, respond to cues, and accommodate unique sensitivities and thresholds. These skills will enable you to follow your baby's lead and to become adept at engaging your baby's attention without overwhelming him or her. This success will help you feel that you are building a rewarding relationship with your baby.*

8:

Feeding Your Baby

The nurses brought me an electric pump and suggested that I start right away. At that point, I really wasn't into it. I didn't feel like a new mother at all, yet they expected me to pump my breasts and start making milk. I hated having to do that. It felt weird. But as soon as I was able to spend a couple of minutes with my beautiful little very premature girls, I decided anything I needed to do to help ensure they would be okay I had to do right away.—Rosa

Feeding is an emotionally charged issue for most parents. It cuts to the core of nurturing care and survival. No doubt we are hardwired to make sure our babies get fed and are well-nourished. Even under ideal circumstances, feeding a newborn baby occupies a substantial portion of new parents' time and energy.

When a baby is in the NICU, concerns about feeding are amplified because physical growth is both a marker of improvement and a criterion for discharge home. Feeding issues are complicated and stressful when a baby needs more time, maturation, or practice before taking to the breast or bottle. Babies with craniofacial anomalies or digestive issues may present other barriers to traditional feeding.

This chapter provides information tailored to the NICU experience, covering the mechanics as well as support around decision making and the emotional aspects of feeding your baby.

Feeding Decisions

Before you gave birth, you probably spent some time thinking about how you wanted to feed your baby. Typically, the choice boils down to formula in a bottle or breast milk from the breast and maybe also the bottle. For babies in the NICU, the options are more complex and can change over time with the baby's medical and developmental course.

Methods of feeding:

· Oral feeding by bottle only, bottle and breast, or breast only

· NG (nasogastric) tube feeding for babies unable to coordinate sucking, swallowing, and breathing

· Surgically placed GI (gastrointestinal) tube feeding for babies who cannot tolerate NG tube feeding

· Surgically placed central IV (intravenous) line for babies who are unable to digest anything

Substances that are fed:

· Breast milk only

· Breast milk and formula

· Breast milk and fortifier

· Formula only

· TPN (Total Parenteral Nutrition) which goes through an IV line, bypassing the digestive system

Depending on your baby's medical course, he or she might move through all or most of these options, and your involvement in these decisions is important. Some options will work well for you and your baby, and others may spur you to explore alternatives. Even if you're told that a certain method or substance is a surefire solution or the way to help your baby grow, *if your intuition or observation tells you otherwise, speak up.* Not all babies respond the same, and your input is valid.

Because of the emotion surrounding feeding, it can be helpful to sort out how you feel about the situation and the available options.

Advantages of Breast Milk and Breast-Feeding

I kept myself going by pumping milk for my son and telling myself that this was one way I could help him.—Sarah

Although many people associate breasts with sex, every nursing mother knows that breasts are also about providing key nourishment for babies. Breast milk has unique properties, essential nutrients, and antibodies that help babies digest, grow, develop, and fight off disease and infection. No formula offers so many benefits. Especially for babies who need intensive care, breast milk has what might be termed medicinal qualities. In fact, if your baby was born before the due date, your body produces milk that is ideally suited, containing the additional protein, fat, and minerals that your premature baby needs.

Breast milk is a gift of nature, and providing it to your baby is one of the few things that only you, the mother, can do. If you were planning on or leaning toward breast-feeding, your baby's condition may strengthen your resolve. If you were planning on formula-feeding, you may be considering breast-feeding, given the circumstances.

It was very gratifying, from very early on, to know that Charlotte was being fed my breast milk, because I knew this would be the best thing for her, and in a way it made me feel closer to her. —Kate

Other advantages to your baby are the skin-to-skin contact and the on-demand availability of breast milk. When it goes smoothly, breast-feeding is *less* stressful than bottle-feeding because your baby can pace the flow of milk, pausing when necessary without choking on the unobstructed flow from a rubber nipple. There are benefits to the mother as well, including:

· Skin-to-skin contact with your infant, which can help you feel close and attuned to your baby

· Infusing a sense of normalcy into parenting your baby

· Increased confidence in your mothering abilities

· Feeling you are indispensable to your baby's health and well-being

· Hormonal benefits that aid in postpartum healing

Formula-Feeding

Although breast milk is best for most babies, not every mother can or chooses to provide it. A mother's milk is not recommended when the mother has a disease that can be transferred to her baby in her milk or when she must be on medication (or is using recreational drugs) that shouldn't be passed on to her baby. Sometimes milk supply is insufficient, such as when a mother is critically ill following delivery or due to the emotional trauma of having a critically ill baby. Occasionally, a mother's hormones or breast tissue don't orchestrate milk production or release. Some mothers choose not to breast-feed because of lifestyle, health concerns, past experience, culture, or employment. Others find the process of pumping unproductive or unbearable.

Although there is agreement that breast milk is medically and nutritionally superior to formula, most newborns can do just fine on formula. But you are likely being encouraged to furnish whatever breast milk you can, for its key nutrients and potential to boost your baby's health and recovery in the NICU.

Staying with Your Decision to Feed Formula

If you had planned all along to feed your baby formula, your reasons may still be applicable and important. If you interpret practitioners' encouragement to provide breast milk as pressure, you may deeply resent these efforts to make you change your mind. It may challenge your autonomy as a parent and exacerbate any guilt or failure you are already feeling.

It is very important for you to recognize that your baby's practitioners are duty bound to educate you about the medical facts and benefits of breast milk for your baby. They are not trying to undermine you, force you to breast-feed, or imply that you are obligated. If you do feel triggered by a practitioner who seems to appeal to feelings of guilt or inadequacy, you can benefit from airing your feelings to a supportive listener. If you conclude, after consideration, that formula-feeding is definitely best for you, say so clearly. The practitioners can support you on this as they recognize that not every mother breast-feeds. Even if you perceive judgment, you can remain steadfast and confident.

Changing Your Mind and Deciding to Breast-Feed

If you had planned to formula-feed, you may decide that breast-feeding is a better alternative after all. You may make this decision gladly yet feel embarrassed and unsure because you are unfamiliar with the mechanics. Breast-feeding is a skill that most mothers have to learn, and even the eager ones can feel self-conscious, awkward, or uncertain in the beginning. Lactation support and practice can help you feel more confident and certain as time passes.

I didn't plan to breast-feed, but the doctor kind of pushed me into it, saying it was the best thing I could do for my son. Once I understood the fact that breast-feeding would be the best thing for my baby, I had no problem doing it. It made me feel more like a mom to him, that I was the only one providing food for him.—Christine

Breast-feeding is even more important for weak and sick babies. It was very encouraged by the staff, and the hospital had lactation consultants to help with all of the set feeding times.—Jennifer E.

If you are resisting but a part of you is wondering *What if?* you may find it helpful to ask yourself these questions to sort out your feelings:

· *Are you resisting because you don't like surprises or sudden change?* Try taking a flexible approach. Consider supplying *some* breast milk. You can attempt a trial of providing colostrum (the valuable, nutrient-packed liquid produced before your milk comes in) and then breast milk to see how you feel about the process. Your breasts will produce these in any event, and your baby will benefit from whatever you can provide. If you give it a try and it doesn't work for you, you can always stop.

· *Are you resisting because you're not sure what your partner, friends, or relatives will think?* Remember, *you* are your baby's mother—and only you can decide whether this is right for you and for your baby. If those close to you object, enlist the support of your baby's doctors and nurses or contact a lactation consultant or a support group such as La Leche League to help you counter objections. If providing breast milk is meaningful and healing for you and good for your baby, others have no valid basis for undermining your choice. You can ask them to respect your decision or confidently ignore them.

· *Are you resisting because you want to feel like you are in charge?* Remember that this decision is yours to make. Don't resist breast-feeding just because you feel compelled to go *against* the authorities. Brashly reacting against authoritative advice is simply another way to relinquish control. Instead, exercise control by weighing the pros and cons, examining your intuition, and making your own thoughtful decision about what's best for you and your baby.

Switching Back from Breast Milk to Formula
If you decide to try breast-feeding despite your original intent, you are to be commended for your courage and willingness to try. Still, you may come upon barriers that even the staunchest breast-feeder would find insurmountable. For instance, if milk production is difficult or too stressful for you, or if you determine that pumping or trying to

breast-feed is simply not feasible, you may switch back to formula. Your decision may add to your guilt and frustration, particularly if you had warmed to the idea of breast-feeding. You may worry about disappointing others or going against recommendations.

Remind yourself that you can decide to return to formula just as carefully as you decided to try supplying breast milk. To ward off others who second-guess you, try gentle hints, such as, "I really value the friends I have who can accept this without trying to change my mind, scold me, second-guess me, or lecture me about how to relax." The bottom line is that you provided what you could. If you still want your baby to benefit from breast milk, ask about obtaining donated breast milk. Also remember that if you are able, you can continue to provide some breast milk even if your baby is mostly formula-feeding.

Deciding to Breast-Feed (and Pump)

With Ayla, after the first day I was able to breast-feed her. It was more difficult than I anticipated, and I felt like I was constantly on display, but it was well worth the effort.—Corin

Breast-feeding your baby may have been the obvious choice for you all along, or you may have decided on it after pondering the options. If you feared you'd be unable to breast-feed because your baby was born prematurely or with a serious condition, you may be relieved to find out that you still can.

Many mothers in the NICU start out pumping their breast milk as the first step toward successful breast-feeding. Most babies are able to feed directly from the breast after they grow, recover, and are mature enough to coordinate sucking, swallowing, and breathing. As your baby matures and gains strength, you can try putting your baby to the breast. After discharge, some mothers will continue to pump for babies who will take only the bottle or who must be tube-fed.

I breast-fed, but we had to start with an NG tube down her nose because she just was burning too many calories trying to eat. Once she started doing a bit better, we tried to breast-feed but had to use a bottle for the same reason she still had the NG tube. She had dropped below five pounds so they had to make sure she was getting calories and not using them all up trying to eat. She eventually figured out the bottle, at which point we added a nipple shield to the breast-feeding, and that helped her out a lot. A few months later, she was able to breast-feed with no help.—Jennifer E.

Despite facing the pump or the challenges of learning to breast-feed in the NICU, for many mothers, providing breast milk helps to soothe the anguish of being unable to prevent their baby's condition or preterm delivery. Your breast milk is the one thing that only *you* can provide for your baby. Knowing that your baby gets so many health benefits from your milk can boost your confidence. Breast milk can also seem like an antidote to the medical technology that surrounds your baby. And learning to breast-feed is one way to reach for normalcy. Though you may resent the awkwardness, the pump, the schedule, the hassle, the struggle, and the mechanical nature of it all, the rewards can be well worth the price. And even if you eventually switch to formula, both you and your baby benefit from your supplying any amount of breast milk.

Despite the fact that I hated being trapped by that horrible machine six times a day for half an hour each session, I knew that keeping it up would only benefit my baby. He would grow stronger because of it.—Christine

Having to pump my breast milk was difficult and easy at the same time—difficult because it made me sad that it wasn't the baby eating normally, and easy because I knew the importance of the nutrition I could provide for her.—Cindy

With Gabe, I pumped every two to three hours around the clock for most of the fifty-five days he was in the hospital. Even though he couldn't feed, it made me feel like I was doing something for my baby. It was the only care I could give him, and I was determined to do it right.—Corin

Breast Care for Breast-Feeding

This section contains basic information for breast-feeding mothers and their partners on breast mechanics, establishing quantity and enhancing quality, and overcoming the challenges of a fluctuating milk supply, pumping, and discomfort.

The Mechanics of Breast-Feeding

Hormonal changes accompany your baby's birth and cause your breasts to start producing milk. For the first few days, your breasts secrete colostrum, a substance high in antibodies and extremely beneficial to babies. Within two to five days, your milk will come in. The engorgement period lasts about forty-eight hours, and your breasts may be uncomfortably full. By pumping, you can establish your supply. Even if you are too ill at first to pump or if you decide not to breast-feed and then change your mind, hourly pumping for a day can reestablish a supply that is dwindling after the engorgement period passes.

When a pump exerts suction (or when a baby sucks) on your nipple, this tells your brain to release two hormones. Prolactin makes your milk glands produce milk. Oxytocin (which also results from skin-to-skin contact and plays a role in uterine contractions during labor) contracts the tiny muscles that surround the milk glands, squeezing the milk down into small reservoirs just behind the nipple. This is known as the milk-ejection, or let-down, reflex. When you sit down to pump, signs of let down may include a sudden thirst, tingling sensations in your breast, leaking nipples, or a feeling of deep relaxation.

Even though you may not be able to put your baby to your breast for many weeks yet, when you provide breast milk by pumping, this is a form of breast-feeding. When you aren't able to be in the NICU for every feeding, your baby can be fed your breast milk in a bottle. If your baby is too sick or unable to suck and swallow, your milk can be fed through a tube going directly to your baby's stomach. If your baby's digestive system cannot tolerate breast milk for now, your milk will be saved for your baby's use down the road. By building up and maintaining your milk supply by pumping, you ensure that your baby will have your breast milk—and you may be able to nurse your baby when she or he is strong enough and can coordinate the suck-swallow-breathe skills that mark efficient nursing.

Establishing Your Milk Supply

At first it was hard. I really had to force myself to begin the milk-production process. Once I got home, it was much easier. I decided to go out and purchase a new electric pump to make things much easier for me. It got easier and easier as the days went on.—Rosa

Start pumping as soon as you can

If you are well enough, you can start pumping your breasts within hours after delivery. Your nurses should give you the equipment, training, and encouragement to do it. If the hospital has a good lactation consultant, use this resource. You can also ask for a referral to a lactation consultant outside the hospital. Speak up if you are not happy with the information or support you are receiving. You deserve to get what you need.

Use the best pump you can

To make pumping easier and more efficient and effective, use a hospital-quality electric pump in good working order with a double pumping kit, which lets you pump both breasts simultaneously. Your hospital may help you obtain one.

Learn the procedures for sterilizing equipment and storing your milk

Ask your NICU for instructions on how to collect, freeze, store, and transport your breast milk. Seek advice on how to keep your pump and bottles clean. Also practice good hygiene. Wash your hands before pumping and keep them clean until you seal the container that holds your milk.

Expect small amounts, especially at first

When you first start pumping, don't be discouraged by scant production. First feedings can be as small as one-quarter of a teaspoon. Practice pumping for five to ten minutes every three hours, and save every priceless drop.

Understand engorgement—or lack of it

Take advantage of the engorgement that may occur when your milk comes in. Pumping provides physical relief from the pressure of the milk building up and reassures you of your supply. Feeling able to produce enough milk can be especially comforting if you have multiple babies.

Some mothers do not experience engorgement. It's not clear why, although some speculate that it might be related to the trauma and stress of preterm birth, emergency cesarean section, having a struggling baby in the NICU, and/or the medications that are used to induce labor or stave off eclampsia. Sometimes the culprit is hormonal imbalance or nonfunctional breast tissue. You are not alone if you do not experience engorgement or if you find that your milk supply doesn't seem to increase, no matter how well you follow the guidelines set out by the lactation consultants. Like many moms, you may find the initial weeks of pumping difficult or unproductive, but as you adjust, you may still go on to successfully supply breast milk and later breast-feed your baby. Whatever the outcome of your efforts, you can pump what you can for as long as you can. It can be a challenge, but you can find a balance between your baby's needs and your own physical abilities.

Pump frequently and completely

Don't be afraid of pumping too often: it is easier to taper an abundant supply than to build up a dwindling one. To establish your milk supply, try pumping every two to two and a half hours around the clock for a couple of days and nights (or eight to twelve times during the day, if sleeping at night is paramount). After your milk supply is established, it's a good idea to pump at least once in the middle of the night. If getting an uninterrupted night's sleep is important, though, go no more than eight hours (give or take) without pumping and then pump at least eight times throughout the day. Whenever you pump, be sure to "empty" your breasts. Technically, there's no such thing as an empty breast-feeding breast, but you can pump out the vast majority of the milk. Doing so extracts the hindmilk, which is highest in fat—these are calories your baby needs. Pump for a minute or two after the flow of milk stops or after it slows to drips.

For establishing and maintaining your milk supply, pump frequently, not longer. As a rule, it is most effective to pump for ten to fifteen minutes every three hours. It is far less effective to spend, say, twenty to thirty minutes every six hours, even though technically you'd be spending the same amount of time at the pump every twenty-four hours. Here's why: First, continuing to pump after the ducts are drained does little to step up milk production. Second, when pumping at longer intervals, milk sits in the breasts too long and a chemical present in the retained milk signals the milk glands to stop production. It's *frequently reducing the pressure* in your breasts that signals your body to continue to make milk.

To build up or increase your supply, simply pump at shorter intervals for no longer than is necessary to empty your breasts. While pumping more often than every two and a half to three hours might sound like a good plan, if it stresses your body, particularly with sleep deprivation, it may be counterproductive. Find the balance that works best for you.

Enhancing Your Milk Supply

As your supply is established, here are additional suggestions for producing ample quantities of high-quality breast milk.

Stay hydrated

Not drinking enough fluids can cause dehydration, which can decrease milk production. To stay hydrated, have a large glass of water handy while you pump or breast-feed so you can quench your thirst. Since NICUs are warm, take a full water bottle with you when you are with your baby so you'll have easy access to what you need.

Eat well, exercise, rest, and relax

Your body needs vitality to produce adequate quantities of high-quality breast milk. Eat a well-balanced diet of nutritious whole foods to maintain your health. Get appropriate exercise as well as plenty of rest to build your stamina and reserves. Do enjoyable activities that relax you. While these directives can seem overwhelming to your already stressful existence, keep in mind that taking care of yourself actually *reduces your distress* in many ways, including helping you make plenty of good milk for your baby. Another way to look at it: healthy habits benefit your milk supply, so you are doing these things not just for yourself but also for your baby. (See the related discussion under "Meeting Your Physical Needs" in chapter 4.)

Avoid milk-tainting substances

Some oral contraceptives, antihistamines, and diuretics can affect your milk, so check with your doctor, midwife, or lactation consultant before using them while producing breast milk. Do your best to eliminate or reduce caffeine (found in coffee, some teas, many soft drinks, and chocolate) and give up nicotine, as well as recreational drugs and alcohol. These substances not only taint your milk but also can diminish your supply. Ask your doctor about prescription medications.

Recognize the effects of diet on your breast milk

Breast milk is affected by the foods you eat. If your baby is irritable or gassy after feedings, he or she may be sensitive to something you ate two to six hours before you pumped that milk or put your baby to the breast. Common culprits are:

- Gassy vegetables, including cabbage, onions, garlic, broccoli, cauliflower, turnips, beans, sweet peppers, cucumbers

- Citrus fruits and juices, including oranges, lemons, limes, and grapefruit, as well as other acidic fruits, like kiwi, strawberries, and pineapple

- Strong spices, including chili peppers, curry, pepper, ginger, cinnamon

- Caffeine, found in coffee, black teas, chocolate, some soft drinks (caffeine accumulates in the newborn and causes nighttime irritability)

- Foods that are at least 90 percent dairy products, such as milk, ice cream, cheese, yogurt, pudding

- Common allergens, such as eggs, corn, corn syrup, soy, wheat, and nuts

Your baby's discomfort or irritability can be caused by food intolerances even if it takes weeks or months to set in. If your baby is receiving fresh breast milk, you can eliminate all the foods on the list from your diet for a week. If your baby is receiving frozen milk, try dipping into a different week's supply or provide as much fresh milk as you can. If you notice an improvement in your baby, you'll know that what you are eating is affecting him or her. Reintroduce the foods one at a time to figure out which are the offending ones. Because dairy products are particularly associated with colic, you could eliminate that food group first and see if doing so brings your baby relief.

As mentioned in chapter 4, eating healthfully, drinking water, resting, relaxing, exercising, and, especially, pumping and spending time with your baby are all *essential tasks*. Put them all on your to-do list, in the top-priority section. Throw away the old list with all that stuff you thought you'd accomplish back when you were naive about what motherhood would be like for you.

Overcoming Challenges to Breast Milk Production

Although breast-feeding is supremely natural, you are not born knowing how to establish, manage, build, maintain, or pump your supply of breast milk. As with most mothering skills, there is a learning curve. Keep the following tips in mind as you master this important skill.

Be persistent

When you are pumping into that clear bottle, you are well aware of variations in your milk supply. If your supply seems to be decreasing, you may simply need to get more rest or respite, drink more water, spend more time kangarooing your baby, or pump more frequently to maintain or build up your supply.

Your milk supply may also fluctuate with your baby's medical condition. For some mothers, the better the baby is doing, the better the milk supply; if the baby encounters an extended bad patch, supply may dwindle. Sometimes when a baby takes a turn for the worse, milk production diminishes overnight. But this lull does not necessarily mean that a mother's breast-feeding days are over.

If you encounter a period of depletion, you can keep your breasts primed by continuing to pump at least every three hours for five minutes at a time, even if you only extract a few drops. If you feel too distressed to maintain your supply, this is a critical time for you to seek lactation support or counseling. When you persist, your supply may build up naturally in response as your baby's condition improves, and you can continue to reap the rewards of breast-feeding.

I'm so thankful to the lactation nurses at the hospital because when Fabian got so sick, my milk production completely stopped. When I was pumping, I think I got two drops out, and they would tell me every day to continue pumping. I hated it at the time. It was horrible, but I did stick to it. I had to write how much I pumped on each side: a drop here, a drop there; a quarter of an ounce here, a quarter of an ounce there when things got better. For three weeks, I hardly had anything coming out. But when he got better, suddenly my milk came back in, and I got home, breast-feeding him completely. It was amazing. To see that he was going to survive and make it and not being scared for his life, that's when the milk started to get better. And I'm so thankful for the support. Without them, I would have never been able to keep it going. —Gallice

Find the routine and rituals that work for you
To enhance your milk-ejection reflex, establish a ritual that conditions your breasts to let down when it's time to pump or feed. First, make sure you won't be disturbed. You might sit in the same comfortable chair or position, sip water out of the same container, and apply the same warm washcloth to your breasts and massage them. Provide breast or nipple stimulation that is comfortable and works for you. Listen to relaxing music, read, or watch television. Take deep, cleansing breaths and imagine being in a beautiful place, perhaps with a waterfall of milk.

Pumping advice often includes the suggestion to look at a picture of your baby or recall holding your baby against your skin. But when you're just getting started, you likely don't have a heartwarming photo or experience to rely on. You can use your imagination, but if visualizing your baby brings up too many anxieties or feelings of grief, this approach may not help. Stacy remembers: "One of the things that irritated me the most was when a lady came in to show me how to pump. She told me to think about the first time I had held my daughter and how well she was doing. All I had seen of my daughter was two very cloudy Polaroid pictures."

If thinking of your baby helps, try imagining your little one at your breast or positive visualizations of your baby growing and thriving. You may also find it helpful to smell a blanket that your baby has slept on.

Many moms talk on the phone, read, or relax in other ways while pumping. Others use pumping as a way to structure their time or to take a break from the chaos of the day. It may help to think of pumping as just a task to accomplish. Find the rituals and routines that work for you.

Seek expert advice for nipple or breast pain
Nipple pain may occur because of the following common reasons.

- *Pump suction.* If your nipples become sore from pumping, try turning the pump's suction down and temporarily limiting pumping time to less than ten minutes until you're not so sore. It may help to put lanolin around the areola before pumping. Ask your lactation consultant or pump supplier for a flexible insert that you can use to take the pressure off your tender spots.

- *Adapting to breast-feeding.* During the first couple of weeks after you start putting your baby to the breast, it is normal for your nipples to be sore for that first half minute after the baby latches on. Some babies have very strong sucks, and some mothers have very tender nipples. If the pain subsides within thirty seconds and your baby is swallowing, you're doing just fine. Your nipples need time and experience to adapt to their new job.

- *Infection or clogged milk duct.* If you experience bright pink, irritated nipples or burning or stabbing pains in your breasts, you may have a common yeast infection called thrush, which is typically passed back and forth between mother and baby. You can both be treated simultaneously to halt the cycle of reinfection. If you experience breast pain in the form of a red, warm, tender area, you may have a clogged milk duct. If the area becomes hot and hard or you also develop a fever or general ill feeling, this can indicate a breast infection called mastitis. For these conditions, consult your doctor, midwife, or lactation consultant for more information, advice, and treatment.

Breast Care When You Aren't Breast-Feeding

If you cannot breast-feed, decide not to, or stop after a while, your body may still produce milk because of the hormones in your bloodstream. Your breasts may become engorged with milk for several days. This can become quite uncomfortable, but continuing engorgement is what signals your body to slow and ultimately shut down the milk supply. You can lessen the pain by pumping just enough to reduce the pressure. This will enable you to taper your milk supply. Don't pump more than you have to or your breasts will step up production again. It's also better to use a manual pump as electric ones are too stimulating and efficient.

Some mothers find pumping too emotionally distressing and prefer to put up with the discomfort. If you don't pump, your body absorbs the milk and your breasts soften gradually. Taking over-the-counter pain relievers or placing cold packs (such as a bag of frozen peas or gel packs) on your breasts may help relieve pain. Wearing a snug bra may reduce discomfort, but don't bind breasts as this can cause infection.

Meeting the Challenges of Breast-Feeding in the NICU

When they were trying to feed him, I felt I was off on the sidelines. I wanted to nurse him. At first, he was too small to nurse, so they had to tube-feed him. Then I couldn't be with him around the clock to nurse him, so he had to learn to take a bottle. I pumped for six months. That's all that I could do. I'm sorry I missed out on breast-feeding, but what's important is that he got the breast milk. I feel good that I did that for him.—Marcia

Most mothers face obstacles along the path to breast-feeding. Expressing milk can be difficult, uncomfortable, time-consuming, or logistically complicated. Establishing and maintaining a supply is quite an undertaking and commitment. It may be some time before you can put your newborn to your breast.

Breast-feeding a NICU baby is a subject that is often neglected. It takes more dedication than anything I have ever done. You must lug around your pump. You must pump every three hours, and you also have to keep track of the time you try and feed your baby too. You can't have empty breasts if you are trying to breast-feed. You are exhausted and stressed, and you are demanding even more of your already-taxed body.

Pumping itself is a process. You take your equipment into the lactation room and you wash your hands, you go and get all set up and start to pump and then try not to fall asleep! You try and think of holding your baby so your body will work, but that thought is stressful since you can't hold your baby so you try other things. Eventually it works. You then have to label your bottles, clean up your space, wash and dry all the equipment and set your watch to do it all over again.

It is depressing. It is stressful. It is exhausting. And it is the best thing you can do for your NICU baby if you can do it!—Jennifer E.

The NICU is not the place to get a great start, but . . . like everything else about the NICU experience, you don't have a lot of choices, do you? Preemies have weaker, sometimes less coordinated sucks; they tire easily; they distract easily (which I thought was more difficult than the tiring); and it's so hard with tension, hormones, and milk-engorged breasts.—Sheila

I breast-fed my older son with no problems. I know what it takes—and believe me, trying to breast-feed a baby who isn't there is pretty difficult. Add to that the fact that your two babies are still in the hospital and you don't know when or if they will be coming home soon. Now that's a task.—Rosa

Grief about your baby's prematurity or condition might also color your feelings. If you feel betrayed by your body, you may second-guess your decision to breast-feed, finding it hard to believe that your body could produce anything useful for your little one. Or if you had imagined putting your baby to the breast in the delivery room, you might feel overwhelmed by the distance you feel from your little one and discouraged when you are confronted with a cold electric pump instead of a warm, hungry baby. Pumping is not what you'd planned.

The hardest part was the day I went home: my milk came in and I was in agonizing pain. I had no idea what to expect. Pumping was a miserable experience that I undertook gladly for eight months because it felt like the only thing I could do for them, but I hated every minute of the actual pumping.—Susan B.

I really had a hard time making myself do it because I just felt so much like a science experiment anyway, with the bad pregnancy, and then the pumping was just so mechanical.—Terri

I felt revulsion at having my milk being drawn from my body by a plastic cup attached to a machine, only to watch a nurse feed it to my son a milliliter at a time through a tube, while my breasts ached to feel his lips and my heart broke because he couldn't.—Leanne

Unfortunately, you may not always receive effective guidance and empathetic support. If your baby is bottle-fed your breast milk, you may wonder if the staff is more interested in your milk than in helping you master breast-feeding. Your desire to breast-feed on demand might not match the staff's routines. When you're trying to assert some control as a parent, it can be frustrating to have to negotiate your baby's feedings. If you had your heart set on breast-feeding but you or your baby simply can't, this can be a tremendous blow. (For more on this subject, see "Supplementation and Bottle-Feeding" later in this section.)

I was pumping breast milk for Alison to get. I hated it. My milk production was not the greatest. I thought of pumping as very unnatural. It emotionally tore me apart. I mentioned the poor milk production to some of the nurses, and they didn't really say anything except get lots of rest and drink lots of fluids. They also mentioned something about relaxing. Yeah, right—when you want your baby home with you, you're still not recovered from the complications, it hurts to sit and hurts worse to get up.—Stacy

I felt resentment. Of course I wanted Emma to have breast milk—it's what's best—but I didn't think the lactation staff understood what an ordeal expressing breast milk would be. They certainly seemed far too chipper about the whole thing.—Diane

Even if you end up succeeding in breast-feeding, the process can be quite trying and drawn out. At first, putting your baby to the breast can be challenging as you both have some learning to do. Preemies in particular can take a long time to learn to coordinate sucking, swallowing, and breathing. Your baby may take two steps forward then one step back. Be patient and give your baby credit for accomplishing as much as he or she does. Comfort yourself by imagining a future in which you and your baby have mastered nursing. Envision it. Allow yourself to hope for it. Then do what you can to try to make it happen.

After I was finally allowed to actually hold her, I felt a wonderful sense of accomplishment. The worst was over, right? But I had to work long and hard to get her to adjust to being held and to even breast-feed (which I was told not to expect at all).

During this process, I held Daphne against my chest, skin to skin, for hours at a time. It took many weeks, including multiple occasions when I stayed in a NICU family room overnight with Daphne, but my determination finally paid off in the end.—Dina

I was informed that due to medication I was taking, I could not give him my expressed milk. I continued pumping but discarded the milk. My husband talked to the doctor, but I didn't want to. I decided that upon my baby's discharge I would try to find a pediatrician who would work with me and allow me to breast-feed. Ultimately, the doctor from the NICU was amenable, so we stayed with him. I met with a lactation consultant who helped me teach my baby to latch and nurse. I could never nurse him exclusively, but he started nursing at seven weeks, and I am so grateful.—Liza

I was absolutely determined to breast-feed my preemie (not knowing at the time how difficult such a thing is!). I arranged special permission with the NICU staff to be able to breast-feed him every time he was bottle-fed, supposedly to try to keep him used to both. He didn't have any trouble latching on to me, though. Well, sometimes he did seem to have trouble, as if he was frustrated and didn't want to latch on. And I'd get all discouraged and depressed. And, of course, the staff didn't really care about making sure I breast-fed the same number of times as he bottle-fed—it was all up to me to push for it to happen. But I kept trying (stubborn mom that I am!). Lots of ups and downs, but we were exclusively breast-feeding by a few days after his due date. Patient stubbornness goes a long way, I think!—Sandy

Here are some suggestions for tackling the challenge of breast-feeding in the NICU and beyond:

- *Discuss feeding options with your baby's medical practitioners.* If you very much want to breast-feed, discuss ways to increase your breast-feeding practice without compromising your baby's progress.

- *Seek out support for and information about breast-feeding.* Talk to other breast-feeding mothers of NICU babies. In addition to lactation consultants, a midwife or doula might be a good source of encouragement and assistance. There is plenty more information available in print and online about the advantages, the mechanics, establishing and enhancing your milk supply, and overcoming physical challenges to breast-feeding. Look for resources specific to parents whose babies are like yours.

I looked everywhere trying to find other people who understood not only what it took to breast-feed twins but how hard it was to pump and bottle-feed breast milk to one and also breast-feed the other one. Especially because they were preemies, their needs and development were different than the typical twins whose parents I came across. It took a long time to find the right place, but I finally did. I got not only support for my breast-feeding questions, but for the whole NICU experience too.—Rikki

- *Recognize that you and your baby form a unique breast-feeding partner- ship.* Every mother has to do a certain amount of figuring out what works best. Look for answers that work for both of you. Problems don't indicate failure—they only indicate the need for solutions.

- *Use the pump to prime your breasts.* For instance, if your baby has trouble latching on to your nipple, you might try using your pump's suction to draw out your nipple before putting your baby to your breast. If your baby is impatient or needs the encourage- ment of instant milk, you can also use the pump or express by hand to get the milk flowing. If your baby is overwhelmed by your milk spurting out at the beginning of the feeding, you can express enough milk to decrease the pressure or volume so that your baby can keep up with the flow.

- *Know that some babies are easily distracted or overwhelmed by external stimuli.* Ask if you can feed your baby in a quiet, darkened room. Experiment with different methods of holding your little one and using a blanket for cover.

- *Practice patience as your baby acquires the necessary skills.* Many babies must learn how to latch on well, work the tongue, and coordinate sucking with swallowing and breathing. Some babies make big strides by working with a speech or occupational therapist. Other babies simply need the tinctures of time and practice.

- *Incorporate kangaroo care into your efforts to breast-feed.* Research indicates that skin-to-skin contact inspires the instinct to suckle. You might try starting your breast-feeding sessions by placing your baby against your bare chest to rest, relax, and soak up your warmth and nurturing. If your baby starts rooting around on your skin, follow this cue and guide her or him to your nipple. Enjoying and relaxing with your little one is a priority, whatever feeding method you use.

It took almost two months for Daphne to learn how to latch and breast-feed. I spent many hours doing kangaroo care and trying to coax her into latching. In the end, my efforts were worth it because she finally got the hang of breast-feeding.—Dina

- *Be flexible.* Make decisions uniquely for your baby—no matter what your sister or cousin or nurse do with their children and no matter what you did with your other babies. Being flexible doesn't mean that you've given in. It means that you are adaptable and responsive to the unique requirements of this unexpected situation.

- *See the feeding relationship itself as meaningful for you and your baby.* Free yourself from society's definition of successful breast-feeding. For you and your baby, successful breast-feeding may mean that your baby takes a bottle filled with your pumped breast milk. Or it may mean putting your baby to your breast for a bit and then providing formula. Don't think in either/or terms. Experiment and adjust. Use the combination of breast milk and formula, bottle-feeding and breast-feeding that works for you and your baby.

- *Recognize that you supply many valuable things to your baby—not just breast milk.* The amount of breast milk you supply and the outcome of your attempts to breast-feed say nothing about your desire to nurture your baby or about your competence as a parent.

Waiting and Stockpiling

They were not even given food for more than a month on the NICU, just IV nourishment. I pumped and froze my milk. Then they started very slowly (a couple of ccs) with gavage feedings.—Susan B.

It can be days or weeks before your baby is given anything to eat by mouth—even by tube—and your breast milk may accumulate in the freezer. You may have mixed feelings about seeing your frozen milk stacked there. It can be a source of pride but also a visual representation of your baby's inability to take this nourishment directly from your breast. You may feel discouraged if your baby isn't able to consume much or digest it yet and disheartened that this milk, made just for him or her, sits idle. You may not be able to imagine a time when that milk will be useful. Seeing those ounces accumulate, you might think about all the good you wish it could do and long for it to have already been in your baby's tummy.

Expressing milk at home just reminded me that I didn't have my daughter home with me. It was horrible.—Diane

But that stock of breast milk in the freezer can also represent a bountiful harvest. You may feel glad that you can provide this treasure. You would never, ever want to see it run out.

It was like a feast of plenty, tangible evidence that I had enough milk for my babies. I would have preferred that they could have gotten it from me directly, but at least they were going to get it at some point.—Rikki

Supplementation and Bottle-Feeding

Whereas the amount of breast milk can be visibly measured when a baby is fed by tube or bottle, intake is not so clear during breast-feeding. Because you're in a medical setting, your baby may be weighed before and after breast-feedings to determine exactly how much he or she consumed. This inadvertently places pressure on you, perhaps leading to worries that your baby is not able to get enough breast milk—either because of inadequate supply or high demand.

Trying to breast-feed her turned out to be quite traumatic for both of us. She would latch on, but after thirty seconds or so she would become exhausted and fall asleep. The nurses would weigh her before and after our breast-feeding sessions, and more often than not she would have lost weight. I was very disheartened.—Rebekah

It is easy to resent the fact that something so natural has to be so closely scrutinized. If only your baby could stay on your breast and nurse on demand throughout the day. In fact, research shows that when mothers are able to provide consecutive hours of kangaroo care to babies who can breast-feed, their babies are able to alternate short periods of suckling with long periods of restful sleep. If you think this could work for you and your baby, speak up.

Still, some babies need the extra boost of supplements. Particularly if your baby was born very early, supplementation with preemie formula or human milk fortifier may help him or her grow. You may resent the implication of supplementation: that your breast milk alone is inadequate. Or on the flip side, you may resent the attitudes of those who second-guess your decision to supplement, especially when it may be a painful decision on your part.

I tried to nurse several times on the unit and many times once we got home, but their doctors and I finally determined that breast-feeding was burning more calories than they were consuming. So I pumped for eight months but never produced a lot of milk. Pumping might have been more successful if I had been able to combine it with nursing, but machines are not as effective as babies at inducing lactation. I felt cheated out of what I had expected to be a nurturing, intimate experience but did the best I could. We also used formula and fortifiers to increase their calorie intake.—Susan B.

Supplements can be provided by tube or bottle. And since you cannot be expected to be available in the NICU around the clock, your baby may receive your pumped breast milk in a bottle. You may be relieved that your baby is being nourished by your milk, even if it comes from a bottle, or you may be concerned that your little one will get used to the bottle and you may mourn the barriers to your efforts to breast-feed. While some babies do learn to prefer the bottle, some research shows that when the mother isn't present to put the baby to the breast, compared to babies who continue to be tube-fed, babies who are bottle-fed may actually do *better* at breast-feeding. Apparently, when babies can practice sucking skills with a bottle, this practice may transfer to better suckling at the breast. Some professionals believe that it is better yet to feed babies with a cup, spoon, dropper, or feeding syringe; this can offer practice eating by mouth but avoid nipple confusion. (Not every baby is prone to nipple confusion, but it is reasonable to take preventative steps if this concerns you.)

Your decisions about supplementation or bottle-feeding may be influenced by research, medical staff, or by your desire that your baby eat a measurable amount, grow quickly, and come home. Some decisions can be medically beneficial to your baby, but they might overshadow your maternal preferences and intuition.

I really wanted to breast-feed her right away. I did keep up the pumping and did eventually get to breast-feed, but they convinced me that bottles were better to start. I really feel bad to this day for letting them take charge because I know now that this is not so. Still, who was I to know? They were the professionals.—Linda

By the time the doctor was ready to stop supplements, I was not able to satisfy Stephen. This is still my biggest single regret. I knew nursing was best for my baby, I knew he was big enough and strong enough to nurse, he was my fourth child so I knew to trust my instincts, and yet I still followed the doctor instead of my heart—and as a result lost out on nursing my baby.—Tracy

Once she had developed the suck-swallow-breathe reflex at around thirty-three to thirty-four weeks, I got enormous pressure from the nurses to give her a bottle. But I wanted to nurse her as long as I could—practice sessions, really, because she was too small to complete a feeding—before the bottle was introduced. This was a major source of tension between the nurses and me. Many thought it was cruel to deny Charlotte the pleasure of a bottle for this period of time. . . . But eventually we had to introduce bottles because she couldn't go home being gavaged, and I think the number of bottles she has had has interfered with her ability to breast-feed.—Kate

It can be quite frustrating—and even demoralizing—if you are working hard to breast-feed but your baby begins to resist nursing, finding it easier and faster to take a bottle, or if your supply falters. If the medical team doesn't support you in your desire to breast-feed, you may feel that your attempts to do what you believe is best for your baby are being undermined. Ideally, your baby can breast-feed when you are present and bottle-feed only when you aren't there or as a supplement *after* breast-feeding.

Take heart. Many babies take to breast-feeding as they grow older or healthier. Some finally take to breast-feeding in the quiet of home.

Providing Breast Milk without Feeding at the Breast

If your baby cannot manage to feed at your breast, resolutely prefers the bottle, or still relies on tube-feeding, you'll need to decide whether to continue to pump. By maintaining your milk supply, your baby continues to benefit from receiving at least some breast milk. You must also decide how important or feasible it is for you and your baby that the tube or bottle contains breast milk only. You can provide breast milk for some feedings and formula for others. You may decide to focus on providing breast milk while your baby is tiny and move to formula later. Or you may find a pumping routine that works for you and continue to feed your baby breast milk exclusively or most of the time.

Even in your disappointment over not being able to put your baby to the breast, pumping can reinforce your involvement in your baby's feeding and give you the lift of knowing that you are supplying your baby with vital nutrients. If your baby doesn't take to nursing, this is not a rejection of you, a reflection on your mothering ability, or your fault. Some babies just have naturally strong preferences or the tendency to resist change, and when they get used to the bottle, they don't want to drink from anything else.

If you were really looking forward to nursing, you will need to grieve the loss of this special way of relating to your baby. Just keep in mind that you can still have a close and rewarding relationship with your baby. You can still experience the satisfaction of providing breast milk and define breast-feeding as just that. You can mimic the intimacy of breast-feeding by cuddling your baby against your warm skin, holding (instead of propping) the bottle or tube, silently letting your baby observe your face or feel your skin, and remaining soothing to your baby during feedings. It may not be the same, but it can still be very rewarding for you and your baby. However you feed your baby, you are nurturing your little one.

I had always planned on breast-feeding my baby, but he definitely changed all of that. I pumped the whole time he was in the hospital (three and a half months). It was the only thing I could do for him, and it made me feel like a mom even when I felt completely helpless. But when it came time to start breast-feeding, he couldn't take in my nipple. It didn't take long for me to give up. I thought he'd had enough struggling to survive. I didn't want him to stress out over feeding.—Sharon

If You Must Stop Pumping or Nursing

Even with the best intentions, efforts, technique, and support, for a variety of reasons, some mothers find that they can no longer pump or feed their baby at the breast. Although breast milk is easier to digest than formula, some babies' digestive systems are so compromised that even their mother's milk is too much for them to handle. Some babies just need time to mature or heal, but other babies will have long-term oral or digestive problems. It can be unbearably difficult to produce milk when it's uncertain the baby will ever be able to be nourished by it.

If you must stop providing breast milk or nursing for any reason, this can be yet another deeply felt loss. You may try for weeks or even months before finally letting go of your hope to provide breast milk for your baby or feed your baby at your breast. But when the costs of pumping or trying to nurse become greater than the rewards, it is quite reasonable to turn your energies toward the many other ways you can nurture your baby. Know your limits and respect them.

Breast-feeding was definitely something I wanted to do, but it was never something that was going to be an issue with me. If I couldn't do it, I couldn't do it, and that was the end of it. And I had gotten to a point with Charlie, after pumping and pumping and trying to get milk for about a week, that I said, "You know what? I have got way more on my head to deal with. I can't cope with this. This frustration is an emotion that I refuse to deal with. So bottle-feed him!"—Jaimee

If you had your heart set on providing breast milk or nursing, you may feel a deep sense of failure, anger, disappointment, or loss that it didn't work out.

It breaks my heart that I was not able to [continue pumping]. I felt very unfulfilled and like even more of a failure than I already did for what had happened. . . . I am tired of feeling inadequate because I chose to bottle-feed my baby. Yes, breast may be best—but I wish that they would make it known that it is not best in all situations.—Stacy

I pumped breast milk for three months for Casey. I felt that he needed breast milk more since he was premature, and I thought it was the only thing I could still do for him. He stopped digesting breast milk when he was three months old and had to be switched to formula. I cried that day—yet another failure to take care of my baby.—Kelly

It is important to acknowledge painful feelings so you can find pleasure in other ways of feeding your baby. Do whatever helps you make peace with the situation. Focus on achieving feelings of closeness during feeding times. You can always put your baby to your breast for comfort without having to produce breast milk. And look at it this way: you didn't fail, you *finished*.

I'm a mother. I want the very best of everything for my daughter. I love her. I would do anything for her. If I had my choice, she would still be breast-feeding. But you know what? I didn't have a choice. My daughter wasn't able to tolerate even a milliliter of breast milk. She was orally defensive, and I had completely dried up well before she came home, despite the fact that I had a really good breast pump.—Brooke

It's really a toss-up whether more mother's tears are shed each day over an incubator in the NICU or over a breast pump. . . . All mothers would benefit from being empowered to take control of feeding their child and doing it in a way that's perfect for the two of them, period.—Sheila

Feeding Multiple Babies

When you have multiple babies in the NICU, you may reconsider earlier plans. If you had believed that you could successfully breast-feed multiples, you might waver when confronted with the need to pump enough milk for several babies for several months. On the other hand, you may look to a breast-feeding relationship to ease the separation from your babies or to provide a nutritional boost.

Multiples present the challenge of doing what is best for two (or more) little ones. It is common for parents to make different choices for different babies. If one baby is more critically ill than the other(s), the mother may devote most of her milk to one infant (or feed from the frozen supply) while supplementing with formula as necessary for the other(s). Similarly, if a mother has been pumping throughout her babies' hospital stay and finds that one baby learns to nurse but another does not, she must decide how to proceed. Does she breast-feed one and pump for the other? Does one get formula? Does she pump for both? Does she stop pumping entirely? Trying to coordinate pumping, breast-feeding, and bottle-feeding can be overwhelming for parents of a single baby. If you are a parent of multiples, feeding can be the most complex and time-consuming task you face—especially if your babies are slow eaters!

It is also normal for you to have mixed emotions about all of the complicated options and the decisions you make. For example, you might have otherwise been content to supplement with formula but now feel enormous guilt doing so for a small, ill, or premature twin. Or you may grieve if one baby cannot take breast milk while the other(s) thrive on it.

Over time, you can continually determine what works for you and your babies as it is the rare set of multiples whose needs and preferences remain identical and unchanging. When you can, keep your options open so that as circumstances change and your babies develop, you can adjust differently for each one. If one baby prefers the bottle, consider pumping for that baby while you put the other(s) to the breast. If you feel you can't possibly provide breast milk for all your babies all the time, give yourself permission to supplement with formula and reassure yourself of the benefits of whatever amount of breast milk you can provide. If one baby does better on breast milk and another does better on formula, meet their unique needs. Don't worry about treating your babies exactly alike. What matters more is that each baby is fed according to what he or she prefers and thrives on.

Points to Remember

· *Decisions about how to feed your baby are emotionally charged. Seek out the information and support you need and stay flexible.*

· *Breast milk is a gift of nature and can be especially medicinal for babies who need intensive care. Providing it to your baby is one of the few things that only you, the mother, can do.*

· *Many mothers in the NICU start out pumping as the first step toward successful breast-feeding. Your baby may be able to feed directly from your breast after growing, recovering, and maturing enough to coordinate sucking, swallowing, and breathing.*

· *To establish or increase your supply, simply pump at shorter intervals for no longer than is necessary to empty your breasts.*

· *If thinking of your baby helps with pumping, try imagining your little one at your breast or positive visualizations of your baby growing and thriving. You may also find it helpful to smell a blanket that your baby has slept on.*

· *If you encounter a period of stress-induced depletion, you can keep your breasts primed by continuing to pump so that your supply can return as your baby improves.*

· *Incorporate kangaroo care into your efforts to breast-feed. Research indicates that skin-to-skin contact inspires the instinct to suckle and babies are able to alternate short periods of suckling with long periods of restful sleep.*

· *Successful breast-feeding can mean that your baby takes a bottle filled with breast milk or putting your baby to your breast for a bit and then providing formula. Don't think in either/or terms.*

· *Take heart. Many babies take to breast-feeding as they grow older or healthier. Some finally take to breast-feeding in the quiet of home.*

9:

The NICU Roller Coaster

I stare down at the gauze over his eyes and the IVs in his scalp, and I remember how people have asked me if I think I'm being tested. No, I don't. A test is something you go through only to see if you can go through the real thing.—Jeff

As you acclimate to the NICU and learn the ropes of getting close to your baby and providing nurturing care, you must also bear the ups and downs of your baby's medical course. Even if your baby's progress is fairly steady, there will be variability and perhaps some setbacks. Whether your baby's course includes deep dives or shallow dips, these downturns can feel distressing and demoralizing because with all your heart, you only want your baby to have upturns.

The NICU is like a roller coaster, and you cannot get off. It is hell. There are good days and really bad days. You live minute by minute in the beginning, then get to hour by hour, then day by day. You are constantly dreading your phone ringing, fearing it is more bad news.—Jody

Many parents use the term *roller coaster* to describe the NICU experience. You may feel as if you are holding your breath. It may be weeks before you can exhale.

It was a roller coaster of good and bad, and it changed by the hour. The second night she was there, we were called early in the morning because she started to run a fever. We raced to the hospital and by the time we got there it had gone back down. They were worried about infection so they put her on a new antibiotic. Then they started the spinal taps. They needed to make sure she didn't have infection in her bloodstream or fluids. In all, Kitquin had ten spinal taps! They never got enough fluid to test, and after the third attempt we only would consent to it if they did it by guided ultrasound. It would seem she was doing better, and they would try to lower the oxygen only to have to turn it back up. Eventually she did get better, though.—Jennifer E.

Even a typical medical course is full of ups and downs. Your emotional journey will correspond, and it can be arduous. The unpredictable twists and turns can leave you wondering what is waiting around the next corner. What new setback, what new apparatus, what new treatment, what new complication, what new struggle lies in wait? The uncertainties can rattle you to the core.

As your baby improves and becomes more predictable, you may feel more hopeful and assured about what's next. Or the opposite may happen: as your baby improves, your emotions may catch up with you, making you feel worse just when you think you should be feeling better. Whatever your experience, it can be an emotional roller coaster for quite a while, even after your baby needs less intensive care.

When she was moved to a bassinet, they lost her preemie pacifier. It must have fallen on the floor and they threw it away, and it was the only one. They didn't have any more. And then I was going to have to drive all the way to stupid [distant town] because that's the only store that carried preemie pacifiers. And I was just furious and angry and upset by this. Just so many emotions all at once. I couldn't even begin to cope with them. And my milk started to dry up. Well, of course, I hadn't had a lot of rest, and it was finally starting to take its toll. She was getting better, and I was falling apart.—Beth

Waiting

Buddy was out of surgery in a few hours. Those were hard hours. Very frightening. Minutes seemed like days.—Ed

Whether your baby has a relatively smooth medical course or a very rocky one, the NICU roller coaster involves a lot of waiting. You're waiting for the doctor to come, waiting for a test result, waiting to confer about a decision, waiting to see what will happen next. You're waiting for your baby to breathe unassisted, to open her eyes, to eat, to grow, to recover, and to respond to you. You're waiting for the chance to hold your baby close. And you're waiting for the day your baby can come home with you. How you feel about the waiting is related to the passage of time, the uncertainties you face, the setbacks that occur, and the balance between your hopes and fears.

Each little milestone was so important. Things most people take for granted, we couldn't. Things you don't even think you'll ever need to consider—like sucking. We had to teach her. Remembering to breathe. There was nothing we could leave to chance. We were in the NICU forever. At least it seemed like it. Babies came and went. Even seasons changed. But our little family held on.—Cindy

Even if your baby's NICU course is relatively short, straightforward, and without crisis, the waiting can be filled with worry, frustration, longing, questions, and impatient anticipation. Especially if your baby's hospitalization drags on, your greatest source of distress may be what your baby has to endure. You may wish that you could take your baby's place—to spare your little one the suffering and to spare yourself the watching . . . and waiting.

Although there are certainly NICU babies that have things much tougher than the boys did, this does not mean they had an easy ride. . . . I was never quite at ease with their continued progression and health.—Craig

The nurses called her a "feeder and grower"—all she needed to do before she could come home was gain weight. Still, my husband and I worried about her constantly. Is she gaining weight adequately? Doesn't that tube they're feeding her with bother her? Will she need the bili lights? Why is there blood in her stool? Do the lights bother her eyes? We asked lots of questions about her condition and visited her as often as possible.—Rebekah

Whether your baby is doing poorly or relatively well, waiting can be agonizing. Isolated from the rest of the world, you are in a place where time seems to stand still and you are powerless to make events happen any faster. You can't, for example, make those test results come back more quickly, speed up that procedure, or quicken your baby's progress. To top it off, when something finally does happen, it isn't always what you were waiting and hoping for.

I cried a lot. The worst for me was the waiting. Every single day we didn't know if he was dying on the inside. Or waiting for test results. I would walk around just hyper, literally shaking and trying to think of things to do to pass the time. Numerous times, we were told, "If this doesn't get better in two days, we'll do more tests." So there's another couple of days of waiting. . . . I did a lot of pacing because I couldn't get the worries off my mind. And the worst part of it was that I did a lot of it by myself.—Stephie

We got to walk with the surgeon and the anesthesiologist to the elevators, and at that point you kiss your baby good-bye and you don't know what's going to happen from there. . . . Okay, now we sit and wait. . . . [Tears] It was probably the longest hour of my life, waiting. . . . The lady from pastoral care came down, and the nurses tried to talk to us, but you really don't want to talk to anybody—at least we didn't. They were trying to be comforting and reassuring, but I didn't listen—basically, I didn't want to be bothered. I didn't want to have anybody try to comfort me. I just wanted to be by myself.—Pam

Waiting takes on a whole new aspect whenever you are told that your baby's condition must be dealt with *immediately*. To most of us, *immediately* means "right now," so when medical action is delayed, the wait can seem interminable. Then if another doctor examines your child and decides that the condition isn't critical, you may not know what to think. Should you relax or get yet another opinion? Whom should you believe? When you've been put on high alert, it's hard to lower the volume on your questions, worries, and impatience. (For more on decision making and weighing opinions, see "Advocating for Your Baby" in chapter 5.)

We followed the ambulance to the Children's Hospital, and when we got there, we waited around forever. So we're just waiting and waiting, and they didn't even have the eye doctors come look at him. And here I'd been told if he didn't have this surgery, he was going to be blind—and nobody was looking at him because they had other stuff they were doing. I just sat there. And then the head eye doctor and about ten other doctors all looked at Josh and said, "I have no idea why your hospital sent him over here—his eyes are fine. This child doesn't need surgery and probably isn't ever going to need it. We're sending him back tonight."

But then after that [back at our home hospital], it was horrible because, almost every other day, they kept telling me he was going to need the laser surgery. For days they were checking him, and then they were checking Evan too, even though he didn't have the same problem. All those days of not knowing—does he need surgery or doesn't he? And questioning everything they were doing. Not knowing who to believe.—Stephie

Waiting with Uncertainty

The doctors said they just didn't know but that she was growing and that was good, but they needed to get her off the ventilator. They tried every ventilator they had. Julie would get off a little, and then she'd have a setback. And if one thing would get better, then another thing would get worse. And this went on and on.—Tim

For many parents, the primary uncertainty is not knowing how their baby's medical course will play out. Especially when your baby is in critical condition, having to wait and see is painful and unnerving. You may feel frustrated that the medical team cannot tell you when your baby's condition will improve. In fact, the doctors may not even be certain about how your baby will respond to a particular treatment. You may have few promises on which to pin your hopes.

After Daphne's first week, we were often told that our baby's prognosis looked good, but we were always cautioned not to be too optimistic. For example, on the day of surgery, Barry and I arrived early to sign various consent forms and to visit with Daphne for as long as possible. Daphne's pediatric surgeon explained the risks of the procedure to us and cautioned that while she was optimistic, "Children healthier than Daphne have expired on the table during this kind of surgery." With that, we were ushered into a waiting room with family to await the outcome. The surgery lasted more than five hours. I will never forget the relief I felt when the surgeon came into the waiting room and announced that the procedure was textbook without any complications. After a while, we were finally able to see our little princess.—Dina

So much of the time, you have to wait and see. If your baby seems to be struggling too much, the doctors won't be able to tell *for sure* what the right course of treatment is. You'll need to wait and see. If your baby is too unstable or sick to tolerate being held, the doctors won't be able to tell you *for sure* when you'll be able to do more hands-on care and snuggling. You'll need to wait and see. In the beginning, your baby's caregivers won't be able to set a *firm* date for when your baby will be able to come home. They may tell you to expect to take your baby home around the original due date or give you a rough timeline, but they won't be able to promise it. And they can't tell you what you and your baby will have to go through in the meantime. You'll need to wait and see. And nobody can guarantee that your baby will emerge from the NICU unscathed.

Scary. Incredibly scary. Like a living nightmare, one in which you don't know where the dark tunnels are going to lead. You just go with what comes and try to make the best of it. When we didn't think we could handle it, we sought somebody to talk to about what we were going through.—Andrea

It was very uncertain. He was given a 50 percent chance for survival, and even if he survived we wouldn't know how he would do. We were told that he could be completely normal, or he could suffer from feeding issues, deafness, breathing issues, pulmonary hypertension, seizures, kidney problems/failure, developmental delays, brain damage, etc. . . . from his condition and the treatments done to save his life. Only time would tell how well he would do. His future was very uncertain.—Corin

Even if your baby is doing well, you may feel on edge, mistrusting that trend until it is well established. Gallice remembers, "For three weeks we didn't want to believe how well he was doing."

James was a feeder and grower. There was nothing medically wrong with him that time wouldn't and hasn't cured. That did not mean that I didn't spend the whole of every night with one ear listening for the phone, my body aching at its emptiness. And when the phone did ring, the fact that my child was doing so well didn't stop my heart rate quickening and didn't change the feeling of dread as I answered that call.—Leanne

If you normally have difficulty tolerating uncertainty, waiting in the dark will be especially hard for you. If you prefer to make rational choices, forming medical decisions intuitively can be unsettling. If you aren't very comfortable with suspense, or if you prefer to have all your ducks in a row and all your loose ends tied up neatly, your baby's NICU stay and medical course can feel torturous.

Living with uncertainty proves emotionally and physically draining for most parents. It's difficult to endure the wait if you can't even count on a bright future at the end. If your baby's very survival is in question, it's hard to know whether to welcome this child or to start saying good-bye. The tension and the conflicting emotions that arise from ambiguity can be paralyzing.

If your baby is declining, you may find yourself wishing for a speedy demise because the suspense and tension are so overpowering that they are threatening your sanity. You're not the only parent to feel this way. Your wishing that the ordeal would come to an end is a powerful testament to how truly difficult this situation is. It is important for you to recognize that there is nothing wrong with your feelings. It's the situation that is so wrong.

When she was three days old, I remember sitting there, just bawling my eyes out . . . saying, "If she's going to die, I want her to do it now. I don't want her to wait a couple of weeks." I felt horrible saying that, but on the other hand, it felt better for me to let that out. And it was true. If she was just going to die anyway, I wanted her to die before I had a chance to really fall in love with her. . . . That was part of it, and another part was that the sooner it happened, the sooner I could pick my life up and move on, instead of agonizing over the next couple of months, *When is she going to die?*—Brooke

Here are some approaches that can help you cope with all the uncertainty of your baby's situation:

- *Know that uncertainties are most plentiful and loom largest early on and during any crisis.* As each situation resolves, many uncertainties resolve as well. Some disappear entirely, some merely shrink, but each resolution generally reduces the scope and number of uncertainties. You may not always like the outcome—and if your child has special needs, there will always be some degree of uncertainty about the future. But as your baby gets closer to discharge, you'll have more certainty to pin your hopes on.

- *Take it one day at a time.* Try to live in the present and not worry about the future. Of course, it is normal to worry to some extent about the possibilities that may unfold, but you can vow to spend less energy pondering events or situations that have not yet occurred, remembering that they may very well never happen. (For more about this, see "Waiting with Your Baby" later in this chapter.)

- *Believe in your own assessment of the situation.* Trust your evaluations of the information you are being given and your appraisal of the doctors' opinions. Recognize the validity of what you observe and know about your baby. Also rely on your parental intuition.

- *Care for yourself.* Get as much sleep as you can; eat nutritious, wholesome foods; and exercise so that you can better withstand the stress associated with uncertainty. See chapter 4 for more on this important coping tool.

- *Take breaks and use relaxation techniques.* Take frequent minibreaks, particularly when you're feeling especially tense. Consciously relax your muscles, releasing the tension in your shoulders, your jaw, and your forehead. Get into the habit of being mindful of your breathing and practice breathing deeply, as this is naturally calming.

· *Seek out support.* Connect with the people in your life who can help and support you. Avoid spending time with people who drain you.

· *Focus on the stable aspects of your life.* Continue (or create) a weekly routine of pleasurable activities, as this gives you something to rely on and look forward to. Routine can be especially comforting in the midst of uncertainty.

· *Realize that anxiety about an uncertain future is normal.* If your child's future remains uncertain upon and after discharge, you can still imagine a rosy future with your baby as you become more comfortable with the questions that remain unanswered. Even if the outcome is full of challenges, you will learn to cope in time, with support.

· *Hold on to life philosophies or spiritual beliefs that help you make sense of this experience.* These beliefs can also reinforce your resilience in the face of uncertainty.

The following suggestions are descriptions of some perspectives that parents have found helpful. Read through them and see if any resonate for you.

· Control what you can and let go of what you can't. Life is a mystery that unfolds, not a problem to be overpowered.

· Take comfort in religious perspectives about why bad things happen. Look for personal and spiritual meaning in the midst of this situation.

· Work toward spiritual acceptance, toward recognizing that you are witnessing a part of nature's cycle of health and illness, birth, and even death. Seek harmony with nature rather than fighting against it.

· Believe that there are higher spiritual reasons for this child to be on this particular journey.

· Wonder if perhaps your baby chose this life to learn lessons that are necessary for enlightenment or the soul's progress. In kind, perhaps you too chose your life for its lessons and enlightenment.

· Adopt a wondering attitude about the future. Instead of specifying your wishes for an outcome, hold onto the idea that everything will unfold as it should and that it is simply not yet time for you to know what will happen.

- Rely on prayer, with the awareness that prayers may be answered in ways we can't always understand.

- Believe in miracles, remembering that sometimes a miracle isn't what we think it should be. Miracles can be found where we least expect them.

Waiting with Unpredictability

He started off pretty well, and I really thought he was going to do very well. Every time he would come off [the ventilator], I would get all excited because it was a step forward. Then he would go back on, and I would be crushed that he was so fragile. He looked so big compared to most of the babies in the NICU, so I expected he would be progressing more quickly.—Tracy

We didn't think there was going to be another problem. I guess we didn't read far enough ahead in the book. So we felt that we were in the clear, and Jacob just needed to grow and get stronger. We were at that stage—and all of a sudden, we have somebody sitting there saying, "In the next two weeks, we'll figure out if your son is going to be blind." It was extremely hard to take. It was almost like the final blow.—Julie

I was very apprehensive when I would walk through the NICU doors. I never knew if it was going to be a good day or bad. Too many times I came in to see them bagging David. It was a very high-stress time.—Jody

The unpredictable nature of your baby's medical course can be the most strenuous and terrifying part of the roller coaster. With each unforeseen crisis, there are renewed feelings of fear, distress, and helplessness. Every setback strikes fresh fear into your heart. Even detours you thought wouldn't bother you can be terrifying when they actually happen.

After a couple of days, Mikey is put into a sort of quarantine status because he tested positive for MRSA, which is an antibiotic-resistant strain of staph infection. Everyone has to begin wearing gloves and gowns while handling anything in Mikey's section. Then Mikey is also a bit jaundiced and put under the lights. Then, they don't want to keep poking Mikey and finding new places to insert an IV. They had been saying all along that that they would eventually need to put in a PICC line, which is a small IV running through a vein directly into his heart. They use an X-ray machine to verify the correct placement of the PICC line. It's a bit of a scary thought and certainly serious. We'd already signed the consent form on the first day, and so the PICC line was put in.—Chip

All these weeks with my friend [whose preemie was diagnosed with ROP], I was thinking, *What's the big deal? It's only the eyes [not life or death]!* Then they tell me that if Josh doesn't have laser surgery that afternoon, he's going to be blind. And all of a sudden, it's *Oh, my God, it's the eyes!* The eyes became everything. I was hysterical. After all these babies have been through, they deserve perfection. They don't deserve blindness. They don't deserve anything bad, you know?—Stephie

If your baby remains in critical condition for a while, waiting can become oddly comforting. As you get used to the current set of medical issues, their familiarity and stability let you relax somewhat. But typically, just as you master one set of medical issues, it's on to new, unfamiliar challenges.

It would be such a relief if your baby's medical course could be displayed on a graph that showed a straight, upward-slanting line representing your baby's steady growth and improving health. And it would be especially comforting if you could see that graph in advance. Unfortunately, many babies experience plateaus and setbacks, and this unpredictable sequence of gains and losses can frazzle even the calmest parents. Parents of babies who experience many setbacks feel especially on edge because they know how fragile their baby's progress is.

Every day was a milestone for Zachary, but at the same time there was always some new threat coming up.—Marcia

We'd get over one thing, and then there'd be another one. Whenever there was a lull, so to speak, we're like, "All right, what's happening now? Something is building up." And there were times we'd be, "All right, this is going too good. There has to be a setback somewhere."—Brooke

One time the NICU called, all excited, to tell me that Josh was off the ventilator—and by the time I got there, he was back on it, so I didn't even get to see him without it.—Stephie

Premature babies in particular tend to have an initial honeymoon period, including some growth and improvement, followed by a setback. Setbacks such as losing a few grams or having slightly increased oxygen needs can be relatively minor from the medical staff's perspective. But to you, these setbacks can feel *major*. Setbacks such as pulmonary hemorrhage or infection, which are generally major from a medical perspective, can feel devastatingly grim.

Whether minor or major, your baby's complications may frighten you, disappoint you, or fill you with grief. Every new difficulty can remind you of the losses you've already endured, and each one starkly emphasizes how *unfair* this situation is. Every setback feels like yet another violation—an inability to hold on to the progress that has been made. If your baby faces serious medical setbacks, the future becomes unpredictable again—and you must wait with that unpredictability.

During Stuart's surgery, we waited forever, when a social worker told us that all was going beautifully. On her heels, though, arrived the surgeon, who told us that Stuart had crashed as they prepared to close. This tiny, terribly scarred boy was not expected to survive the next twenty-four hours. Yet he did—slowly, painstakingly, with many setbacks and battles. He was to be moved several times from conventional vent to the oscillator to the jet ventilator. He needed the same surgery yet another time. . . . Yet come home he did.—Susan C.

When your baby was admitted to the NICU, you may have been told to expect many ups and downs—that these alternating setbacks and improvements are a NICU thing. Fortunately, experience helps you become familiar with the treatments and the often minor and temporary nature of setbacks. As you adapt to this new definition of *normal*, restore calm by reminding yourself that your infant's bumpy medical course is typical. And even if the course becomes atypical, major setbacks don't necessarily rule out a good outcome.

Here are some actions you can take that may help you to get through this unpredictable cycle of two steps forward and one step back:

· *Record the dates and details of your baby's progress and setbacks*—
weights, feedings, conditions, illnesses, treatments, procedures,
caregivers' assessments, being held, kangaroo care sessions,
being put to the breast or bottle, reactions to you—whatever
facts, observations, and experiences you feel are significant.
Doing so can help give some order to the chaos. It can also clarify your memories of what you and your baby have gone through
and help you to see how far your baby has come—ups, downs,

and all. Many parents treasure this record as a testament to their endurance and to their baby's triumph. (When a baby dies, this kind of journal can become a treasured keepsake that affirms the baby's existence and importance.)

· *Ask for the explanations and information you need when your baby has complications or setbacks.* Being told "It's just a preemie thing" or "This is typical" may reassure some parents, but if that explanation doesn't comfort you, ask for more details.

· *Seek out parents of NICU graduates who had issues similar to your baby's.* You can find these parents through your unit social worker or your hospital's parent-to-parent support organization (if the hospital has one). If there are no local avenues, try the Internet— many parent networking sites have mentoring programs. Hearing about another infant's ups and downs—and especially seeing that the family came out the other side—can be very reassuring. It's also comforting to talk with someone who understands.

· *Give yourself time to adjust to the variability.* It's natural to feel discouraged or distressed by small and hourly variations in weight, feeding amounts, or oxygen needs, especially in the first days or weeks of your baby's NICU stay. Even when setbacks are insignificant or "typical," you'll be thrown by them. Trying to distance yourself from your baby's variable status is not realistic, but in your own time you'll learn to ignore the hourly or daily details and focus on your baby's big picture and the progress made over longer stretches of time.

· *Accept that you may not get used to your baby's ups and downs.* Even though the NICU roller coaster is normal, every downturn can be frightening, and you may protest the ride with every fiber of your being. It's natural to be buoyed by good news and crushed by bad. That's especially true when the downs aren't so minor.

· *If your baby is making great progress and you want to celebrate, do so in ways that reinforce your joy and hope.* Commemorate your baby's gains with a trinket, a picture, or a note in your journal. Remember to take pictures of the firsts. Even if you fear that your baby will be intubated again, pictures of your little one's face without a ventilator tube are still to be cherished.

Waiting with Your Baby

Sometimes, waiting with uncertainty and unpredictability can take the place of being with your baby. This is understandable. Until you have some answers, you may dwell obsessively on what the future might bring. You may focus on your worries, or you may believe that your life will begin again only when you and your baby leave the NICU. Unfortunately, waiting in this way makes it impossible to stay emotionally in the moment with your little one. Instead of parenting in the present, you're focused on the future.

There is another way to wait—and that is waiting *with* your baby. Of course, concern about the future is part of being a responsible parent. But waiting with your baby means focusing mainly on the present. While you wait, you watch and see everything that is happening with your infant. You keep vigil. This is not a passive process. Here are some suggestions for waiting with your infant:

- Worry only about what's happening *today*.
- Learn about your baby's *current* medical conditions and treatments.
- See your baby as an individual and a member of your family.
- Notice your baby's preferences and personality.
- Learn what you can do *now* to comfort and care for your baby.

Waiting with your baby makes waiting rich and meaningful. When you look back at this time, you will know that you were very much a part of your baby's life during this ordeal. By waiting with your baby, you are laying the stones on your shared path through life.

Balancing Hopes and Fears

When Lauren, my daughter, was born, I guess I never even thought babies survived at that low of a weight, so boy, did I have a lot to learn. But in the beginning, I was scared of everything. . . . The neonatologist told us that she might have learning problems due to prematurity. It scared us, but he did use the word *might*—not *will.*—Shirley

Hoping for the best and fearing for the worst is like straddling a fence. Fear may dominate your emotions, but simultaneously clinging to your hopes can improve your balance. Striking that balance isn't always easy, but it can help you adjust to whatever may happen—and can help you wait *with* your baby.

Though at times your hopes may be going up in smoke, remembering your dreams and wishes helps you hold on with optimism.

Optimism can help you cope with much of the uncertainty and unpredictability that is natural during a baby's NICU stay. Being surrounded by hopeful practitioners, family, and friends can also help keep you afloat in a sea of fears and ambiguity.

When we visited Neil the first time—me wheeled there on a gurney, an hour after his birth—the first thing the nurse attending him did was congratulate me. I didn't see much to be congratulated on. My body had just committed the ultimate betrayal and kicked out my baby far, far too soon. Yet congratulations are so much better than an "I'm sorry"—and being congratulated made me start thinking that maybe there was something to be happy about, that maybe things weren't quite as bad as they seemed.—Tara

Maybe when I was in that mixed-feelings state of not wanting to cope with that whole situation, maybe at that point—I've sort of forgotten about it because it's embarrassing—but we didn't know if he was ever going to be a normal baby. He was not there; we did not want to admit it. But people were so reassuring. I think that gave us right away all the optimism we needed, and it was transferred to him, and then we felt pretty good about him. I found him so cute. I realize that he was not the most beautiful baby for other people, of course, but for me, he was the cutest baby in the world.—Gallice

Optimism isn't blind to reality, however. With *realistic* optimism, you can acknowledge your fears and face the difficulties even as you hold onto hope. This balance of hope and fear makes parenting a powerful job.

The one thing with Banning that I fixated on—and I knew I had to stop—I was fixating on his weight. And he got down to a point where he was one pound ten ounces from three pounds six ounces—and it was like, I can't ask anymore because, every time, he's losing weight, he's losing weight, he's losing weight. I've got to focus on something positive. So I would write things in his journal, the things that I could see that he was doing, the progression, his milestones, no matter how small they were. If he had taken an extra ounce of milk that day, it was so exciting. So I wrote a lot.—Pam

When the going is rough or in the face of monumental uncertainties, the balance may shift toward fear, overshadowing your hopes. Wishes can seem impossible, and you may hesitate to express or even think about your hopes under the guise of making the worst outcome easier to bear. But dwelling exclusively on your fears can keep you from connecting with your baby and doesn't make the worst any easier to endure. (See also "Dealing with Fears" in chapter 6.)

So look deep inside yourself and you'll find those hopes and dreams you had during the pregnancy. They don't just disappear when your baby is admitted to the NICU. They are still a part of you. Allow your buried dreams to slowly emerge into the light.

In addition to these buried dreams, as your baby's hospital course progresses (especially if it is difficult), new hopes will evolve. At first you may continue to hold on to elaborate dreams for the future, but when you realize that these are unrealistic or distant, you may gradually revise them to more achievable goals. You may begin to feel satisfied with small increments of progress as your baby attains one small goal at a time. For example, at first you may say to yourself, "I just want my baby to breathe unassisted." Then if your baby's lungs are taking a different path than you'd hoped for, you might say, "I just want my baby to have good results on the ventilator." Shirley put it this way: "I just wanted her to be healthy. . . . I would worry about the developmental stuff later."

As your baby improves, you may gather the courage to reclaim some modified form of your original wishes. You may hope for larger things, such as breast-feeding or taking your baby home, healthy and free of equipment. As your baby's medical path becomes clearer, it's easier to allow yourself to hope, even if that means rethinking the future. Although you will still grieve for what you've lost, you can also rejoice in the adjusted dreams that are coming true.

At any time, you can also build hope by finding special meaning in what happens around you or your baby. Perhaps your favorite nurse postpones a vacation, and you take this as a sign that the universe is working in your favor. Perhaps you find comfort in a gentle snowfall, a mother bird nesting in your eaves, or a shooting star. Others may dismiss these details as superstition or happenstance, while you, caught up in the mystery of birth, find yourself more open to the wonders that surround you.

The point when I realized things would probably be okay was when I came to the NICU to find my son, who was very heavily sedated, lying on his side with his hand cupped over his nose and mouth—an unusual position impossible for him to get to on his own—and the nurses said they hadn't positioned him like that. This was the same position my grandmother (who had passed away when I was in junior high) always slept in. I felt at that moment that she was there with him, watching over him, and that things would be alright.—Ami

I started to look for omens. It obviously goes to show my state of mind at the time, but if I didn't see kangaroos on the drive to the hospital (we have lots of bush and lots of 'roos), I'd think it was some sort of bad sign. My mum also had a plant that she was obsessive over. When I had Ngioka, the plant was sick. She was convinced that she had to keep the plant alive and then Ngioka would survive. Another mum had a thing about parking spaces (which were at a premium at our hospital). If she drove into the car park and got one, it was going to be a good day.—Jo

As discussed in chapter 4, you can also build hope by becoming aware of what you tell yourself. Instead of obsessing about how awful the situation is, dwell on a mantra such as "This too shall pass" or "In life, the one constant is change." Even when hope is hard to find or when it appears so frail that you're afraid to lean on it, hold on to your faith that all will turn out for the best. Replace doomsday scenarios with optimistic thoughts. Take to heart the positive signs you observe. Remember that many NICU babies do well and yours can too.

Some parents find it easier to focus on optimistic thoughts after their baby has gotten past a certain point: perhaps making it to a particular gestational age, or after getting off the ventilator, or when negative predictions are proven wrong. If, deep down, you believe that in the end everything will be okay, trust and focus on that feeling.

Every hour there was a different emotion with each of the children, but we always tried to stay positive and we always thought that they were strong, and they were as relatively healthy as they could be at that point, and that they were just going to get through it—that it would be a long haul, but that they would get through it.—Betsy

My fears and my worries were all before he was born. After he was born, I never remember thinking, even one time, *He's not going to be okay.* I really was convinced that he was [going to be] fine; nobody led me to believe any differently. I didn't think that he would have any neurological problems. I just really thought that everything was okay.—Jaimee

Up to that point in time, I was just kind of living with the idea that she was going to die. The doctor said, "She's going to die," so that's going to happen, right? Then [when they told us she wouldn't make it through the night], all of a sudden, I had this weird sort of certainty, where I knew she was going to make it. And she was going to go, "Ha ha, fooled you!"—Brooke

Although your optimistic thoughts may not change your child's outcome, they may very well affect your child's quality of life. Instead of holding back your emotional connection with your baby, you can invest with optimism. In the face of uncertainty, positive thoughts are free—it's the negative ones that can cost you dearly.

You may always have concerns about your child. But instead of imagining future catastrophe, put that worry energy into picturing an optimal future—not a perfect or even a typical future, but one that is the best it can be. Visualize that whatever challenges lie ahead, you will have the strength, the courage, and the wisdom to cope and to seek the paths that will bring your family the most happiness and contentment. Whatever happens, assume that your child will be blessed by destiny.

When Medical Practitioners Dash Your Hopes

Pronouncements from medical practitioners can strongly affect your emotional state. Reassurances are comforting, but pessimism is devastating. Sometimes you want to hear honest assessments; sometimes you don't. The safest setting in which to hear assessments is during an extended conversation, when you can ask questions and get the support you need. The worst time is in passing, at your baby's bedside.

One well-meaning doctor gave us an update on our son's condition after a tough week of complications. As he finished, he said, "You know, he might actually make it," as though it were a slim possibility. Not making it had never crossed my mind. My faith, hope, and certainty that he would survive were the only things getting me out of bed every morning. That seemingly positive comment devastated me. I cried for over an hour.—Laura

Some practitioners may urge you to have realistic expectations by informing you of all the harsh possibilities or inappropriately sharing their own feelings of hopelessness or anxiety with you. In your state of vulnerability, it's difficult to ignore these comments from well-meaning but misguided practitioners, and they may be unaware of the pain they cause.

Your high hopes are simply your parental wishes for your baby, not necessarily unrealistic expectations. Of course you hope all will be well. Of course you want your baby to survive and thrive. Hope (and even denial) helps you cope. You might remind certain practitioners that it's far easier to be brave when you don't know about all that could go wrong! Especially if your baby's medical course or prognosis is uncertain, you need the medical team's assistance to find a balance between hope and fear.

It is the special caregiver who can offer hope without making promises. Susan C. explains her reactions to the very different comments of two practitioners:

The chasm between the acts of kindness and the acts of cruelty was deep. Three days after the death of our firstborn, his twin underwent life-threatening surgery. For days I asked questions of every professional who came near us, questions designed to elicit hope. No one could offer any. Everyone was understandably guarded and careful. One quiet afternoon, as I sat watching, waiting, asking nothing of anyone, one brave doctor knelt down next to me, put his arm on my shoulder, and said, "It's okay to hope, you know. Some of them do make it." On another, quite later afternoon, just after we had emerged from a second, unexpected bout of NEC, I sat next to my baby's bedside, tears seeping down my cheeks, feeling incredible relief. Remarkably, he had turned another corner. Inexplicably, a nurse felt it necessary to advise me: "Don't relax now. You will be dealing with this for years. Even if he does recover from this, you will spend years rushing in and out of the hospital dealing with strictures and other medical complications. It will never be over."—Susan C.

Acquiring realistic expectations for your baby is a drawn-out process that always includes hope. Don't let others' remarks discourage you from having hopes and wishes.

When Hope Shines More Brightly

If your baby starts out in critical condition, you may have many days or even weeks of high anxiety. As your baby's condition improves, it can be difficult to change gears. It can be a challenge to start thinking of your baby as a grower and feeder instead of as a medical case that must be watched closely. It's like shifting from a roller coaster ride fraught with peril to the relatively smooth ride of a limousine. You can still expect bumps in the road, but no one's life is in danger.

As your baby's discharge date approaches, you may still find it hard to believe that the limo is for real and your hopes are coming true. Learn to trust that your baby is on the road home and work on letting your fears recede. Doing so will free you to put your energy toward getting better acquainted with your baby and skilled at any special care. When your hopes burn consistently brighter than your fears, relax and enjoy the feeling.

As my son became more stable, I tried hard to keep up and make the transition to being a mom of a stable baby instead of a critical preemie. . . . It was a more disjointed process for me than what my husband experienced, but the three of us did come out the other side feeling extremely close to one another.—Maureen

As you and your baby head toward home, if your baby's future development remains unknown, your hopes are tempered by uncertainty. But because infants are so resilient and unpredictable, your baby may do relatively well. This is a hope to hang onto. If your fears about delays or disability are eventually confirmed, hope still endures, even as you continue to grieve—and cope, adjust, and heal.

When Hope Changes Direction
What happens when the parents' worst fear becomes reality? When a baby is dying, hope doesn't disappear. It simply changes direction from hope that their baby will live to hoping their baby will die peacefully, surrounded by love.

Parents may hope for the chance to hold and caress their baby free of the tubes and lines. They start to envision their baby spending the final minutes or hours tenderly cradled in loving arms. They can plan to hold their baby skin to skin; mothers can hold their little one to the breast. These desires to protect and be close to their precious baby are an extension of their earliest hopes, when they thought the path led toward home.

It was pretty clear to me he was dying. I asked the doctor whether or not she thought there was any hope. She said, "In my professional opinion, no." So I said, "Then take him out of the incubator, I want to hold him." And it was the first time I held him. He couldn't maintain his own body temperature yet, he wasn't strong enough to be taken out. . . . [tears] And I held him for maybe an hour, and I rocked him and I told him how much I loved him, and he died in my arms.—Micki

When hope changes direction, heartfelt dreams and worst nightmares all loom large. This intense combination of opposing images is both natural and necessary. The passion of the parents' hopes and fears reflects their profound relationship with their baby. And even as they grieve, they move toward healing transformation.

Multiple Realities—Multiple Roller Coasters

When you have more than one baby in the NICU, you have more than one set of hopes and fears for recovery, feeding, growth, health, and development. You have multiple medical courses to keep track of, each with a unique pattern of progress and setbacks. You may find it nearly impossible to catch your breath between the alternating dips of these simultaneously running roller coasters. Parenting multiples in the NICU can be a gargantuan and dizzying task.

Because of pulmonary hemorrhaging, they couldn't bring Daniel back easily, but he finally seemed to stabilize again. We had just seen our first trauma using emergency procedures. And we were pretty scared about that. In my mind, I remember thinking [Daniel's survival] was a very iffy thing. I didn't know what his outcome was going to be, and when the phone rang at 3:30 in the morning, I thought they were announcing that Daniel had died. I was sure. But no, they were calling to say that Shayna had begun pulmonary hemorrhaging. So it was frightening and it was ugly. I remember Debbie hanging up and screaming and crying, "I can't take this, I can't take this!" It was pretty horrible, about as awful as it gets.—Mitch

If your babies' hospital course is filled with complications, there is always *something* that has just happened, that is threatening to happen, or that one of your babies is still recovering from. Anxiety is your constant companion. You might feel as if you have not been able to relax since before the dawn of time.

I would go back and forth because when one would be sick, then the other would be okay. And then it was not only, *How can I do this, be there for two babies?* but I could never enjoy myself because if one baby was doing okay, the other baby was inevitably really sick and about to die. So for months, there was never a day when I could even, like, just let my shoulders down and collapse and be okay. They were so sick, and there were so many things that were going to kill them.—Stephie

If you're extremely lucky, your babies will follow similar medical courses, but inevitably, there will be differences. You'll still have to keep pace with each of them separately, and you may anxiously compare them with each other. How much weight is each one gaining? How much supplemental oxygen does each need? Any apneas or bradycardias? You want your babies to thrive individually but also together, as a unit. And you hope that the healthiest of them is a harbinger of how the other(s) will fare.

With multiples, you may also have a special set of worries about the future. You want each baby to be okay, but you may also worry about how their outcomes may differ. If one of your babies is disabled or developmentally delayed, not only will you mourn for that child, but you may also fear the loss of that mystical bond between siblings who are twins, triplets, or more. If one has significantly more limitations than the other(s), you might worry that he or she will be left out. The dichotomy of mourning and celebration may be ongoing. And given that parenting healthy multiples is a challenge, you may wonder how you will possibly manage to care for a medically fragile or disabled child in the mix.

Here are some strategies that can help you deal with the multiple roller coasters:

- *Keep a small notebook for each baby.* Use these notebooks to jot down each infant's daily events, milestones, and medical issues as they occur. Separate notebooks can help you to keep the stories straight, and you'll worry less about missing or forgetting something in the midst of the chaos. If you want, each notebook can also become a journal—a place for you to write about your feelings and thoughts for each child and situation. You'll be glad to have these records to bolster your memories and help you make sense of your journey.

- *Assume that your babies will have unique medical courses.* Just because one of your babies has a certain frightening complication doesn't mean that your other baby(ies) will develop it.

- *Be prepared for the ups and downs.* Remember that one baby's ride may get bumpy just as another's smooths out. Knowing that this seesaw effect is common can make it a bit less distressing.

- *Keep perspective.* Rest assured that you will be able to catch your breath down the road. Take one day at a time and remember to trust the journey.

- *Focus on progress over the longer term, not on daily differences.* Your babies may have medical courses that are very different day by day, but in hindsight their overall picture may look quite similar. Avoid focusing on the daily differences. Look instead at their weekly progress. Even when the overall picture is different in the

short run, your babies may have very similar (and excellent) outcomes down the road.

· *Grieve both the obvious and the subtle losses associated with having
multiple babies.* If your identical twins are struggling with different issues, own the feelings you may have about them not sharing
identical outcomes. If your triplets are kept apart, acknowledge
the feelings you may have about their being unable to snuggle
together the way they did inside you. These acknowledgments
will help you cope and move forward.

Making Comparisons in the NICU

The next morning I went in to see her, and there was a set of twins in the NICU.
They were tiny, smaller than Kit was, but they could breathe on their own. Their mom
came in with the lactation consultant while I was in the back of the room looking at
my baby (less than six feet away.) She was allowed to hold her babies and even
try feeding her babies, and all I could do is cry and look at my daughter. I felt very
cheated and very, very jealous. "This is not how it should be" is all I could mutter as
I watched Kit's stats on the monitors.—Jennifer E.

In the NICU, you are surrounded by babies and their parents, but
you may hesitate to make contact with them. Early on, you may be so
focused on your baby that you are unaware of the others. But as your
baby stabilizes, you may look around and compare. You may wonder:

· Do these other parents understand what I'm going through—
even though our situations are so different?

· Is it normal for me to feel competitive about whose baby goes
home first with the least medical equipment? Do these other parents feel the same competitiveness toward my baby and me?

· If I talk to parents whose babies are doing better than mine, will
I envy or resent them? If I talk to parents whose babies are doing
less well than mine, will it be too depressing? Will I incur their
envy or resentment?

· If I talk to parents who are focused on their fears, will I be able
to hold on to my hopes? If I'm overwhelmed by my fears, can I
tolerate parents who talk only about their hopes?

Even in the NICU I felt inadequate, especially around more experienced NICU
parents. It was the only place I felt somewhat normal, but even then . . . I just felt
like a freak.—Diana

Seeing other kids in the NICU posed problems, since we weren't supposed to compare. Some other kids weren't doing as well as our girls. It was tragic. It was very depressing and made us recognize how limited any parent's control is. On the other hand, I remember that triplets were born and released after just a few days. I remember Rikki thought it was unfair and that she had let the girls down by not holding them in longer.—Dwight

All these other preemies were so sick, and I had one of the only ones that was doing really well. I felt embarrassed that mine was doing so well, and I felt so bad for them. I was so happy, but because of them I felt ashamed that I was so happy.—Gallice

Sometimes appearances can be deceiving. For instance, beautiful full-term babies can have catastrophic and fatal conditions that are not visible. If your baby looks like the picture of health by comparison, whether your baby is doing well or not, you may worry about disheartening the parents of tinier, sicker-looking infants.

Visiting Ellie in the NICU was surreal because here was our big, almost ten-pound girl lying in the bassinet, filling it up from head to toe. We couldn't help but chuckle that she was almost too big for the thing. Looking around the room were these tiny premature babies who looked sick and unhealthy. Other than all of the tubes that Ellie was hooked up to, she was this big, beautiful, healthy-looking baby. I remember feeling guilty about that and wondering what other parents thought who saw her next to their babies.—Angie

Still, despite any uncomfortable undercurrents, talking with other parents in the NICU can benefit you enormously. These conversations let you establish your credentials as parents who understand each other's emotional ordeals. As you share information about your children, you can form supportive connections. In fact, when you are a newcomer to the NICU, you may feel an odd sense of comfort when you see new babies like your own arrive. New admissions mean that you aren't the only novice struggling to acclimate to the NICU and grappling with harsh realities. But as time passes and you grow more accustomed to this place, it may hurt you to see new parents arrive. Your heart goes out to them as you remember what a struggle those early days were. The longer your time in the NICU, the less you'll care about the situational differences, competition, envy, resentment, and whether the talk focuses on hopes or fears. What will matter most is the common ground of parenting a precious baby in the NICU.

It was hard, going in there every day and passing by the babies that were smaller than him. . . . But by the same token, we were sharing the same heartbreak of not being able to take a baby home with us, going through the experience of being on that unit, and the grief and agony and joy of going through the hurdles.—Vickie

Finding out how other babies are doing can give you some perspective about your child. You can feel fortunate for the complications your baby has avoided. When you learn how babies farther along than yours are faring, you can begin to imagine what might lie ahead and prepare yourself for the possibilities. The flip side is that when you look at babies who aren't doing well, you may feel terrified about your baby's future.

Making comparisons is inevitable and natural. It can help to remember, though, that every baby's course is unique. Another baby's roller coaster isn't necessarily a gauge of how your baby will fare. Even though another baby's progress is faster than your baby's, your little one's outcome may be just as good. Comparisons become more pointed when other preemies die or when other preemies go home.

When Other Babies Die

You could tell when things were upbeat, and you could tell when things were going bad because people would talk in whispers or quieter tones or there'd be times when the nurses would be crying.—Tim

The hardest part of NICU life was seeing some of the babies die. You sympathized and mourned for them, feared for your own child, and were secretly thankful it was not you.—Laura

Whether or not your unit encourages contact between parents, it is likely that you will get to know some other families whose babies are in the NICU. Even if you do not know each other's names, you will recognize one another. If a baby is not doing well, the parents and the medical staff will often reflect this reality—the unit climate may seem grim, more fearful. And as you sit with your baby, you are faced with stark evidence of what could have happened—or might still happen—to your little one.

I think one of the saddest experiences was the second day after Andrew was born. . . . I went with another NICU mom to go see our babies, and I just remember looking at her baby, thinking, *I feel so lucky. How did I get this, a baby who had a better chance than her baby?* Then I went back to another room, and I wasn't there ten minutes and the nurse came and told me that that mom's baby had just died. . . . I think that was the first time that I realized the seriousness of having a premature baby. I didn't realize that if there's one thing a preemie will do, it will keep you guessing. A baby may be looking good right now and in ten minutes be coding. I think that was the first time I actually cried after Andrew was born, realizing what we might be in for.—Vickie

When another baby dies, you might grieve right along with that baby's parents. Knowing how painful it is to have a critically ill baby, you identify closely with those parents. You recognize the depth of their bereavement. You can hardly bear to imagine being in their place. If you yourself have experienced the death of a baby, your grief may be triggered anew. You aren't just identifying with those parents; you've been there. And you can only hope you won't find yourself there again.

Our closest friend in the NICU lost her son after six months, two weeks before our son was discharged. How do you express your feelings of such deep loss? How do you comfort someone who has lost something you still have? How could we possibly understand what she was going through? How do you look at a beautiful little baby in a doll-sized coffin? How do you put him in the cold, dark ground in the pouring rain? All she kept saying was that he was getting wet. . . . After his death, we hit our breaking point. We needed to get out of there. We pushed, and two weeks later we took our son home.—Laura

I'm so upset. . . . Nathan's father was one of the pallbearers, and he watched as they lowered Nathan into the ground. He was so brave to do that. But then, that's what being a parent is all about, I guess. Always watching over your baby and making sure that [he's] safe, whether it be warm and comfortable in an incubator or ensuring that his coffin is set down softly and gently.—Leanne

Especially if your baby is in critical condition, a death in the NICU may prompt an eerie feeling that your child could be next. This reaction is natural, but remember, one child's outcome has no impact on another's. Also keep in mind that most NICU babies survive—neonatal intensive care works most of the time. If you've been afraid to bring up the possibility of your baby dying, another baby's death can give you an opening to discuss your fears with your baby's medical team. Ask how your baby's situation differs from the other child's so you can get some reassurance.

When Other Babies Go Home

Whether you spend days, weeks, or months in the NICU with your baby, you are bound to see other infants who are getting ready to go home. Discharges can give you some hope for the future—babies really *do* leave this place. But discharges can bring up a variety of painful feelings as well:

- *You may harbor intense sadness, envy, even anger.* You want to take your baby home, not just watch others take their babies home!

- *You may feel impatient, as if you and your baby will never get out of here.* Watching babies come and go is so hard—especially if the babies going home were admitted to the NICU way more recently than yours.

- *You may wonder whether your baby's discharge will be similar.* Will your baby be that healthy or look that robust? Will your baby also be accompanied by monitors and medical devices?

- *You may feel competitive.* If a baby with continuing medical needs is discharged, you may wonder why your baby can't go home as well.

- *You may feel fearful.* If a baby with clear medical or developmental needs is discharged, you may worry whether you could care for your baby at home with needs like those.

If you wonder whether your baby's discharge may be complicated or delayed, ask. While your baby's practitioners can't look into a crystal ball, you can request detailed information about what they are thinking and how they are formulating your baby's unique prognosis.

What to Remember about Comparisons

If you feel uncomfortable about your impulse to compare your baby with others in the NICU, it may help to keep these ideas in mind:

- *It is normal to compare yourself and your baby with others in the NICU.* Comparisons are part of getting acquainted with the landscape and forming relationships. As you get to know other parents, you'll feel surrounded and comforted by this community.

· *Making competitive comparisons may signal the need to work through your losses.* When you find yourself comparing your baby competitively with other NICU babies, recognize that you may need to acknowledge and work through a particular loss or injury to your parental identity and confidence. For example, you might be struggling with having a baby who still needs oxygen while surrounding babies are on room air.

· *Each baby is different.* Comparing your baby to others can provide perspective but will not necessarily give you an accurate view of what is in store for your child.

· *Maintain some separation from others' heartbreak.* If you are especially sensitive and empathic with others' heartbreaking situations, calm yourself with this mantra: "It's not me. It's not my baby. Right now, we're doing okay. It's not us."

· *Celebrate your child's accomplishments*, even if other babies have not reached that stage. Other parents may envy you and your baby, but you also give them hope for the future.

· *Your experience is valid!* No matter how early your baby's birth or how complicated or straightforward the hospital course, your experience of loss, trauma, and disorientation is valid.

When we were in the NICU, we saw so many come and go while we waited to see if our survivor would survive. I couldn't identify with people [who were] there so briefly, dealing with a temporary, resolvable problem concerning their baby(ies). I couldn't understand how someone could fall apart while dealing with premature infants (especially multiples) who were comparatively healthy, who would all go home soon. Truth be told, I felt a sort of contempt, not to mention raging envy, at their reactions to the less daunting challenges that they faced.

And then I saw people lose their only child, both their twins, all of their triplets. I saw tragic, beaten parents leave that godforsaken NICU with no one, with nothing to show for their suffering. And I realized that I was to them what the others were to me. I realized that suffering comes in degrees, yes, but whatever degree is thrust upon you seems unbearable because it is the worst you have known. I realized that any parent dreaming of a healthy pregnancy, a normal delivery, a beautiful child—the parent that each of us is at the beginning—any parent who ends up in a NICU, for whatever reason, for whatever period, has something to grieve. And our grief expands to fill whatever void it marks in our lives.—Susan C.

Making Medical Decisions in the Gray Zone

On the NICU roller coaster, when a baby's condition is unstable or poor *and* the prognosis is unclear, this is known as the gray zone. An unclear prognosis means that the doctors are uncertain as to whether the baby will benefit from intensive care. Some babies, when coaxed by aggressive intervention, will cling to life for a time, only to die anyway after much suffering. Other babies will pull through but continue to be challenged by medical conditions and/or developmental delays in the long term. Still other babies surprise everyone and do fairly well after a time, perhaps with negligible or only mild challenges. When a baby is in the gray zone, it's unclear which of those paths he or she will take.

Outside the gray zone, the prognosis is clear (whether good or grim), and doctors are decision leaders, confident in pointing to either intensive care or hospice care. But in the gray zone, because the prognosis is unclear, doctors invite the parents to become the decision leaders. The neonatologists share what they know and discuss with parents the specific burdens of treatment and how benefits and outcomes remain speculative. Because the parents are most closely connected to their infant and the ones who will bear the consequences, the medical team follows their lead.

These are grave decisions that are a matter of life and death. Should medical staff intervene aggressively, or is it best to let nature take its course? Choosing between intensive care and hospice care is an agonizing decision to make and an immense parental responsibility. It involves assessing the severity of the baby's problems, poring over the options, considering the potential benefits and harm of aggressive intervention, changing minds a dozen times, or choosing to rely on the doctors' wealth of professional experience and recommendations. After the decision is made, parents must face the outcome, whatever it might be.

If you have to decide how aggressively to treat the most devastating complications of your infant's condition, you may feel the most protective of your baby and the most connected to him or her. What a crushing time to feel the full weight of parenthood.

At one point, when he was about two days old, they told us they didn't think he'd survive through the night. They asked me, if he stopped breathing completely, did I want him to be resuscitated. Before he was born, I automatically said that yes, I wanted him to be saved. But after he was born, I tried to think about him and the pain he must be in and how it might be better for him if I just let him go. But I finally decided I couldn't do it. We had to sign papers saying that they could try to save him. I felt terrible, like I was causing my baby all of this pain. But I couldn't let him go. It was something I really agonized over.—Jennifer A.

As Geoffrey was born, not breathing, looking so pitiful, I wondered if we should have done a DNR and just let Geoffrey pass. He was obviously not comfortable and looked so little and frail. The guilt I felt was with the question *Were we being selfish and putting a baby through all of that so we could have a baby and me a son in particular?*—Shaw

If you decide to try or continue intensive care, you are betting that the benefits will outweigh the risks or harm. If you decide to decline intensive care, your instincts as a parent are leading you to protect your baby from invasive and painful procedures and a life of suffering. Whatever you decide, you make what you believe is the most compassionate choice for your baby's situation. You make your decision with the best of intentions and with the deepest love.

Some parents reach for a trial of aggressive intervention, only to question their decision in hindsight. For the parents whose babies survive but at a price, they emerge from the NICU saying, "Never again."

Somehow, we were reconciled to his death yet couldn't bear to allow it to occur without extending him every possible chance. We consented to surgery, something I'll always regret, but only in hindsight. Soon, we were holding our tiny son as he died in our arms. . . . If only I had known what I know now.—Susan C.

I honestly don't know what I would do if I went into preterm labor again. I might not run to the hospital. I hope I never need to find out. Sometimes I think you need to let nature take its course. Alex suffered a lot with all his surgeries. I can't imagine life without him, even though it would be a lot easier.—Mo

Indeed, some parents say in hindsight that the right decision would have been to let their child die as a newborn rather than put him or her through a painful life. As Suzanne points out, even though there were moments of joy, she believes the suffering was too high a price to pay.

If I faced this decision again, I don't think it would be as hard to decide. I wouldn't blink an eye about stopping life support, or not beginning it on any baby who had little or no chance for survival, or when survival would probably mean enduring a life of continued suffering. I'd be sad and I'd grieve, but I'm not willing to take those odds. I'm not willing to have my child take those odds.—Suzanne

Neonatal Hospice

What happens when a baby's prognosis is unclear and parents turn away from intensive care? What happens when a baby's prognosis is clearly grim and there is no beneficial treatment? This section offers you a window into the what-if that preys on many parents' minds. It can be a difficult read, but it offers reassurance by illuminating this path and the compassionate options that exist.

Andrew was able to meet Ellie just a couple of hours after she was born, and he was sure he felt her squeeze his finger . . . Later, when I went into the NICU, the nurse gently turned Ellie's head toward me so I could see her since I was sitting low and couldn't get out of the chair. When she turned Ellie's head, Ellie opened her right eye a crack and looked at me. Those were the only responses we ever got from her. What a blessing that she would give her mommy and daddy! When we held her later, there was no additional response. She didn't cuddle in, didn't squeeze fingers, didn't respond to touch. We never heard her cry. I know now that we had lost her long before we made our decision not to keep her on life support . . . As difficult as it was, we ultimately made the right decision for our daughter.—Angie

Long gone are the days when neonatologists felt obligated to use the technology even when all it did was induce suffering or prolong dying. State-of-the-art neonatal intensive care includes knowing when it's in the child's best interests to withhold or withdraw intensive treatment. When there is nothing more that intensive care can do to save a child's life or extend it without inducing suffering or dependence on artificial life support, treatment turns to palliative care and hospice.

Palliative care reduces suffering and is appropriate for all babies in the NICU. But in the context of hospice, palliative care focuses on making the baby completely comfortable by removing medical technology, eliminating pain, and supporting the parents and family as they spend time with their dying infant.

Sometimes this path is recommended by the doctors who can unequivocally state that a baby is dying and there is no fix. Other times, when a baby's outcome is uncertain but looking grim, this path is chosen under collaborative decision making between the parents and medical team. For parents, their hearts, minds, and gut instincts inform this decision. Seeing their baby's suffering, sensing that intensive care will only lead to more suffering, and knowing that they themselves would not choose this kind of life, it becomes clear that their courage lies in letting go.

I was told I needed to think about what I wanted to do if there were complications. If he coded, what did I want to happen? The doctor said, "We can work on a kid for forty-five minutes, but at that point there can be so much damage, especially with a child his age, that what you save may not be worth saving—for him, for you." So I said, "I want him to have quality of life."—Micki

I remember thinking, *I can handle this. You know, she just lies in her bed, we can G-tube-feed her, she's got oxygen, she's not in pain. I could do this forever. It's okay.* And even before that crossed my mind, I thought, *No, it's not okay, it's not okay for her. It's no life for her.*—Suzanne

When hospice care is invoked, parents can see their baby's face and body without the mask of intensive care. Parents can hold their baby without the encumbrance of technology, and they don't have to worry about oxygen saturations or other vital signs. Some parents are able to take their baby home to die. For many parents, the hospice decision is confirmed by the sense of freedom and peace that surrounds them and their baby.

They called and said that he was going down quickly. So I rushed over there and I got to hold him like any baby. It was so neat. He was just so beautiful and so perfect. It was weird too. He was dying but you don't really see it. Then they took him away, and then they took the respirator stuff off, and he died right away pretty much, so I got to hold him some more.—Charlie

With my son Gavin, I am glad I was able to hold him while he left this life just to be able to let him know that I was there for him. . . . I remember holding him, when they took off the vent, and he looked at me as I started to cry. His look was almost as if to let me know that he was gonna be okay. It's a look that will be burnt into my memory forever.—Jamie

The last time we held him was when we took him off life support, which was the most difficult day of my life and was a very bittersweet moment. I wish I could have held him forever.—Corin

When she died, oh, her face changed dramatically, from this tortured, slack, no-tone [look] to just so peaceful. And I literally really think I could see her spirit lifting, and I was like, "Go for it. Go, baby." . . . All I could think was that she was out of her pain, out of her suffering.—Suzanne

Some people wonder whether seeing and holding a baby makes grief more painful—whether it causes parents to become "too attached." But, of course, the parents' bond has formed already, and being able to nurture and soothe their dying baby offers rich and cherished memories. In fact, whenever possible, taking a baby home to die can be similarly healing, as it offers more time, privacy, and the ability to soak up the baby's essence and do whatever nurturing parents want to do.

We told him stories and made promises. I still owe him a day of kite flying, bubble blowing, and a baseball game. . . . I held him, and we spoke to him and stroked him, and I did get to rock him to sleep with no medical staff looking on. We lived two hours away from the hospital, and this was the first time we spent days with him. It helped us say good-bye.—Ed

If a baby dies in the hospital, instead of relinquishing the body to the morgue, parents can take their baby home and provide after-death care themselves, right up to the burial or cremation. As part of the green burial movement, this compassionate option is another healing opportunity to continue nurturing their baby and gradually realize that their baby is indeed gone, making relinquishing the body more natural.

If you must travel this path, you can find more information and support online at www.NICUparenting.org.

I feel his presence much of the time and feel very strongly that he is involved in our lives. Yoni will always remain a part of our family.—Micki

I sang to my son, right before he passed away, "Now I lay me down to sleep, I pray the Lord my soul to keep." And now before I go to bed every night, I say that, to keep him knowing that I'm here and I'll see him someday. This way, when I die, he'll know where to find me.—Charlie

Decisions about Long-Term Care

God didn't do this. This is not God's plan, nor is it his will. It just happened. What I have decided is that God wants to help me through this by guiding me in making decisions. This may mean that eventually Alex goes into foster care. . . . Sometimes God does give you more than you can handle.—Mo

When a baby's condition has been stabilized and is no longer critical, but the baby continues to require significant and ongoing specialized care or medical equipment, parents face agonizing decisions about long-term care. When home care is not feasible, parents might choose to move their baby temporarily to a rehabilitation hospital or a long-term care facility. When an institution is the best place, parents can still be very much involved, and this can be a permanent solution for some families. If parents decide that neither home nor an institution is the answer, they can relinquish their child to a medical foster home or an adoptive family who can manage complicated medical needs or severe disabilities. This placement can happen straight from the NICU or down the road.

If you face decisions about how to meet your baby's significant and ongoing special needs, just as with life-and-death decisions, you can rely on your devotion to your baby's best interests, your careful consideration of all the available options and information, and what your mind, heart, and gut tell you. Know that your decision is based on love, not rejection. Acknowledge your limitations honestly, and remember that thoughtful, realistic decisions are responsible and healthy. There is no right or wrong choice, but simply what you believe is best for your baby, you, and your family. Also keep in mind that most decisions are not written in stone. As needs and situations change, you may be able to reevaluate. Finally, accept that difficult decisions entail painful feelings. Feeling badly doesn't mean that the decision is wrong. Whatever you decide, you will have losses to grieve, cope with, and recover from.

The Extended NICU Stay

When treatment, recovery, or growth is complicated, the discharge date remains uncertain. If your baby's NICU stay is much longer than expected, your hopes may have been raised numerous times, only to be dashed by many sudden deteriorations or crises. Without a clear timeline, your baby's hospitalization can feel like running a never-ending marathon. The ongoing separation from your baby and the disruption to your life can become difficult to tolerate.

I didn't realize until weeks into their hospitalization how much the NICU environment along with their ongoing hospitalization were wearing on me. I lost it one morning. I can't remember what triggered it, specifically. I just remember feeling like we were all on a forced march with no end in sight.—Rikki

Balancing your hopes and fears over the long haul becomes more challenging. You know that a long stay in the NICU does not always end with a triumphant homecoming. Some babies are not discharged home but to a long-term care facility. Others spend many months in the hospital only to die. You may wonder if this will happen to your little one.

Pacing yourself through a not-just-temporary NICU stay is challenging. You may agonize about the amount of time you are spending at the hospital, especially if the demands of older children, distance from the hospital, or other stresses pull at you. If you work outside the home, you must allocate parental leave—how much to spend at the hospital with your struggling baby and how much to set aside for homecoming.

As the hospital stay lengthens, you may find that you start to feel distant from your baby. This is a natural way to protect yourself from the blows of repeated disappointments or extended uncertainties. Although you cannot completely avoid the hurt, occasional distancing can sometimes help you to survive this endurance test.

As you search for balance between hopes and fears, home life and hospital life, and connection and disconnection, guilt is natural. You wish that you could do everything for your child—but real life intrudes. It is common to feel that every aspect of your life is suffering. Although this balancing act is very tiring, establishing a routine can give you some welcome predictability and some sense of normalcy. (See other coping strategies in "Waiting with Uncertainty" earlier in this chapter.)

Someday, when you can look back on your baby's NICU stay, you will do so with wonder. You'll realize that when life is most challenging, you simply do what you have to do. It wasn't an easy time and you may have some regrets, but you'll be able to look back at the bigger picture with pride. You did the impossible—and you did it well.

Points to Remember

· *Most babies follow a medical course that is a roller coaster ride of ups and downs, triumphs and setbacks. Parents experience the same bumpy, unpredictable ride.*

· *Waiting, especially in the face of uncertainties and unpredictability, can be frustrating and unnerving. As you settle in, you can learn to wait with your baby and to find richness and meaning during this time.*

· *Maintaining your balance between hope and fear isn't easy, but working at it can help prepare you for whatever may happen—and help you wait with your baby.*

· *Comparing your baby with others in the NICU is an inevitable part of establishing a much-needed connection with other parents and gaining perspective. Neither you nor your baby is a contestant in the NICU. Each baby is an individual on a unique path.*

· *With two or more babies in the NICU, it's common for one baby's ride to smooth out and another's to take a plunge. Keep individual journals for each baby and focus on overall progress instead of hourly or daily variations.*

· *If you face or have made life-and-death decisions for your baby, know that your love and devotion guide those decisions. In time you will be able to make peace with your decision, let go of what might have been, and accept what is.*

· *If your baby has an extended NICU stay, it can be particularly important to establish a routine that injects balance and respite into your life.*

· *Despite the difficulty of riding the NICU roller coaster, when you look back at this time, you'll see that you prevailed and even grew. You may have some regrets, but you'll recognize that you did the impossible, and you did it well.*

10:
Discharge and Homecoming

Suddenly, when the day of discharge came close, I felt confused because I longed for it so much, and still I wasn't prepared. I felt that taking him home could be dangerous, considering germs, and I didn't trust my ability to take care of him. I was very happy that we could pack our things and go home but knew I would desperately miss the contact with the nurses.

After the doctor told us we were going to get to take Sarah home the next day, I walked around in a fog. I was thrilled, excited, scared, and generally nuts.—Cindy

Discharge and *homecoming.* These two words are loaded with meaning for parents in the NICU. Day after day, perhaps week after week, with a lump in your throat, you try not to notice new parents being escorted out the hospital door, taking their babies home while yours remains in the NICU.

In the beginning, even if discharge is just around the corner, it can seem faraway and elusive. If your baby is extremely premature or requires lengthy treatment and recovery, discharge may seem impossible.

Still, you eagerly anticipate the day when the term *discharge planning* will be directed at you and your baby.

The night before Ryan was discharged, I was sitting there with him and Elizabeth [Ryan's twin], who had already been discharged and saying good-bye to all the nurses—we all cried tears of joy! I remembered early on seeing the nurses parade around with a baby ready to go home and thinking, *Will that ever be us?* When it finally was us, it was incredible!—Sara

In many ways, the feelings associated with discharge and homecoming are similar to those felt by parents of "regular" newborns. But in addition to the typical worries and adjustments, you must accommodate your baby's very real medical needs and attend to potential developmental concerns. You may also have mixed emotions about bringing home *this* baby—who's not the "typical" baby you had imagined during your pregnancy. Although being home at last with your baby can be a joy and a relief, you may also feel disorientation, anxiety, doubt, and renewed grief. This chapter offers strategies for coping as well as tips for preparing yourself and taking over the care of your little one with confidence.

Finding a Pediatrician

One of the main tasks in preparing for your baby's discharge is to decide who will follow your baby's medical care beyond the NICU. Selecting a pediatrician, general practitioner, or other specialists and therapists can be comforting because it ensures that you and your baby won't be adrift or isolated from medical support after discharge.

But your selection process is more complicated now that your baby's requirements might be different from what you expected. After the NICU, your ideas, questions, and concerns about care are bound to have changed. You may also have a clearer sense of what you need in a relationship with any medical practitioner. You certainly want someone who is knowledgeable, thorough, responsive, available, and reassuring without being dismissive. You will want a physician who respects your role and considers you a teammate.

I remember thinking when he came home and got sick, *I don't know how to deal with this. They did.* There was a real sense of fear. I remember calling my pediatrician and apologizing. And he said, "You are the one mom in my practice who gets to be a hysterical mom. Don't ever try to do it yourself. Call me. We'll get past this stage, and things will settle down."—Kathy

When deciding on a pediatrician—or any other practitioner—here are some issues to consider:

- Is this practitioner in independent practice or part of a group? How is on-call and vacation coverage arranged? How do you reach the doctor in an emergency?

- Does this practitioner see your vigilance as a healthy adaptation to having a fragile newborn or a sign of pathological anxiety? Will this person honor your job as parent and partner in your baby's care?

- Does this practitioner value your input and boost your confidence in yourself as a parent?

- What is this doctor's approach to collaborating with other physicians and specialists? Does this fit with your ideas and your baby's needs?

- Who will coordinate medical care if your baby must see multiple specialists?

- What is the practitioner's stance on breast-feeding? How much support and encouragement can you expect if you are committed to breast-feeding but still struggling?

- Is this practitioner specifically experienced with infants like yours?

- What is this practitioner's attitude toward developmental follow-up?

- Do you get the impression that your questions or concerns will be taken seriously rather than brushed off?

- What sort of support do you feel you need as a parent? Does this practitioner appear to be interested and able to provide this type of support—or refer you to other sources of support?

- What does your intuition tell you about how well you and this practitioner can work together? Do your styles of relating mesh well? Does this person seem warm and open to you?

Choosing a pediatrician and other practitioners can be a challenge for any parent. It's okay to make a decision and then switch if the fit is not good. There are many physicians, nurses, specialists, and therapists who work very well with NICU babies and families, and you shouldn't have to settle for less. You and your baby deserve to get the extra care, reassurance, and support you need.

I do remember calling, saying, "His oximeter reading is __. His heart rate is __." I asked the doctor months later, "What do you think about a parent like me, giving you all of these numbers?" He [told me], "You're just like the parent who calls in and says, 'He's breathing real fast. His heart is racing.' It's the same thing. You're just giving me the numbers. Don't worry. You're not an abnormal mom."—Kathy

It's important to find a pediatrician who knows about preemies. They say it doesn't matter because once they're home they've left the hospital and left all those things behind. But it's important. If it's important to you that your friends understand, it's a hundred times more important that your pediatrician understands.—Marcia

Transferring Back to Your Local Hospital

When the NICU is far away from home, many parents experience a wrinkle in discharge: the baby is first discharged to a local hospital.

If your baby was admitted to a distant NICU for higher-level care, you may have felt grateful for the top-notch attention but stressed by the distance. Now with this transfer, your attitude may flip—you're grateful to have your baby closer to home but stressed by adjusting to a new place. And the transfer itself can be nerve-racking.

The actual transfer was scary. Both babies were loaded into the same incubator with tons of equipment and one NICU nurse. We followed them down to the ambulance bay and watched as they were loaded into an ambulance for a fifty-mile ride, mostly on big-city toll roads. I almost panicked as the ambulance pulled away. They had never been outside the NICU before, let alone careening down a toll road at sixty-five miles per hour.—Julie

Moving to the local nursery entails a significant adjustment—to the level of care, the staff, and the protocol. For instance, you may feel concerned that the local unit lacks the technology of the higher-level NICU. It's important to remember that your baby doesn't require all those bells and whistles any more. Much of the technology you came to see as comforting is no longer necessary.

You may also miss the doctors and nurses you came to know and trust. Will this new crew give your baby the same careful treatment? Of course, you can expect them to be just as careful, even though they may appear less concerned about your now-thriving infant. As long as your baby is doing well, consider a more relaxed environment to be a good sign. Plus, as a matter of course, you are likely to have freer access to your baby.

Soon enough, you'll be acquainted with the new landscape and the medical staff. If you want the team at the other hospital to communicate with this team about your baby's care plan, kangaroo care, feeding, or your level of involvement with your baby, speak up.

Medical practitioners are generally eager to share expertise and do what benefits the babies and families in their care.

You'll certainly appreciate the shortened travel distance, the ease with which you can spend time with your baby, and the extra time for tending to priorities.

Getting used to the new NICU was very hard. Our local hospital is only a Level II NICU, and they just weren't used to dealing with babies who had my trio's history. I felt better knowing that the neonatologist at our local hospital had studied under our neonatologist at their birth hospital, but it seemed I knew so much more than the nurses. The first day was a frustrating round of evaluations from neonatologists, respiratory therapists, anyone even remotely responsible for Clare and Emily's care. I felt they were being used as guinea pigs because the staff in the local hospital rarely had the opportunity to care for micropreemies. The gals were exhausted and cranky for days. Things were more lax here than at the large hospital. Since Clare was only on a tiny amount of oxygen, they didn't take it as seriously as they should have. Luckily, I was holding her when she had an apnea episode. (They were doing periodic weans at the time.) Scared the heck out of everyone. After that, there was a respiratory therapist sitting bedside during any wean. But lax also worked in our favor. Aunts and uncles as well as grandparents were finally able to visit the gals. Clare and Emily were showered with attention and someone holding them practically every hour of the day. It made me feel better knowing they had so many visitors because I was still occupied with Jacob, who was still at the birth hospital an hour away from home.—Julie

If this transfer was eagerly awaited, it may feel like a triumph. But if this transfer is made for insurance reasons, you may feel angry and scared, wondering if cost is trumping your baby's safety. If you are worried, state your concerns, ask questions, and protest vigorously if you are not convinced that moving to your local hospital is in your baby's best interests.

The Transition to Discharge

I don't think anyone is emotionally prepared to bring her baby home. I remember watching other babies being discharged. The parents would walk in to the NICU and the nurses would say, "Would you like to take your baby home today?" I was not going to have any of that. I needed preparation. I told the staff that as soon as there were even rumors among the docs that one of the babies would be going home soon, they had to tell me so I could prepare.—Susan B.

As time passes and you witness your baby's growth and resilience, you may contemplate your baby's discharge with a mixture of hesitancy, impatience, apprehension, and eagerness. The thought of taking your baby home is a thrill, but leaving the relative safety of the hospital and going out into the dangers of the real world may give you pause. Mostly, you may feel anxious and unprepared. Still, you can't wait to have free access and hold your little one *whenever you want*. Will your baby be coming home this week or next? If a discharge date has been set, you may feel overwhelmed with anticipation about having your little one home.

Especially if your baby's NICU stay was lengthy, approaching discharge can be like returning to a wild part of the NICU roller coaster. Even though your baby's graduation from the NICU is exciting, in some ways you may dread it.

Looking back, I think that despite our protests that we wanted them home as soon as possible, we got very dependent on the order and expertise represented by the NICU setup. We were confident and skilled at being proponents for our children but not ready for a primary caregiving role. I also think we got used to the lifestyle—as inconvenient as it was—of having our schedule of visiting them and leaving our parental responsibilities at the door of the NICU. What made it even scarier was that we surprised ourselves by hearing out loud how vociferous our objections were in reaction to the news that they'd be coming home.—Dwight

For us, since we had two other kids at home, we were not that eager to have him home as soon as possible. For me, the longer he could stay in the hospital with good care in a pretty safe environment—of course, hospitals can be a source of infection and all sorts of bad things, but I saw it as a safer place than our house full of germs.—Gallice

Until your baby's caregivers begin to discuss discharge dates, you might not realize how nervous and vulnerable you feel. You may not even recognize your hesitancy until your baby is finally turned over to you. Still, in the push and pull between wanting your baby to stay in the NICU and wanting your baby to come home, home wins.

When it finally came close to time to take Sean home, I became really nervous. On the one hand, I wanted my baby home more than anything. It seemed like it had been forever since I had given birth to him. On the other hand, I was scared. What if something happened? What if he stopped breathing and I panicked and forgot what to do? What if? What if? What if? (I'm a worrier by nature, anyway, so I was just awful at that time.) But I finally decided I could do it. I figured God wouldn't give me this beautiful, strong-willed boy, let him grow, and then when I got attached and brought him home, take him away from me. So home we went.—Ami

I nearly passed out while they were going over the discharge instructions, I was so overwhelmed. I was scared to take her off the monitors and leave the care of the hospital, where I knew they could help her if something went wrong. I was so incredibly nervous walking out of the hospital but overjoyed as well. When we got her home I finally felt like I could bond with my baby knowing no one was watching or evaluating. I could kiss and talk to her and finally felt like a mommy.—Corin

It was not until we unhooked her from the monitors that I realized how scary this would be. Thus far, she had been supervised around the clock. Her vital signs were monitored at every moment. Suddenly, it did seem too soon! I was afraid that she would stop breathing at home and we would not know. But more than that, I wanted her at home with us. I could not wait to lay her in a real crib! As I carried her out of the hospital, it began to feel right.—Renee

Practicing Care

Fortunately in many hospitals, preparation for discharge involves several steps that build your parenting confidence. As your baby stabilizes, you participate more and more in your infant's basic care. You gain practice diapering, bathing, and feeding your little one—with any needed guidance from the nurses. By the time you take your baby home, you may feel like a pro.

Many hospitals have what they call a step-down or transitional unit for babies whose primary needs are to master feeding and to continue to grow and heal. Babies in step-down are often cared for less by nurses and more by parents. A step-down unit is a calm, encouraging environment in which you can become even more familiar and comfortable with your baby's particular care.

If the hospital doesn't have a transitional unit, you can ask to take your baby into a separate room so you can parent in private, without the hovering and watchful eyes of staff. Some hospitals encourage nesting, where you can spend a day and a night or two in the hospital with your baby. This can feel like a test of your abilities, but it's really a chance for you to gain confidence as your baby's sole caregiver while you have the security of the medical team nearby for consultation.

Before going home, we spent the night in the NICU's parents' room—against medical advice, as we were told to go home and get one last good night's sleep. But I wanted to take care of Molly for the first time knowing that the nurses were right down the hall. I don't think any of us got any sleep that night, so we were exhausted by the time we got home.—Susan B.

The doctor said we could take him home if we stayed overnight in the hospital. Yeah!!! We got everything ready, and I was so excited I forgot to wash my hands when I got him. The nurse wheeled him in with his crib into the little room. She instructed us finally on how to care for him. I felt a little scared when she said that even a cold could put his life in danger, but I hardly listened because I was just in bliss holding him.

That night I did kangaroo care all night long. We didn't even use the lame crib they wheeled in for him. I was so excited. I changed his diaper every three hours and fed him whenever he wanted it! I was feeding him on demand and I was proud of it, although the nurse seemed to be surprised. I was most afraid of them thinking I was unable to care for him, though. But I didn't need the nurses' help at all the whole night! After that, I was very confident that I could take care of him myself and I could hold him all I wanted and cuddle with him all day and all night.—Ruby

The day before he left the NICU, we had all kinds of training to complete, and that night I had to stay with him alone in a room to prove that I could do it. I was so nervous that I would do something wrong and they wouldn't let us take him home that I barely slept a wink. When we walked out of the NICU, I couldn't believe they were actually letting us take him with us, and I shed a few tears.—Mindy

Some hospitals encourage transitional steps like these, whereas others are not physically set up for such experiences or are not philosophically inclined to provide them. If you do not have the chance to experience these transitional steps or if your opportunities to practice caregiving are limited, you may feel especially anxious about bringing your baby home. After all, you may wonder, if you're not considered competent enough to take your baby from the nursery to a private room or participate in caregiving, how could you possibly be qualified to take your baby home from the hospital?

I was completely unready for coming home with her. I suppose you are never emotionally ready to come home with a child, but I wasn't even close. I didn't feel like I could handle her. You feel like everyone must be able to see how incompetent you think you are. You feel like you have a big neon sign over your head flashing "Incompetent mom, incompetent mom. I don't know what I'm doing. Take this child away from me!"—Beth

But even with plenty of practice, the thought of discharge home may be frightening, especially if your baby has ongoing medical needs. How can you be sure that your baby won't have another downturn while in your care? If your baby requires ongoing monitoring or treatment, how will you continue that kind of care at home? Even if your baby had a fairly easy course or is going to be discharged with a completely clean bill of health, you may feel a bit apprehensive about being solely responsible for your infant's well-being. What if you are not protective enough and something terrible happens? How will you even *know* if something terrible is happening? After your baby has been surrounded by medical professionals and technology, it can be hard to imagine that everything will be okay under your watchful eye alone.

When she got to the point where it was obvious she was okay and coming home, I was afraid of new motherhood. I mean, it took two shifts of nurses to care for her around the clock. How could I do it alone?—Kelli

I was afraid to not have the monitors. How do we know she is okay without a machine telling us she is okay?—Jennifer E.

As we drew close to the discharge date, not so much with Shayna's but surely with Daniel's, I knew he was going to have an apnea attack and turn blue on me one night, and I would have to do infant CPR. It felt comparable, I think, to standing at the edge of a platform about to do your first high dive, your first bungee jump, your first skydive. I was trying to psych myself up: "Okay, you can do this. Pay attention." They made us go to an infant CPR class. It was required, and I took it very seriously. I needed to know this because I felt that Daniel was going to need to be resuscitated once or twice by me. So did I feel like a parent? Not really. I felt like I was going to have to be the doctor, not the parent.—Mitch

Gaining Confidence in Your Caregiving Abilities

The last night, I roomed in with him in an isolation room, and what bliss it was to have him all to myself! Of course, the nurses were still coming in to check his vitals, but he was mine! The next day, amid much fanfare and video cameras, we took Stephen home. It felt so good to walk into my house with him in my arms. I sat on the couch and just held him and held him for hours. Finally, I could make the decisions on when or how to feed him or bathe him or dress him!—Tracy

Many factors can build your confidence. In the relationship-centered NICU, you are able to feel close to your baby. You have plenty of hands-on caregiving experience. The medical practitioners have confidence in you. As the NICU discharge date approaches, your baby has shed the need for intensive care and complicated technology. Your baby is responsive to you.

I got to room in with her in a private room the night before she came home. That was really special. They wanted to make sure I was comfortable with her home apnea monitor. We spent the night just cuddling. I thought how lucky I was that I already really knew my baby, whereas moms who have a two- or three-day-old baby are rooming in with a stranger. We had ten weeks under our belts and knew each other well. That was nice.—Kelli

Some parents feel confident in spite of a unit philosophy that doesn't encourage parent participation or a reluctant medical practitioner who lacks faith in parental competence. In the face of such doubt, confidence may be borne of defiance and impatience. You may be more than ready and pushing unequivocally for discharge.

The doctor explained his concern that it was too soon, that she needed to become more adept at bottling. He told us how hard they had all worked to ensure her survival and how they hesitated to send her home too early. I told him, simply and forcefully, that I had also worked very hard for the same things and that it was time for me to become her mother. I explained that I had risked my very life to bear her—and that we felt she would thrive at home. Our family physician was contacted, and he agreed to assume responsibility for her release from the hospital—and we took her home!—Renee

But most parents feel a mixture of confidence and apprehension. Even if the medical team is assuring you that your baby is ready for discharge, you may wonder if *you* are ready. But going home is exactly what you need to do because more time and experience caring for your baby is what will rebuild your faith in yourself as a strong and capable parent.

Here are some strategies that can build confidence and soften apprehension about parenting successfully at home:

- As your baby grows and improves in the NICU, imagine what it would feel like to leave the hospital with your own little bundle in your arms. Visualize being a calm and nurturing presence for your baby at home. Specifically envision holding and feeding your baby and all the soothing techniques you can try during fussy times. Visualizing success boosts your ease of attaining it.

- You may be especially anxious about your baby's homecoming if the attitudes and expectations of the medical team have not encouraged confidence in your ability to parent your tiny baby. But remember that hospital policy and unit attitudes are unrelated to your actual competence and readiness to be home with your baby. Some units simply keep parents at bay until discharge.

- Your *own* anxieties also do not reflect your actual competence. Your fears may be borne of inexperience and perhaps reflect the wound you suffered when you could not protect your infant from the condition that sparked the need for intensive care. The antidote? Assert yourself as a protective parent in the NICU. State your preferences about how your baby is handled; participate in feeding, diaper changing, bathing, dressing, and soothing; and take part in decisions about your baby's medical care.

- Whatever your situation, if you think you would benefit from more hands-on experience with your baby, ask your primary nurses about it. You might tell them that you feel unsure about your abilities and would like to practice certain caregiving tasks while they watch you and give you feedback or suggestions. Let them know you need to experience being the primary caregiver for extended periods in the NICU while you are still able to rely on their presence and consultation. Most nurses take pride in their abilities to teach and coach parents and would be glad to have such an eager pupil.

- If you have any questions about your baby's care, medical needs, future risk factors, or follow-up, ask them. Ask questions a second time if you are not sure about the answers. Inquire about written resources, and get instructions or information in writing, if that helps you. Don't be afraid to go back to the neonatologists and nurses to clarify anything you don't understand.

- When you find out that discharge is imminent, you may be tempted to spend *less* time in the hospital. You may be preoccupied with setting up the baby's room, stocking up, and arranging for additional help. You may try to clean house, run all your errands, and tie up all your loose ends, much like any parent whose due date is fast approaching. Although these nesting activities may seem pressing, be sure to spend enough time nesting at the hospital with your baby. Your homecoming will benefit much more from a greater acquaintance and practice with your baby than from a clean house and a stocked nursery. Remember too that cleaning, preparing, and shopping are practical chores that eager friends and relatives can do for you. Do only those home-nesting tasks that are most meaningful for you.

· Even if you have returned to work or live far away, try to spend as much time as you can with your baby in the days before discharge. Ask a primary nurse to be available, if necessary, while you take over your infant's care. Even if your NICU does not offer a formal transition process for the shift from hospital to home, you can create one for yourself.

· Request that any necessary training or specialized instruction take place several days before discharge. Trying to learn critical-care tasks at the last minute is likely to make you feel anxious, unprepared, and unable to retain the information. When you train in advance, you have time to absorb the lessons and the chance to ask questions and practice.

· If you are breast-feeding, see if you can stay overnight in the hospital to establish around-the-clock feeding for your baby before discharge.

· Even if you are not breast-feeding, ask if your hospital can accommodate you and your partner staying with your baby for one or more nights before homecoming. Think about doing this a few days before discharge so that you can still have one final full night's sleep before the big day.

· Remember, you can always call the NICU to ask questions or get reassurance after you and your baby are home.

Discharge with Multiple Babies

I was filled with mixed emotions when my babies came home! First of all, Karlianne came home two days before Alycia. I actually felt a little guilty for being so excited about Karlianne coming home.—Michele

Even after Ashley came home right before Christmas, it wasn't the same. I still had one other baby at the hospital and was still cheated out of being able to bring my twins home together from the hospital.—Rosa

Bringing home multiple babies involves extra challenges and compli-cations. Often, babies are discharged on different days. If this hap-pens with your babies, you may feel alternately relieved and distressed at the thought. Your joy at the homecoming of one baby does not negate the yearning you still feel toward the other(s). It's so hard to leave anyone behind.

My daughter was discharged first, ten days after my due date. We were so excited. It felt wonderful to finally bring her home, but in many ways it was much harder to have one baby at home while the other was still in the hospital. I felt terribly torn. —Susan B.

I was so torn. I was thrilled Sara was coming home, but I felt guilty that Zane and Carter were still in the hospital.—Jill

They were next to each other in the NICU for a long while, and then Riley got to come home. And then it was like—tugging on my heartstrings here again—Banning was saying, "My sister leaves, and I'm here all by myself." You know? And then I'm thinking, *Oh, he's going to think we abandoned him and that I love her better because she got to come home first.*—Pam

Derek came home more than a week before David. That was very hard. On one hand, I was so happy to get Derek home and go to my house and not an RV, but on the other hand, I felt like I was deserting David. When David came home, I finally felt like a complete family.—Jody

While staggered homecomings can make you feel torn and in limbo, there are advantages to you and your babies. Different discharge dates can

- reduce your anxiety about discharge,
- let you ease into homecoming one step at a time,
- allow you to get the hang of each baby individually,
- build confidence in your ability to handle all the caregiving, and
- give you the chance to gradually adjust to being at home with multiple babies.

Pam, who earlier acknowledged the difficulties of bringing home one baby at a time, talks here about the advantages. Then Betsy reflects on how appreciating the nurses' devotion helped her let go of her guilt when her triplets were discharged separately, a month apart.

Having a previous child, I know what it's like to take care of babies. I know they need a lot of attention. I was happy because [the twins] could come home one at a time, and I wasn't overwhelmed with both of them. And I could get to know Riley [at home] for those weeks because I knew her, but she wasn't like she was mine. And when Banning came home, it was the same thing. . . . So I was happy they got to come home one at a time just so we could do the bonding and getting to know each other.—Pam

Dylan's nurse was almost like his mother. I knew that she was constantly there taking care of him, giving him baths, brushing his hair, just doing the things that he needed her to do. He had that nurturing, and everybody would ask me, "Doesn't that make you feel weird?" No. I'm so happy that I can walk away and know that she's there and that he's being taken care of.—Betsy

If your babies are discharged on the same day, you're spared the emotional rending, but it isn't necessarily easier. Homecoming with more than one baby is a juggling act, with setting up, accommodating needs, learning preferences, and adjusting *multiplied*. If a part of you is dreading the onslaught, this is only natural. It is especially important for you to enlist some type of home assistance, whether from family, friends, community outreach, or employed help.

Discharge with Medical Equipment . . . or Without

Some babies are discharged without clear ongoing medical or developmental needs. Other babies go home with monitors for detecting breathing or heart rate irregularities. Still others are discharged with medical devices—for example, supplemental oxygen by cannula, a colostomy or an ileostomy, a gastrostomy tube or button, or a tracheotomy and a home ventilator. Leaving the hospital with equipment— or without it—prompts a variety of feelings in parents. Naturally, your reaction to how your baby is discharged reflects your attitudes toward your baby's medical needs. It can help you to be aware of your attitudes so you can make sense of your feelings and reframe or mindfully accept them.

Monitors

Home monitoring holds different meaning for different parents. If your baby is being sent home *with* a monitor, you might wonder if the hospital is discharging your baby too soon, in too fragile a state.

Although you may be eager to have your infant home, the technical gear may be worrisome. Monitoring can also seem like a burden, bothersome and tedious. As always, if you don't feel comfortable with your baby's discharge, talk to your baby's doctors about your concerns.

In contrast, if your baby is being discharged *without* a medical monitor, you may be relieved or see this as reassuring proof that your baby is robust enough to come home. Or perhaps you are reassured by NICU technology and *want* your baby to be sent home with monitors. You are accustomed to alarms alerting you to spells of apnea or bradycardia. You're used to knowing your little one's exact oxygen saturation levels. You've depended on technology to tell you whether your baby is okay or not, and you may not trust that you can monitor your baby's condition by observation alone.

If you found monitors comforting in the NICU but your baby is being discharged without them, it's because the medical team believes that your baby no longer needs constant monitoring. It might take a while for you to feel reassured, especially if the NICU has monitors on your baby until the moment of discharge. It's okay to ask for monitoring equipment at home—even if you use it only for a few days to help with the transition. It's a legitimate request.

Before she came home, she passed the sleep test, and we were not required to bring her home on a monitor. Nevertheless, for our own peace of mind, we did anyway. It only lasted for a few days: the alarm would only go off occasionally when she was nursing, and I could see that she was fine, so by the end of the first week we returned the machine. Basically we just got tired of the wires and carting the thing around.—Diana

Before or after discharge, if you have come to depend on monitoring for peace of mind, talk to your baby's doctor about weaning your baby *and* yourself. Ask your baby's practitioners to explain specifically what to look for so that you can practice focusing on your baby rather than the monitor. Finally, when you can see what they see, you can trust these professional assessments of your baby's growing resilience. Acknowledge what's behind the practitioners' confidence in your baby, and allow yourself to feel confident too.

Another factor to keep in mind is that every baby is different, and neonatologists vary in how they make this judgment call. So resist comparing your baby's discharge plan with another baby's. Also keep in mind that monitors do not offer some sort of magical protection. They don't *prevent* problems, they merely point to them, sometimes with a hypersensitivity that is less than helpful. If you have concerns, talk to the medical team about the pros and cons of having a home monitor for *your* baby.

Medical Devices

My husband took over the arrangements for the nurses and equipment, which included apnea monitors, oxygen, ambu bags, and nasal cannulas. It was a big job, not to mention keeping track of the insurance and paperwork. We felt pretty thrown into caring for the equipment as well as the babies, even though we had nursing help at home.—Susan B.

Medical devices are more intensive than monitors and typically treat short-term (but sometimes long-term) problems with breathing, feeding, or digestion. The decision to discharge a medically dependent baby is multifaceted. Getting out of the NICU reduces the risk for infection, and babies tend to thrive at home under the parents' care. Even though medical devices are required, intensive care is not.

For some parents, finally being able to take their baby home supersedes their feelings about the medical technology that comes along. Bringing the hospital home with you might even seem appealing after months of bringing yourself to the hospital. Especially if your baby's survival was uncertain, coming home with medical devices may seem peripheral to the big picture. In fact, this equipment can represent a safety net, as it did to Lara, who brought home her baby with a nasal cannula and oxygen tanks.

It's funny, but Gracie probably could have been off the oxygen a good month or so before we took her off it. Our pulmonologist, a wonderful, intuitive sweetheart of a guy, knew that I had to be weaned as much as Grace did. He had told me that we would do a sleep study once she came off, but we never did because it was abundantly clear she was ready once we decided to do it.—Lara

Other parents feel betrayed when medical devices accompany their baby home. Especially if you were told your baby would eventually recover without complications, coming home with equipment feels like a disappointment, tarnishing the joy you expected to feel. You probably assumed that your baby would graduate from medical devices before, not after, graduation from the NICU. Mostly, you want the medical intervention to be *over*.

I was absolutely devastated at the idea of bringing the twins home on oxygen. I had really believed that by the time they were ready to go home, they'd be ready, and I could leave the hospital behind. I wanted to go home, but not like that, not with the hospital following me. It took away some of the thrill of discharge. It was like a heavy cloud over us.—Rikki

David came home on oxygen and an apnea monitor. I hated both but understood that he needed them. People would look at us when they saw David's oxygen and sometimes made comments that were hurtful.—Jody

Bringing home a medically dependent baby can add a layer of grief to hospital discharge. You may also wonder if the need for medical devices is strong evidence that your little one is too fragile to be discharged into your care.

The most emotional and worried that I got was in reaction to the idea that we would be bringing the girls home while they were still on oxygen. It seemed very risky and seemed to require too much from us. We may have secretly believed that we were supposed to be handed children that required no special medical assistance, that the kids would stay in the NICU as long as they were "abnormal" or "catching up," and that we would get them to take home only when they were all done needing any special help. The fear that they were not ready for life outside the NICU and that we would fail them (or that the act of being released would fail them) was palpable.—Dwight

Your adjustment can depend on how you feel about the medical equipment itself. These devices can aid your baby's continued growth and survival. They also offer the reassurance of knowing you can feed your baby a measured amount through a tube or provide oxygen as necessary. But it can also signify to you that your baby could become a chronically ill child, one who will never be like other children. The sight of a feeding tube or nasal cannula may remind you of a sick relative—or the NICU—and trigger grief and fear. The thought of bringing your baby home with a gastrostomy tube or button may fill you with dread. Or you may alternate between assurance and anxiety.

With homecoming, you hope to join the ranks of "regular"

parents with their "regular" babies—but ongoing medical needs make this seem impossible.

I wanted to leave the hospital like other parents with their new babies. I was devastated that I'd have oxygen tanks in my house and that my babies wouldn't be like other babies. I felt like a failure. I was embarrassed. I had been assured that they'd be off oxygen by the time they came home, so I also felt angry and betrayed. What made it even worse was that [the NICU staff] didn't get it that I was devastated. Like I was just supposed to be glad that my babies were coming home. I was grateful, but I was also afraid of what it meant.—Rikki

If you are grieving your child's discharge with medical equipment, you might get little sympathy or even be afraid to mention your mixed feelings to anybody. You don't want to appear ungrateful for your child's medical progress and homecoming. You don't want others to misunderstand your feelings, criticize you for having such high hopes, or consider you selfish or rejecting. But your mixed feelings are only natural, as this situation violates your expectations and dreams for a completely victorious homecoming.

When we brought Carter and Zane home to join Sara, Carter was on oxygen and monitors. I was very resentful—I couldn't carry Carter like I could the others. I hated the equipment, and I know Carter hated being connected to it. But it was his lifeline, and I had to come to accept that. It was very difficult.—Jill

Coping with Your Baby's Ongoing Medical Needs

I still feel very strongly that the NICU does not prepare you for coming home, which maybe isn't their job, but it would have been nice to talk to some other micropreemie parents to prepare me for what was to come. Because about five days after discharge, David stopped breathing, and my husband and I had to perform CPR on him. Thankfully, he came back and once again we were back in the hospital. He was discharged the next day, but it still haunts me to think about it, and it's been over a year now.—Jody

Here are some coping strategies:

· Mindfully acknowledge and accept however you feel. It's normal to feel glad that your infant is home and to feel upset that your little one is still fragile or encumbered by equipment. It is natural to wish that your baby didn't require home nursing care— and normal to wish that you didn't have to become an expert at disabling alarms, setting up a feeding pump, or CPR. Isn't having an infant supposed to be less technical than this?

It was a blur because I had one baby home and another in the hospital. At first we had eight hours of nursing a day, then sixteen. We always had two different nurses each day, often more. We would go to bed with one nurse on shift and wake up to someone new. Keeping the shifts scheduled was tough. Many of the home nurses we loved, but some were just fillers, here one day never to be seen again. It was also hard having strangers in the house so much of the time.—Susan B.

· If you feel uncomfortable with the idea of taking your baby home with monitors or medical devices, say so! Share your concerns and do not settle for "Trust me" statements. Ask specific questions about your reservations. As the parent, you have every right to understand their reasoning and the basis for their medical assessments.

They almost let us take him home without a suck. I wanted this baby home more than anything, but I was very uncomfortable with that. I was [gavage feeding] in the hospital, so I knew how to do it, but I was not going to take it on at home. I knew that Charlie had apnea, and I knew that we were going to have to come home with him attached to an apnea monitor. I was not, on top of that, willing to do the feeding part. Just having the monitor was really scary.—Jaimee

· Ask your baby's doctors for a prognosis so you can prepare yourself for what's in store. For most babies, medical devices are temporary, offering a necessary boost for the first days or weeks at home. For some babies, medical devices are necessary for several months or years until they grow out of the need. For a very few, it's permanent.

· Strive to reframe your attitude about the medical equipment. See it as an assistant to help you meet your baby's complex needs. See it as a representation of your baby's will to live. See it as a marvel of technology that allows your baby to thrive at home.

· You, your baby, and your family will benefit if you can enlist and accept others' help. A good home health care agency can provide immeasurable assistance and support, and your insurance may cover these visits. Often, public health nurses and occupational, respiratory, and physical therapists will come to your home. See about getting a case manager to coordinate your baby's care. Your hospital social worker and your pediatrician should be able to guide you to resources.

We had home nursing and opted to always have them at night so we could sleep and be rested to care for them when there were no nurses.—Susan B.

- For friends and relatives eager to assist, make lists of all the chores, errands, and financial/medical paperwork that must be done, and learn to delegate. It is so important that you get the ongoing emotional, logistic, and financial support you need to care for your medically dependent baby.

- If you equate medical devices with life and safety, you may need to be emotionally weaned from them at the same time your child is physically weaned. If you are reluctant to let go of technological support, you can ask for the extra information and reassurance you need.

- If you mourn having a tethered baby, give yourself time to adjust. You may be angry and protest at first, but as you gain confidence and get into a rhythm, you'll find that you can adapt. And as you get to know your baby better, you'll be able to see your child rather than the tubing and devices. If your child is weaned from this equipment, you will still have those victorious feelings you long for. If not, your child's ability to thrive is the victory.

Homecoming, at Last

I will never, ever forget the moment when we brought Anton to the car. I walked along the corridor leaving the NICU, carrying Anton in my arms. He was dressed in the smallest available winter overall, and he was so small, it almost felt like there was no baby in all those clothes. When we went through the door and got outside, I suddenly looked at the outside world with new eyes. The air was so cold to breathe. . . . I felt the security from the NICU was over, and now Anton had to face reality, even though we would do our best to keep him away from the greatest dangers as long as possible.—Inkan

After days, weeks, or months of intensive care, picking up your baby at the hospital, buckling her or him into the infant car seat, driving home, and walking in the door can be a surreal experience. It's also one of those events you'll never forget, a delicious and memorable occasion.

Bringing him into our home was like taking the deepest, most cleansing breath of fresh air you ever could. My whole head cleared and my body tingled. We settled in, and the three of us cuddled all together for the very first time. It was bliss.—Laura

Actually having a baby home was so incredibly joyous! All I wanted to do was hold her and look at her and just plain enjoy being a mommy for the first time since I had given birth to her. Finally, there was no one telling me what to do and when to do it with her. I could hold her whenever I wanted, for as long as I wanted!—Sara

We didn't tell anyone he was home for a whole day so that we could have him all to ourselves. We would fight over who got to hold him.—Ruby

Of course, like most other parts of this journey, homecoming can be emotionally overwhelming. You may readily admit to feeling excited but not so readily admit to feeling grief, anxiety, and unease. Terri puts it this way, "It was satisfying but also very strange." Once the initial rush of excitement has passed, many parents describe an array of mixed feelings.

It felt both miraculous and scary. Just two months earlier, we did not even know if our child would survive. Yet, now, despite all of the difficulties we still had ahead of us (dealing with her physical impairments, etc.), Daphne was in my arms as we walked out of the NICU for good. However, that cold, sterile, noisy place had been the only home she had ever known, and we were somewhat anxious about our ability to deal with all of her needs without the twenty-four-hour support of highly trained medical professionals.—Dina

I really had some funny feelings that day [of baby's discharge]. They lasted about twenty-four hours. By the next day or a couple of days later, most of those feelings had passed, and he was part of the family.—Richard

Being so tired really dulled the emotional experience. More than a joyous occasion, we were relieved to not have to make the drive to see her anymore. The first thing we did when she came home was eat lunch and take long naps!—Mary

You probably consider your baby's discharge an end point of sorts. Exiting the hospital with your baby in your arms feels like a grand finale. But as soon as you drive off, that feeling of closure is quickly replaced by the awareness that homecoming is a new and significant chapter of this journey.

It simultaneously felt amazing and somewhat scary to finally be home with her. This was where my baby belonged. While I will forever be grateful for the technology and medical know-how that permitted my daughter to survive, I couldn't help but think how my nice, quiet, warm, familiar home was so very different from anything my daughter was used to. Daphne had spent her entire life to that point in a very bright, sterile, noisy room in an isolated part of a hospital where most people she interacted with wore scrubs and lab coats. So, as happy as I was to have Daphne home with me, I was also somewhat worried about her ability to adjust to living at home.—Dina

The Emotional Fallout

I thought I was prepared, but they really do not prepare you to be home with micro-preemies and all that entails. Also, you are not ready to deal with the level of emotions that hit you when you leave the NICU. For so long you are pushing down those feelings to be able to be strong for your babies. Once you are home, they come out big time. I was later diagnosed with PTSD from the NICU experience.—Jody

Like most parents after homecoming, you may experience some degree of emotional fallout, including

- feeling unsettled,
- dropping your emotional guard,
- reclaiming your parenting freedom and responsibility, and
- recognizing that your adjustment is ongoing.

Feeling Unsettled

Now that you're home with your baby, you might expect to feel only joy and celebration, yet you may also feel unsettled.

It was nice—and it was scary—having her home. It was the hardest thing I've ever done in my life—even harder than having her in the NICU, because you're on your own. I got home with her, and the first thing I wanted to do was go back. I was thinking, *This isn't right. I don't want to be here. I want to be back there. It's safe in there.*—Beth

The scariest part was sleeping. I wanted to watch her 24/7 and make sure she was okay, but obviously we had to sleep. The first few nights, my husband and I took turns staying up just to make sure she was fine. It was hard to believe that everything was going to be okay.—Corin

I was a bundle of raw nerves, jumping at every noise. I was scarred that something horrible would happen to them because of my ineptitude.—Rikki

Feeling unsettled has many sources. You may feel somewhat disoriented. As much as you longed for this time, having your baby at home feels so different, odd even. You've left behind trusted caregivers and your baby's first nursery. And it's all up to you now. The anticipatory anxiety you felt before discharge has followed you home. As Mary says, "We were relieved and happy to bring her home, but I was somewhat anxious that our round-the-clock source of information wasn't as accessible."

Something I didn't expect was a feeling of emptiness when we got home. We had spent the last ten weeks with a whole family of people taking care of this baby. There were all the doctors and nurses, and we were just two of the people helping out. And all of a sudden it's, "Here's your baby. Take him home, and you're not coming back unless there's a problem."—Richard

I felt a deep sense of loss leaving the NICU. It had been my home for more than three months. Just by the act of taking Jacob out those doors, I no longer belonged. When Jacob was just a couple of weeks old, we returned to the hospital for a day of doctor appointments. The NICU allowed me to use the refrigerator on the floor to store Jacob's bottles. When I walked in to get them, I felt like an intruder, a total stranger—when just two weeks before I had belonged there. When so much of your emotions are wrapped up in one experience, it's unsettling to be set free.—Julie

We plopped her down on the floor in her car seat and stared at her and said, "Now what?"—Sandi

It can be unsettling if the uncertainties haven't entirely disappeared. There may still be medical issues that remind you of your baby's tenuous beginning and questions about developmental outcomes that prod you to watch your baby vigilantly. You may feel pressure to provide "perfect" care, to minimize your baby's exposure to germs, and to maximize your baby's progress. You try to find the delicate balance of being protective without being overprotective, vowing not to let your baby's exceptional start turn you into a hovering or fearful presence. Gallice recalls her baby's homecoming, which was quickly followed by a return to the NICU with a serious viral infection.

The boys were so excited. They were really wild and crazy, and it was hard to hold them away from the baby. They were running around their room and holding him and picking him up, and it's crazy now when I look at it. We were not comfortable at all about letting that happen, but you know, we wanted it to be a happy event, and not start saying, "Now be careful. Don't touch, don't, don't, don't." We wanted them to feel comfortable about this homecoming, not to fill it with negatives and don'ts. The baby should not be a big don't. And we wanted to make it a normal life and not consider him as a sick baby. Now we would do things differently. Probably they did get too close to him. Now I would really put him in quarantine if I had to.—Gallice

It can be unsettling to reach for normalcy in a situation that is not quite normal. Though you may be tempted to override your protective urges and turn away when you become anxious, that can pose real dangers to your baby. It's important to find a balance between your baby's very real needs for protection from germs and overstimulation and your need for your baby to fit in to your family life. Trust your instincts. Germs aside, you may become all too aware of how much you have been looking forward to making up for lost time with your baby.

When we brought Sara home, I didn't feel completely like a parent because Carter and Zane were still in the NICU. Once we were all home, I thought I had to make it up to them—try to hold them for all the days I couldn't hold them. My actions were out of love but also out of guilt that I couldn't be a mother to them like I wanted to when they were in the NICU.—Jill

I shudder to think what this must mean, but one of the first things I wanted to do when I brought her home was to take photographs: posed pictures in frilly dresses with pink backgrounds. It was a disgusting obsession and very unlike me. I think I wanted to pretend her preemie experience had not happened.—Renee

You're simply not the carefree parent you imagined being. Coming home can be quite intimidating and overwhelming, and you may remain vigilant for a while. As Susan B. recalls, "I was most afraid that something terrible would happen while I was sleeping." But considering what you've been through, your desire to be a protective, appreciative, conscientious parent is only natural—and an asset.

The usual things that bother new parents—colicky crying, lack of sleep, fussiness, begin stuck at home—these things seemed like nothing to us. We were just so grateful. We were happy to hear them cry because it meant they were doing what they were supposed to be doing.—Susan B.

Dropping Your Emotional Guard

At a time when you had imagined putting your baby's traumatic birth and NICU stay behind you, you might be surprised to discover that the emotional journey isn't over yet. In fact, after your baby is home, you may begin to grieve fully for what you and your baby have lost.

We said our good-byes to the rest of the nurses and made our way home—a family at last! We got home and put both babies in their cribs, and I cried for hours! Relief, fear, pity—*Why me?*—Sara

It was very emotional. [That day] I cried the whole way to the hospital. I cried the whole way home. I think it was a little bit of everything. I was bringing him home, which was so emotional. A lot of it was a relief to me—like, it was over, it was done, he was out of the hospital, he wasn't hooked up to anything except this apnea monitor. And there was definitely a piece of it that was a little scary. You know, this is still kind of a young baby, and I kept thinking to myself, *He's still not supposed to be here.* This is still really early. But most of it was relief—I was so glad that he was coming home. . . . It was very emotional and actually very nice.—Jaimee

Many parents notice that painful feelings bubble to the surface just when life starts to feel more stable or relaxed—because they are in a place where they can afford to drop their emotional guard. Especially if you cruised through the NICU stay without too much turmoil, you may be shocked to suddenly feel despondent or overcome with emotion. But it is human nature to experience intense feelings only *after* the initial danger has passed. Fathers in particular may feel they can finally afford to express their emotions without undermining their ability to support their partner. Jaimee talks about how her husband finally allowed himself to cry the day they brought Charlie home:

Seeing my husband cry was really, really hard, but I knew it was because he was so happy that the baby was home. I felt like he knew that now I knew that this baby was mine and was safe and I had nothing to worry about—and so it was the same sense of relief. But for a very short second, I got upset because I thought, *Oh, my God, he's afraid.* Since then, we've talked about it, and he said, "That's the whole reason why I could never do it before. Because you would never understand that it was me just being able to have feelings too, and you would think that I was worried."—Jaimee

It is also normal for the memories and regrets to come rushing to the foreground. You may sort through your experiences, examine them, try to make sense of them, and try to find meaning in them. These are all-important parts of grief work. Particularly if you had multiple babies and one or more died, homecoming can trigger your grief.

I attended a national business meeting the October after their birth and Spencer's death. (I brought Stuart and a grandmother to watch him while I was in meetings.) I remember the grief I was feeling. I didn't realize it at the time, but I was steeped in grief. I should never have tried to carry on so normally, attending meetings and attending to business as if I were normal and everything were all right. I couldn't focus, couldn't concentrate, and couldn't care about the things being presented to me. I sat in meeting after meeting chronicling in my head all that I had been through, trying to give it some order, some sense, some meaning. At one point, I even took an unused deposit slip from my checkbook and wrote down each thing in the order that it had occurred. I carried that slip of paper around and stared at it during the meetings, trying to comprehend it all, remembering.—Susan C.

You may experience a variety of the emotions associated with grief. Perhaps you are wracked with anxiety over your baby's condition, even though the doctor tells you your little one is doing fine. You might feel sad and sentimental, missing the support and camaraderie of the practitioners in the NICU. On the other hand, now that you are no longer under the thumb of the NICU, you can afford to feel angry about the ways in which you weren't able or allowed to parent your baby. And when you are feeling frustrated or inadequate as a parent, you may feel intense guilt, sadness, or regret and then wonder what's the matter with you.

Particularly if you repressed some of your feelings while your baby was in the NICU, you can expect to start feeling them—and perhaps even be flooded by them. But even if you did a fair amount of grieving all along, more feelings will likely tumble out when you're finally in the comfort of your own home, cradling your precious infant in your arms.

As you settle in and relax little by little, you'll have the energy and time to deal with your emotional backlog. Take the opportunity to move through your feelings when they come up. Keep in mind the source of these intense feelings. Look back and acknowledge that your baby's hospitalization was a traumatic crisis.

Homecoming has been a huge relief. . . . Most of what I feel is very happy, but there is an undercurrent of pain from this experience. It's just below the surface, and I know I need to find ways of working through it so it won't always color parenthood. I felt it recently when I took Charlotte to the lab at the community hospital to check her anemia. I stood by her on the table while the lab tech prepared to draw her blood, and when the lab tech began rubbing the alcohol wipe on Charlotte's foot, Charlotte howled loudly. The lab tech was so shocked and kept saying, "I haven't even stuck you yet!" I knew that the smell of alcohol—so present in her memories of hospitalization—made her afraid. It saddened me to think of how Charlotte spent the beginning of her life in such an environment, and I'll never really know how it has affected her.—Kate

I just have a constant dull feeling of fear that I can't pinpoint. It is particularly challenging when my baby is sick. When my baby is sick, as he has been with teething, a virus, or a cold, I automatically fear the worst internally. Externally, I appear calm and under control, but internally, I must actively convince myself that it is just a cold, just a virus, just teething, or some combination and his symptoms are all normal and will subside. It has also been difficult for me when I've seen my friends' experiences with the NICU. At those times, I tend to relive our NICU experience, but with a renewed sense of dread and a reality check in terms of what could have been. Recently, a friend had an emergency c-section at 34 weeks. Her baby was in the NICU, developed an infection, and ultimately passed away. While I was trying to be supportive of my friend, I was internally struggling with my own feelings related to my son's NICU experience. I got a strong dose of reality and realized how much I had minimized my son's infection while in the NICU. At the time, I didn't think of it as particularly serious. I just thought that he'd be cured by the antibiotics and it was fairly simple. Only in retrospect, do I understand the gravity of the situation and how dangerous an infection can be to a newborn. All I wanted to do was hold my son and hug him. I have gotten into the habit of holding him while we sleep.—Liza

If your baby has ongoing special needs or if you have multiple babies who demand vast amounts of your emotional resources, dealing with your emotional backlog can be a longer process. But whenever joy meets despair, you can face them both. Acknowledging your feelings and getting support will free you to cultivate a loving, close relationship with your baby(ies). It's never too late to unburden yourself.

Reclaiming Parental Freedom and Responsibility

After being closely supervised in the nursery, you have not only the *freedom* to decide what to do with your baby but also all the *responsibility*. This realization is both exciting and frightening.

First, there's the exciting honeymoon period, where you're delighted with your twenty-four-hour access to your baby. Then reality and exhaustion set in—and the honeymoon fades. The challenges of parenting build up, and it sinks in that twenty-four-hour access to your baby means being on duty twenty-four hours a day. As much as you have endlessly longed for the chance to care for your child, actually *doing it* endlessly can be exhausting. You are covering all the caregiving *and* all the shifts. While this new arrangement has its advantages, it can also feel formidable.

For the first few weeks, we walked around the house like elated zombies and wished someone could have dropped by to pick up an afternoon shift so we could get some sleep.—Sherilyn

Unfortunately, during this exhaustion phase, when you need support the most, you may be getting the least. Your baby's first follow-up visit comes and goes, any support the NICU offered is a distant memory, and you may still be isolated from all your germy friends and relatives. You may also feel oddly disappointed or let down—after all those weeks of fantasizing about being home with your baby, all you're doing is feeding, soothing, changing diapers, and, if you're lucky, sleeping.

Monotony and sleep deprivation are challenges faced by all new parents as caring for any newborn is a full-time job. But if you have multiple babies, a premature baby, or a medically fragile baby, you may feel especially overwhelmed. Small or neurologically immature infants and infants recovering from or in the midst of treatment for a medical issue tend to require a great deal of soothing and feeding. Add hypervigilance to the mix, and you are toast.

We'd be lying in bed, the closet light would be on, and Daniel would make noise in the bassinet. I would get up and lean over and open my eyes wide to get used to the light and stare at his face and determine what color he was—so that was the kind of sleep I was getting.—Mitch

If you are really, *really* lucky, your baby will sleep a lot, eat well, soothe readily, and generally fit into your life and your home. But for the vast majority of NICU graduates and their parents, adjusting to home is much more complicated.

The day finally came when she was to go home. I didn't feel prepared because she only weighed three and a half pounds. I knew that for sure something would happen at home and that I wouldn't know what to do. Once home, I was glad and hoped that things would get better. But boy, was I wrong. Just the opposite. It was even worse.—Rosa

I was terrified. My babies were so tiny—both under five pounds. I had no idea it would be so much work.—Erica

Shayna came home first. She was cute—she was this little doll. She was always swaddled in her blanket. We'd get up, give her a bottle. She was not that hard. Then Daniel was discharged, and that was an entirely different story. He was uncomfortable, and he screamed and screamed and screamed. It was tough. And once there were two of them at home, within thirty-six hours we were wiped. There was an unbearable amount of sleep deprivation and not just for a bad couple of days, but when it continues for a week, it's hard to function. It was really hard in the beginning.—Mitch

Homecoming with three tiny babies can only be chaotic. Both Clare and Emily came home on apnea monitors and medication for apnea. Jacob came home [later] with no equipment but with lots of medical care needs and extreme feeding issues. Between weight checks, follow-up visits, and Jacob's specialists, we were packing up babies and equipment to visit some doctor at least twice a week. Moving three babies from place to place is hard enough, but then to lug equipment! It made for some interesting times.—Julie

Even with just one baby, becoming a round-the-clock caregiver takes practice and some adjustment. It requires effort to get acquainted with your baby(ies) on your own terms, to learn how to meet various and varying needs, and to listen to your instincts.

Consider the following ideas and tips for making the transition from parenting in the NICU to parenting at home:

- Try to remember that despite the traumas of your baby's condition and hospitalization, your parenthood has expanded over the weeks and months since your baby's birth. You may not have really felt like a parent until you brought your baby home, but recognize that you were a real parent all along, even though your role has now expanded.

- While you and your baby are settling in together at home, you already have a lot of experience and coaching under your belt that most new parents don't get. Your lack of confidence may have very little to do with your abilities, being more a reflection of the trying transition from hospital to home and your adjustment to being the one in charge.

- Settling in can be a tumultuous and emotional process, but you will adapt and prevail. Find value in the path you traveled to arrive home with your baby.

- Preoccupation with your baby is an integral part of your ability to be a nurturing and protective parent. Your concern for your baby's well-being is what energizes you to instinctively meet his or her needs.

- When concern turns to anxiety, it can deplete your caregiving and parenting energies. That's why it's so important to get support from others for your emerging parenting instincts. When you begin to feel overwhelmed, having the backing, encouragement, and collaboration of your partner, your pediatrician, and your relatives and friends can help you feel energized instead of paralyzed. Create a circle of close friends and advisors who can support you and your efforts.

- Trust the process of learning how to best care for your baby. Look again at the ideas you had about parenting before the NICU and see if those goals still feel good to you. If they do, figure out ways to make them work; if not, modify them.

- Flexibility is fundamental to honoring any baby's needs as every infant is unique. Perhaps you had hoped to carry your baby in a sling. Babies on oxygen or monitors are tougher to carry in a sling, but you can do it, and your baby will benefit from the close body contact. Or maybe you had never considered wearing your baby, but after experiencing (or reading about) the joys of kangaroo care or attachment parenting you might like to try this approach. You may decide to co-sleep, as much of the world's mothers do with their babies and young children. You may breast-feed longer, reaching for the worldwide average time of four years. Experiment and discover what works best for you and your baby.

- To ease your baby's adjustment to home, you can try to simulate the familiar NICU. For instance, many NICUs are active at night, so after babies go home, they tend to sleep better at night to light and sound. If this works for your baby, you can dim light and sound slowly over a week or more. Also try keeping the daytime softer, quieter, and calmer at first so your baby can be awake without being overstimulated. You might play a CD of soothing ocean waves or womb sounds at low volume for background noise.

- Naturally, friends and relatives may be eager to offer the strategies they used with their healthy term babies. Their ideas may or may not be appropriate or effective. Thank them for thinking of you, then take the advice that fits and discard what doesn't.

- Continue to advocate for your baby. Hear your internal voice and trust yourself to evaluate what your baby needs to settle in and thrive. You know your baby better than anyone else does. Others are entitled to their opinions, but you are blessed with your knowledge.

The early days after Daphne first came home from the NICU were very difficult adjustment days. Daphne refused to sleep and had trouble even relaxing the first night at home. We had set up a crib in our bedroom so that Daphne would be close to us. There was a mobile and an activity box in the crib similar to the ones she had in the NICU. The problem, we soon learned, was that it was just too quiet and too dark for her. The NICU was very noisy and well lit at all times. Ultimately, we learned that she could remain calm with background noise from a white noise maker or with music playing and if we used a special lamp to direct light into her crib.—Dina

During the first year, Ali got a number of very resistant bacteria in her urinary tract and had to take a few medicines that she hated so intensely that each day was marked in four-hour battles, followed by hours of tears and sadness. I used to hate that I was forced to do this to her. I still can't quite describe the depths of my angst and despair. I was tormenting her, and it didn't seem to really help. I so worried about permanently damaging my relationship with this particular child, who has always been so intense and stubborn yet fragile and reluctant to show affection.

I let her nurse well past her third birthday, something I never intended to have happen, yet a bond and emotional release for both of us prevented me from taking any action that wasn't totally lead by her. I took a god-awful amount of criticism about her lengthy nursing. I even wondered myself (quietly and privately) if perhaps I'd lost my always-tentative grip on sanity . . . but for me, this was my way to prevent permanent damage to my maternal relationship with my daughter.—Sheila

Above all, rather than focusing on the burdens of responsibility, cherish the freedom. If you take joy in holding your baby close, celebrate it. Become the kind of parent you want to be, even if it's outside the box. Surround yourself with people who understand this and who rejoice with you. Your desire to hold, protect, be close, be responsive, and repair your relationship comes from a positive instinct to nurture, which benefits both you and your baby.

I didn't feel like he really knew who I was until after he was home. It was the way he would look at me when I picked him up and the way he would snuggle into me.—Sharon

I just wanted them near me all the time. I was very idealistic. I was never going to leave these babies. I was never going anywhere without them—lots of nevers. It was actually a very long time before we left them with anyone. . . . We just had the intense need to be with them and heal. Just the thought of being able to hold my baby whenever I wanted to—I said: "I'm never going to put them down. Once I get to hold them, I'm going to hold them forever." And then like after two days, "Okay, we can lay them down here a little bit now." But we were very much like that. Once they were home with us, we were glued together.—Stephie

I started to enjoy him more and to get into lots of kisses and cuddles. Before then, I'd always been affectionate only up to the point where his muscle tone increased, and then I'd quickly stop. But he always had that "More! More!" look in his eyes. And I definitely had the "More! More!" feeling in my heart.—Anne

An event after Molly's homecoming highlighted and strengthened my feelings for her. Six weeks after she came home, I found myself crouched in a parking lot with my daughter while a tornado passed over. I held her tiny body beneath me while hail pelted us and the wind threatened to snatch her from my arms. It was a terrifying experience! But I discovered, incredibly, for the first time, that I wanted my girl to live. I fought for her life in that parking lot, and things were not the same after that.—Renee

Your Ongoing Adjustment

We did speech therapy, OT and PT, lots of developmental follow-up. It just was. It became our social life, visiting doctors and therapists. We were so lucky. Most of the dire predictions never came to pass, so we lived in crisis, but also in gratitude.—Susan B.

Breast-feeding was challenging without the consultant right there, but we managed it. It was also a challenge to just leave her alone. To this day, I wake at every noise she makes and she still, at age two, has yet to sleep through the night on a regular basis. She was very, very set on her every-three-hours feedings that the hospital had her on.—Jennifer E.

Basically, the boys had to be in a bubble for two years to avoid catching colds, which would delay the lungs growing good tissue. That was very isolating and hard. Friends and family really didn't get it. They think since they are out of the NICU that everything is fine. They don't understand when we can't have visitors, and we have to ask them to get shots before visiting. They think it's really not a big deal and that we need to get our boys sick to build their immune systems. Many friends and family thought we were overreacting and overprotective. They still don't get it, and I think they never will.—Jody

As you begin to settle in after homecoming, you may finally start to feel more like a *real* parent, but you may also feel frustrated by how distant "normal" still is. You might wish that you could forget the whole NICU experience and start fresh. Now that you're home, you want a "regular" newborn period. You want your baby to have a "regular" infancy. You want to be a "regular" parent. But as you soon discover, just because your baby is home doesn't mean that your baby's exceptional start is completely behind you. You're likely still dealing with the medical and developmental aspects and definitely with the emotional aspects.

I had several family members tell me that we will have other big things in our lives and to just get over this. Really? What is bigger than doing CPR on your child? It gets to the point that I don't talk to people about a lot of things since I know they just want to hear everything is great and nothing else.—Jody

I feel that it's important that family and close friends understand how the NICU experience can affect a parent. That being in such a stressful situation can cause lifetime scars, even after the child is better, and that time does not heal all wounds.—Jennifer E.

When Isaac was four years old, I heard a speaker (a psychologist) at my twins group who talked about something called assumed disability. She said it was something that often happened in conjunction with or subsequent to an actual disability—perhaps a devastating illness or injury—and a parent or caregiver ascribes limited ability to a child that might not be true. A lightbulb went on. I realized that

I would ask Molly to get her shoes, and she would, and then I would ask Molly to get Isaac's shoes, and she would. I realized that both Molly and I were enabling Isaac. Poor guy, I went home and pulled the rug right out from under him. Until that time, I had assumed that he needed help with everything, mostly because he was so compliant and so willing to accept help. He never had the usual toddler defiance, that need for independence. Since that point on, I have tried to be vigilant. I also learned that Molly was Molly, and that it was tough enough to grow up without having to worry about your twin. I became vigilant about that too, fighting the urge to rely on her help for him and not allowing teachers or friends to use her as a surrogate mother or as an excuse not to push Isaac.—Susan B.

It's important to remember that your adjustment and recovery from the NICU experience can span the NICU stay, homecoming, infancy, and even early childhood and beyond. As you settle in and reorient, as you drop your emotional guard and move through more feelings, and as you reclaim your parenting freedom and responsibility, you will continue to process your experiences, heal the wounds, and grow as a parent. You may even discover that in some ways, your journey is more precious than being a "regular" parent. Stay open to the emotional riches, whenever they appear. Revel in your gratitude.

Because Daniel was small, anytime there was an opportunity to try to feed him, we would. He would always wake up between 11:00 PM and 1:00 AM, and I would always get him—and you know what? I didn't mind getting him. The fact was, when he started getting bigger, I loved getting him. I'd bring him down, I'd turn on the light over the kitchen sink, and I'd give him a bottle. I used to hold him real high on me, and I'd just put my cheek on his while I gave him his bottle, and I just thought he was the sweetest thing in the world to give a bottle to. So I didn't mind getting up.—Mitch

As for my parenting the boys when they came home, I was elated. I didn't care if I had to have bottles in my hands twenty-four hours a day, which it seemed like I did. I needed to make up for lost time and to finally feel like these babies were mine.—Stephie

Caring for my tiny babies became a full-time obsession. But it was, and still is, a labor of love. When their care would start to overwhelm me, I'd think of how extremely lucky I was to have all three of them home with me.—Julie

For many weeks, I prayed that Daphne would simply just survive. After her repair surgery, I was so overwhelmed with joy to learn that she could pass solid waste, and (while I realize that it may seem strange to others) I felt like I was witnessing a miracle every time my daughter had a dirty diaper. Bathing Daphne was also very fun for me. In the hospital she had only ever received sponge baths. Now, I was able to introduce her to baths in a basin and, later, with me in the bathtub.—Dina

I was walking with my baby in the stroller outside. It was March, and the sun was shining, and I could smell spring in the air. I tried really hard to feel like any mother walking with her baby, and I think I looked like one, but I was crying all the time, remembering my terrible fear only a couple of weeks before. I was so happy that I was walking there, in this sunny moment, with a little healthy son. This was so much better than I had ever dared to hope for. It was probably much more intense than the moment a "normal" mother gets her baby on her chest right after delivery. This was my moment, and it was two months after delivery. But it was a moment that only a mother of a premature baby would understand.—Inkan

Bringing home your baby is momentous. It is a triumph for all of you. You traveled through a grueling phase of this journey and made it home together. Now yours are the able hands that cradle your baby. Yours are the eyes that assess your child's well-being. Your intuition and judgment are what count.

Every time I see Daphne make the most minute, noticeable progress in her development, I am filled with thanks, pride, and joy. If she doesn't gain weight fast enough, or fails to drink appropriately from a bottle or straw, or gags because of her various oral motor delays, I cringe and fear that I am failing her. But, when she recently made extremely fast progress in her physical development (after months of minutely slow progress due to internal scar tissue adhesions that were finally surgically removed), my determination to do whatever I can to help her was reinforced.—Dina

No matter how much you long for normalcy and only want to look ahead, moving toward the future does not mean discarding the past.

I know for us breast-feeding for four years turned out to be a real salvation. At age six, Ali still talks about when she nursed. From the language she uses and the times she recalls it, I know it's fundamental in the way she thinks of me. I'm glad, because I'd hate to think of Mom being conjured up by the thought of vile antibiotics being forced down her throat as a baby.

I go on each day believing that my children will take all of the experiences of their childhood into consideration when deciding how they feel about their mother

. . . and that as long as I continue to lead with my heart, in the end it will be all good.—Sheila

Points to Remember

· *Discharge preparation is a process that can help you gain confidence. Just as your baby must go through several steps to be considered ready to leave the NICU, you also have developmental steps to take as a parent before you can feel ready and able to take over your baby's care completely.*

· *Before you leave the NICU, find a pediatrician to collaborate with. Doing so will reassure you about your baby's continued care.*

· *Practice caregiving, even rooming in with your baby before leaving the hospital, so that you feel confident about being in charge of your baby's care. Ask for repeated opportunities to do this if you think more practice would help you.*

· *If your baby will be discharged with monitors and/or medical devices, you may have strong feelings about this situation. If you believe your baby is still too fragile to come home, talk to the medical team about the reasoning. If you want the reassurance of monitoring equipment at home, inquire about this as well.*

· *Your baby's discharge is a truly momentous occasion. In the midst of celebrating, it is also normal to experience emotional fallout, where you feel unsettled and bereaved, excited and exhausted, worried and impatient.*

· *Become the kind of parent you want to be, even if it's outside the box. As you gain confidence and trust yourself to evaluate and provide what your baby needs to settle in at home and thrive, you can reap the fruits of your parental freedom.*

· *Your desire to hold, protect, be close, be responsive, and repair your relationship comes from a positive instinct to nurture, which benefits both you and your baby.*

11:

Your Healing Transformation

There are lingering reminders, subtle differences between my son and his younger, full-term brother, between my son and his three-year-old peers, differences that remind me daily of the battle he fought, the battle he fights. Language comes slowly to him, comes stiffly from him. Sensory difficulties interfere with his ability to feed himself, to tolerate textures. And his scars . . . oh, his scars.

I am unable to adequately articulate the fierce protectiveness I feel toward this child. Daily I am humbled by the strength, the sheer grit he has shown, continues to show. And I love him with a depth and passion previously unknown, unimaginable to me.—Susan C.

Like any significant life event, your baby's birth and need for intensive care is not something that you simply get over. Naturally, your baby's exceptional start continues to touch your life in many ways, directly and indirectly, obviously and subtly. You may wonder whether you can ever completely heal the grief and trauma of this journey.

Just when I think I've done okay, something happens and I realize I've still got far to go. Our daughter, Hannah, really has done remarkably well. Even so, I still feel traumatized to some extent by the experience.—Stephanie

Healing doesn't mean forgetting or brushing away the lessons learned. Rather, it means moving forward with what you've gained. It also means becoming better, not bitter.

This final chapter holds some thoughts and words of encouragement about adjusting, healing, and moving on.

Evidence of Your Healing

Early on, when your grief takes center stage, you may remember only the negative aspects of this journey. But after a time, even if you've been shaken to your core, you can come to value your experience—not for the suffering it caused, but for the positive aspects, such as how you've grown and the good that you've harvested because of it. Eventually you'll be able to say, "You know what? I *got* something from that." This is evidence of your healing.

Still, for months or years after your baby's birth, you may have moments of intense sadness, anger, fear, or regret. Old jealousies and yearnings may stir when you hear of another parent's ease with childbirth, witness a woman whose belly is ripe with pregnancy, or see a newborn babe in arms. In particular, you may be deeply affected by other losses in your life as well as by outside events that hit close to home. Catalysts that reactivate your original trauma are opportunities for you to work through deeper layers of grief and to reach for more healing. As you move forward, you'll be less overcome by pain and more able to experience the joys, yet more evidence of your healing.

As time goes on and my boys grow, my perspective shifts and changes. I'm better able to compartmentalize my emotions and prevent the sorrow from those years ago from tainting the pure pleasure I feel now in having witnessed my once–critically ill preemies become funny and smart and beautiful children. It can still be difficult, though, to separate then and now. When I see an ambulance with its lights turning and siren blaring racing down the road, I instantly bite my lip and have to hide my panic. I wonder if the passenger is like my little one when he was tiny and had to be raced back to the NICU for a second course. But then I look over and see him thoughtfully doing his alphabet puzzle, and the anxiety eases.—Maureen

I still have fears, but I try to see it as something I have learned to cope with. In the beginning, I could not talk about it without crying—the first second I opened my mouth—and now I can talk about it almost without crying. I guess you heal. No matter what you have to deal with, your life continues, and you go through a healing process.—Gallice

Nathan wasn't one of my son's close friends, but his death has hit me so hard. It has been almost like a turning point. It seems so awful, but that one event has opened up places inside me that have been dark for years, five and a half years to be exact. There seems to be so much now that's bursting, demanding to be written or spoken, and I'm surprising myself with how I'm coping with it all. It's difficult when an idea or a feeling emerges. I feel that I have to put pen to paper to remain calm. It's very odd. But each time I write, part of me heals just that little bit more. At times I almost feel still, peaceful . . . not very often, perhaps only once or twice, but it feels good to know that I can reach that place.—Leanne

I still feel jealousy sometimes. But it is so hard to put it into words because I think we push that away as a "bad" feeling. But it is so normal, so understandable. I tend to understand it as part of my grieving process and then move away from the jealousy/anger/resentment place and move under that to the real sadness and loss that fuels the jealousy.

And I am feeling the jealousy less often, and being grateful more often, and not needing to compare so much because my boy is my angel, and I couldn't want anything but what we have right now—so much love.—Maren

Other evidence of healing is when you can look back and instead of an unrelenting flood of emotion, you feel only a small stream or perhaps just a trickle. *Looking back* no longer means *going back.* Your baby's birth date becomes more clearly a celebration and a time to recognize your gratitude.

It wasn't until everybody started singing "Happy Birthday" that I just lost it. I just couldn't believe it was a whole year that had passed. Tom and I just looked at each other, but here they were, eating cake, smashing their fingers in it.—Betsy

Conor's going to be four in two weeks. We had an early birthday party for him this weekend. It was a wonderful day. But even so, I had to hug him, smell him, and cry because I'll never get over what we've faced and what we continue to face.—Laura

I get more emotional around Charlie's birthday because I know it was a much harder place to get to. . . . Around his birthday I say, "Oh, my God, look at him. He makes me laugh and he's so funny. He's so wonderful and cute." I love him so much, and I can't help but think that I really almost didn't have him.—Jaimee

It's hard to believe those scrawny, tiny, funny-looking babies I had seven years ago today are now rambunctious, maddening, hyperactive, lovable, robust seven-year-olds. I only had one bad dream in the days leading up to this last birthday, so that's a great improvement over the previous years. And in the dream, it wasn't me having the preemie; it was the woman in the next bed. Whatever would Freud say?—Joyce

Still more evidence: as your emotions lighten up, you also change how you talk to others about what happened. When your baby's need for intensive care is such a big focus in your life, you may feel that nothing short of the whole story will do. But as you adjust and acquire perspective, you become more selective about how much and with whom you share the details. You can value your journey privately, without the urge to tell everyone your story. It can be liberating to be able to say simply, "Yes, she's small" or "He has strengths and weaknesses, like any child," and leave it at that. And when you do share your story, you can talk matter-of-factly about your child's birth, hospitalization, and development.

You may also notice a change in your reaction to medical practitioners or the follow-up team. At first, you may feel exposed and inadequate when professionals are scrutinizing your child, and you may discount your own observations. Over time, though, you will come to appreciate and trust what *you* know about your child. Gaining this confidence is more evidence of your healing.

The turning point is very clear for me. It came when we went through a second round of developmental testing when Lars was around twenty-one months old. I disagreed with some of the results, but instead of getting angry, I realized that no one else knows Lars like I do, and I don't need anyone else to tell me that he's okay. Wow. It was around that time that I finally began to have a deep sense of his wellness. Strangely enough, his bout with respiratory syncytial virus just increased my confidence in his basic health instead of bouncing me back into sick baby mode.—Kris

Letting Go of What Might Have Been

From my own experience I can tell you that the blues can still find me, the guilt can still creep up when I'm not looking, and the sense of responsibility is constantly present. Even some of the old fears surface and try to drag me under. Parts of these emotions are attributable to being a preemie parent, parts are simply because of being a parent, period.—Maureen

As you grieve, you let go of idealized images of what should have, could have, or would have been—and realize that all deliveries have their disappointments, all new parents have their struggles, and all babies have their imperfections and temperamental idiosyncrasies. With time and experience, you can come to appreciate your "real parenthood." The circumstances of your baby's early months fade into the background, and you focus on what you have, instead of on what you missed.

I had had such a picture in my mind my entire life, it seems, of how happy I would be when I finally had a baby. I can remember thinking this as a very young child. And how great the moment when you first met your baby would be. Well, of course, with a preemie it was far from the moment I had waited for all my life. Since Bronwen's birth, I have been struggling with feelings of being cheated, being angry that I didn't get the birth I had planned, angry at what my baby had to go through, and on and on.

I have been getting a little bit better with this kind of thing lately, but today something wonderful happened. I had a moment where I looked at Bronwen and I realized that I do have all those things I was hoping for so long ago. It was a perfect moment. I saw her and thought, *Isn't my baby wonderful? I love being a mom!* and none of those other feelings were there to mar the moment. Of course, I have thought those exact same things before, but today it was different because there were no negatives coming up behind, like, *Yes, but maybe it could have been better!*

My dreams have come true, just not exactly when I thought they would.—Nola

You also learn to appreciate your child's unique mix of strengths and challenges. Instead of wondering *what if* your child had been spared that ordeal, you can focus on who your child is now.

In so many ways, I think Macy's most amazing qualities somehow may have resulted from her preemieness and/or the battle that it required her to wage. I will always wonder what she would have been like if she had been full term, but I cannot imagine her being any smarter or funnier or more energetic or more athletic or more anything that is desirable in a child. My view as her mother is of course clouded, but I think she is just the cat's meow. I can truly, honestly say she might have been different had she been full term, but she couldn't possibly have been better than she is.—Christi

If your child's delays have more clearly become disabilities or if there are ongoing medical problems, you will always wish that she or he could have an easier path. But as time passes, this wish will take up less and less space in your life or in your relationship with your child. Instead of expending energy thinking about what didn't happen and doesn't exist, you learn to embrace reality. In fact, your child may inspire you the most, by his or her ability to accept what can seem to you to be entirely unacceptable.

So many times people comment on my positive attitude, and I want to scream, "What choice do I have?" This is how it was and is, and nothing can change that. And Stephen has fought and fought to come as far as he has and still has more fights ahead. His example is what keeps me going. He deserves a mommy who can laugh and smile with him. Who will play and be silly. Who will always be there to help him and support him. I do cry in my time late at night, after all the others are in bed. [But] my positive attitude is a shield of sorts. It lets me get through the day with my miracle and return his joy, smile for smile.—Tracy

There are some times when I think about it. But I don't cry because they were born premature. I cry because Jacob has special needs. But it doesn't happen very often anymore. It used to happen so often when things were up in the air.—Julie

Moving On in the Face of Uncertainties

Clare's and Emily's issues are pretty much gone. We're still on the lookout for learning problems, but they're doing great in school so far. Jacob's problems are severe and eternal. It's not a matter of integrating his premature birth but more his disabilities into our lives. When I look at Jacob, I no longer say, "He's a preemie," but rather, "He's a little boy with multiple handicaps." And we're still floundering with issues of disabilities. No one person can take our hands and lead us to the right decisions for Jacob. Our intense love for Jacob gets us through each day.—Julie

If you're raising a child whose future is still uncertain or looks challenging, you may wonder how you can move on when you don't know where you're going. Although you may not know exactly how your child will develop, you do know how she or he is today, and you can probably guess where your child is headed tomorrow and perhaps next week. Staying focused on current realities can help you cope.

Unfortunately, even the current realities are not always clear. Doctors don't yet grasp all of the ongoing effects of prematurity, serious neonatal illness, or various congenital conditions, and they can't always give you definitive answers. But as you learn to trust your intuitions and find medical practitioners, therapists, and teachers you can collaborate with, you can know what is knowable and move forward rather than perseverating on what's unknowable and remaining stuck. Just as your child's growth will unfold over a lifetime, perhaps in unexpected ways, the same is true for your coming to terms with your child's special needs.

I remember the turning point very clearly. It was just this past summer. After our trip to Denver, when Stephen was so much healthier and able to do more, I felt as though we had gotten over the hump in his care, so to speak. Even this winter, when he did have a brief return to his illness, I felt that it was a temporary setback and not part of a permanent pattern.

Oddly enough, it was the [respiratory specialists] in Denver who also helped me be more at peace with the idea that he will likely have long-term delays and possible mental disabilities. They were the first who would actually look me in the eye and tell me that Stephen might be mildly retarded. All the others have talked around it. It was hearing it straight out that allowed me to begin to assimilate it and learn to adjust my life to it. Until then, the most frustrating thing has been that *delay* implies a lag that will be made up. I kept waiting for Stephen to catch up. Now that it has been put into terms implying a permanent situation, I can deal with it as part of life and not wait for an ending that won't come.—Tracy

I am in the process of finding a sense of peace about raising a special needs child. Yet I am completely at peace with the child. We have a quiet snuggle each morning when I wake him up for preschool, and the weight of him in my arms, against my chest, the flutter of his eyelashes as he struggles awake, his breathing, yawning, stretching—they are miraculous to me again and again. I am in awe of this little being in my life.—Susan C.

It just was. When your babies are born at twenty-four weeks and one and a half pounds, you know you are in for a long road. In many ways, those months in the NICU prepared us for what was to come. I think it would be much harder to have a full-term baby who had health or developmental issues. At twenty-four weeks, you expect struggle. At forty weeks, you expect perfection.—Susan B.

Talking to Your Growing Child about the NICU

My daughter likes to see pictures from when she was in the hospital. She gets really upset if she doesn't see my hand there or something of mine right by her. She's like, "Why weren't you there, Mommy?" "I couldn't be. I'm sorry!" Those times hit me pretty hard—not being able to help it.—Marcia

From the time he was born, I was real honest with him. When I would hold him and talk to him, I would tell him everything. I don't know if he knows or understands [tears], but I told him everything.—Pam

It's normal for children to be curious about their birth and infancy. They want to know how they arrived and how their parents reacted. When they see photographs or tiny baby clothes, they want to hear the stories behind them.

You will want to be able to talk to your growing child about his or her birth and NICU stay. These experiences shouldn't be a secret or something to be tiptoed around. Your child deserves to hear about this extraordinary beginning. However, you want to be able to tell the story in a way that is reassuring to your child and doesn't trigger intense feelings in you.

If you're overwhelmed at the prospect, first try writing down what you'd like to convey. Be sure to include anecdotes about the pregnancy, delivery, and hospitalization, and include how it felt—how exciting, how scary it was—and also how much hope and love you felt. Writing down your story without censoring the information or your emotions gives you the opportunity to organize your thoughts and consider how to talk to your child. Getting your feelings out on paper, especially your guilt and regret, can help you stay calm and positive when you have this conversation.

Offering reassuring explanations and answering questions in a comforting manner helps keep your child from being troubled by what you say. Reassure your child that the doctors and nurses took excellent care of his special needs and that you pitched in whenever and however you could. Explain that she slept most of the time (rather than lying awake, missing you) because she was so busy growing big and strong. If you're looking at photographs, point out the equipment that helped him grow and explain how most of the wires were just stuck on with tape, and there was medicine so it didn't hurt. Remember always to convey the deep joy you feel about having your little one in your family.

In general, describing your child's early experiences with a measure of pride ("You did so well!") and nonchalance ("You sailed through surgery!") encourages your child to take those NICU experiences or complications in stride. Try to avoid relating your horror or heart-wrenching emotions. As Sheila observes, "It seems that both Kate and her friend, also a preemie, are very comfortable with their unique journeys, scars and all."

Finding Meaning in Your Journey

When you can find meaning in your journey, you can feel less victimized by what has happened to you and your little one. You can see a deeper purpose, and you don't feel so much that you've been randomly chosen or that you suffered needlessly.

One way to find meaning is through understanding what has happened and why. Gathering information and answers can help you feel a sense of mastery over what occurred and retain a sense of control. Even if no one can tell you why this happened medically, the more you learn, the better you can put together an account that makes sense to you and that you can live with.

There's also a spiritual side to finding meaning. Over the years, as you look at the big picture, you may acquire a sense of purpose. You may conclude that you endured these experiences for a reason that has to do with the path you and your child were meant to take. The twists of fate can seem less cruel and arbitrary when you feel a sense of destiny or higher purpose.

I am still convinced that everything will work out as it should, even if I don't understand why something happens at the time. I also have faith that I was given a tremendous gift from G-d, who needed a home for Daphne and knew that I was up for the challenge, even if I sometimes don't feel so confident that I am doing everything I can to help her.—Dina

Finding spiritual meaning in your journey can be an important part of integrating your experiences into your life. You may find meaning through certain philosophies or religious beliefs about life and fate. You can also find meaning in your discovery of treasures, your deepened appreciation, your resilience, and your personal growth.

I'm very energetic. I'm very impatient. I'm a doer and a mover, and I like to get things done. With Erin, my life has come to a complete skid. With the boys [it's], "Hey, let's go upstairs and watch TV," and [snaps fingers] we're there. But with Erin you've got to get her out of her wheelchair, and when you get upstairs, you've got to strap her into some apparatus—it's a whole process. To go anywhere with her, to do anything with her, to go to a movie, anything, it's a slow, slow, tedious process. With my wife, who's the most patient, loving person you could ever meet, it's no big deal for her—she adapted. This is something that I think God wanted to give her the day she was born. It was like, "This woman here, she could raise a child with cerebral palsy." So when she got older, she got a child with cerebral palsy. Me, he probably said, "This boy needs to settle down. We need to slow him down a little bit, so let's give him this child too, and he can develop into a person who can slow down by being with her."—Charlie

Finding Treasure in Adversity

Here's my cousin having one [healthy child] after another. The worst is that they just don't realize how blessed they are. They take it all for granted. And in that weird little way, I think that perhaps there is a little bright side to having a preemie because no one else but a preemie parent will understand the amazing joy I feel when James does such a simple thing as smile at me.—Teresa

As time passes and your grief softens, you may find solace in what you've gained because of your child or this experience. Any treasure you've extracted certainly doesn't make this ordeal something you would wish for, given a choice. Still, recognizing anything positive can help you come to terms with this experience and integrate it into your life in a way that adds value. Many parents hold gratitude for healthier perspectives and stronger, deeper family relationships.

Her birth brought us closer in the sense that we realize she is a part of both of us and we regard her as a miracle. I think that was one of the first times we were able to sit down and really tell each other what we felt. Not only that, but we were able to lean on each other.—Jackie

I think Neil's prematurity brought us closer together as a couple and a family. Leaning on each other as the only people who really understood what we were going through made a huge difference, and we went out of our way to be kind to each other.—Tara

I'm more positive about everything the children do. Everything has such a big meaning to me now. Everything they say, everything they do. If they do something wrong, it doesn't count as much anymore. I see the positive side of things more. I'm grateful we can be a tight-knit family.—Gallice

This pregnancy and birth were real eye openers. I felt compassion for every woman who ever gave birth. My relationship with my husband has also deepened and grown.—Ruby

It's made our family stronger. I also don't dwell on the small stuff. I've seen the rough part of life. I've seen what these children have had to go through, and I think that in the day-to-day situations it's going to work itself out. It's not a life-threatening thing. If it's fixable, it's okay.—Betsy

I think the NICU stay ultimately helped me connect with my son. I gradually developed a stronger bond with my son without the responsibility of caring for him in the middle of the night. After he came home, even though I was exhausted, I had already established a bond with him and was grateful to be able to get up in the middle of the night to care for him. I also gained experience, confidence, and support while he was in the NICU and felt much more competent to care for him when he came home. Plus, prior to my son's birth, I was adamant that he would sleep in a crib and be in his own room fairly early. My son is now a year and is still in my bed. My husband had always wanted him to sleep with us, but until I was apart from him, I hadn't considered it.—Liza

You may undertake new, meaningful pursuits. A natural extension of your experience is to offer support to other parents you meet.

When I've talked to people who've been through it, I know exactly what they've been through. You know you can help someone like no one else can. That's very rewarding.—Vickie

The university recruited a doctor who is well known for his work with children who have pervasive developmental disorder, autism, and the like. He is putting together a committee of medical people, therapists, school people, and parents to work on developing a community-based center to provide services to the children and their families. I am excited that he asked me to participate. I am hoping this effort might help me develop the sense of doing something with all that we went through, just as I have found writing about my experiences for this book so helpful.—Susan C.

I started a nonprofit organization to give back to others in the NICU in memory of my son and in honor of my daughter. It helps to know that I can help others who go through the difficult NICU experience and offer a little comfort.—Corin

Uncovering silver linings is something others cannot (and should not) do for you, as it lacks empathy and tries to fix your pain. If others are offering you their insights or pointing out your blessings in disguise, you can gently inform them that you appreciate their attempts to help but you must discover treasures for yourself, in your own time.

Some might think I had a dream lifestyle—no kids, some money, the ability to come and go as I pleased. But there was a problem. My relationship with Susan was less than rock solid. I felt like we were husband and wife, but that we were just roommates much of the time. I did my thing. She did hers. And sometimes we did stuff together. It's as if we were two pieces of bread with no peanut butter to really hold us together.

I needed the peanut butter. I just didn't realize that the peanut butter would show up in the form of children.—Jack

Weaving Treasures into Your Tapestry

When you begin to grieve and adjust to your baby's exceptional start, you take the coarse, unwieldy threads of your feelings, identity, and relationships, and you reluctantly begin weaving them into your tapestry. At first, up close, all you see are the cruel knots, the unconventional colors, and the messy, uneven pattern—and you are repelled. You may wish you could do the rough parts differently, or cover them, or remove them. But after a while, you can take a step back, see your tapestry as a whole, and appreciate how those rough spots fit into the big picture. They're complicated and show the struggle, but they make your tapestry richer and more interesting, and you are pleased with the overall effect. By accepting those parts, you aren't denying the pain, betraying the difficult realities, or relinquishing the need to continue adjusting. But part of healing and moving on is allowing the threads to have their place and acknowledging their value to your tapestry. Instead of turning away from the rough patches, you treasure them. From this comes peace.

After much reflection, I find that I do not feel like I am in a different place now than I was two years ago, than I was six years ago. What is different is that I have stopped trying to escape this place and begun to understand, accept that this is the place in which I am now and forever rooted. At first, then for years, everything for me was about the shock and denial that I could be the mother of a dead son, that I could be the mother of a surviving son who might not be normal, a son who might be marked differently but as indelibly as I was from the experiences we survived. My efforts to understand this reality, to organize it, to label it, to change it, to control it, were all born from a drive to escape the place I found myself in. I never expected to be in that place, so surely I could find a way to make sure my stop there was a brief one. But the place grew in me, and I grew in it, and finally I could see that separating me from it was fantasy.

The thing—finally—is, I have what I have. I am the mother of a dead son, a different son, a dear son. I have three very different boys who root me differently to the very same place. A certain kind of sorrow will always filter my experiences, as will a certain sort of appreciation, a depth of experience and understanding I could not have gained any other way. All of which I'd still give anything to have been able to avoid, but the gifts of which I can finally begin to embrace along with the pain.

Every day, in some way, I miss Spencer, the wonder of what might have been, the unanswered questions, the aching over the missing space in every aspect of our family. Every day, in some way, I marvel at Stuart; I am continually catapulted between the heights of pride and appreciation for who he is, what he has survived and accomplished, and the depths of fear for the unknowns in his future, the hurts yet to come. Every day, in some way, I am healed by Justin, so transparent in his adoration, his heart so kind, so open. There is something hard and raw about living this gamut of loss, grace, fear, hope, wonder, risk, awe. But there is something also, something powerful and peaceful, about looking it all full in the face and sitting down squarely in the middle of this place.—Susan C.

Vulnerability, Appreciation, and Hope

We all have our hurts, our losses, our isolations. If we don't have them now or haven't had them in the past, we can rest assured that they are coming. One of the biggest ways that I am different than I was, one of the challenges I now face daily, is learning to live effectively and fully with that knowledge.—Susan C.

Over time, you can learn to accept and cope with feelings of vulnerability to life's adversities. You protect yourself when it's possible and adopt philosophies about why bad things happen. All of this can help you let go of what you can't control and focus on what you can.

I know I believe in miracles now, but every time I meet someone who has lost a baby or a child, I also realize that we were nothing except just plain lucky. Every child is a miracle; every loss of a child is a tragedy. Any sense of fairness or control is an illusion.—Susan B.

You can even come to value this sense of vulnerability because it keeps you in touch with your child and with your own emotional landscape. With vulnerability come awe and appreciation—and gratitude that it wasn't worse.

I guess one thing that I've hung on to, to try and make sense of this, is just—appreciation. I've been reading a lot of philosophical stuff over the past few years about appreciation. I just try to appreciate the fact that my husband and I have a beautiful daughter who is small but healthy! I have just tried to keep the perspective of being thankful that Hannah's challenges are (hopefully!) only temporary—that she does not have a permanent disability.—Stephanie

It's very easy for me to see how bad things could be. . . . Even with Emily's cerebral palsy, it's always possible to compare her with children who have much more severe cases and be grateful—again, relatively.—Diana

Having a premature baby has made me grateful for even the tiniest things. I realized how thankful I was for modern medicine and for all of those people who had decided to become doctors and nurses. I was thankful for every gram T.J. gained and every breath he took. It really made me grateful for the little things.—Claire

I know I would have loved them if they were full term, but I don't know if I would be in awe of them or so appreciative of them. They are my heroes, and they showed me that miracles are possible. That's a gift too priceless for words.—Stephie

Even though you may maintain a sense of vulnerability, you learn to balance your fears with hopes. As your grief subsides, you become more open to optimism—and you find encouragement in unexpected places. If your baby is struggling with delays or disabilities, you learn how to attend to even the smallest rays of hope.

When Macy was about a year old, I had a bittersweet experience while looking at some photos of my husband's family. I came across one of him as an infant, and it looked so much like Macy at the same age that I just burst into tears. Peter found me there, still crying, much later and asked with alarm what was wrong. When I was finally able to talk, I blubbered, "And she looks just like you did." He was confused, and then bemused—"Why is that something to cry about?" But he never did understand why it made me so emotional. Somehow seeing the physical similarities told me that she might not be scarred forever by her preemieness, that she just might be okay after all. It was one of those odd healing moments.—Christi

There have been many turning points. I look at them more like stair steps instead of corners because each small turning point takes us further upward (and some downward). When I saw Jacob yawn and stretch like a normal baby at two months old, I finally truly believed he'd live. Watching Clare and Emily grow up. Learn to walk, talk, make friends. Their first day off to school. The first time Jacob laughed out loud, said "I wan cook," yelled "Go Bulls!" during the playoffs, his hero worship of Michael Jordan. Watching Clare and Emily in the classroom, seeing the spectacular drawings they do, listening to them explain the world in their own voices.

Stepping down when Jacob had his first seizure and being thrown into a whole new world of worries. Watching him balance on his own for the first time, only to throw himself off balance by clapping so hard for himself. Looking at the pure joy on his face the first time he rode a bike; the pure terror as he realizes he's slipping into another seizure; and the satisfaction, after babbling the same phrase over and over, when we finally get it. Our despair as we watched him waste away in just a few weeks and have to finally make the decision to place a G-tube, and our thrill when he finally breaks thirty pounds at six and a half years old. My angels as flower girls in my friend's wedding, watching them walk down the aisle hand in hand and having my breath taken away by their unbelievable beauty. Holding each of my children's hands and marveling at the perfection and grace of movement in a hand whose palm used to be the size of my thumbnail.—Julie

Finally, you can appreciate how your children come together in ways that benefit them all. Many parents report that their other children profit from having a sibling who needs special care, and their baby's development profits from these sibling relationships.

As Vincent grows up, I realize that one of the best things you can give a disabled child, if not the absolute best thing, is a sibling or two. Jessica is a fantastic friend and support to Vincent, and it really comforts me to think they'll always have each other (with luck).—Anne

Gregoire and Jeremy are more aware of children with disabilities. They don't look at it as being [strange]—it's part of their world. They're not shocked by it. It's good. It has helped them. They know that some children are different, some children can be sick. They know that children can die . . . and [that] they are lucky they are healthy. And that children with disabilities can have a nice life and do nice things. They know there is hope and happiness with these children.—Gallice

Resilience

I've had people at work who say, "If it were me in your situation, I couldn't have done that. To come back to work and just turn it off and go to work and then go home and deal with your problems at home, and then come back to work, turn it off, do your work." They just respected the strength I had to do that. It was very hard to do, and yet I just did it.—Charlie

You and your family may have been through more than you ever imagined you could survive. With each jolt, each scare, and each disappointment, you might have wondered whether you'd be able to get up again and move forward. At first, you might have decided that you *had* to get up for your baby's sake. As time passes, though, you may begin to see that you get up again and again because you *want to* and because you are resilient and stronger than you ever believed possible.

By the time my son came home a little over a week later, my daughter had been readmitted because she turned blue due to her heart defect. But none of the challenges have been as traumatic or scary as those early life-and-death days in the hospital. Even my daughter's heart surgery seemed like just one more hurdle. The rest has just been tweaking. I just look at them now (nearly twenty years later.) I didn't screw up too badly. Everyone's alive and no one is in prison, so that's good.—Susan B.

Resilience doesn't mean smiling through the pain, instant forgiveness, or undying gratitude. It means feeling your grief, disappointment, and discouragement, plus having the internal wherewithal to take a deep breath and rise up again—holding tight to whomever or whatever helps you feel strong and steady. Resilience means seeing yourself as able to bend when necessary, to hang in there, to adapt, to bounce back, and to carry on. Resilience is surviving what you must.

But resilience is not just getting through, it's also becoming vibrant again, perhaps even more so than before.

They don't show that many signs of their prematurity. It's just their past and our past. We certainly went through a long trauma. It was a tough experience, and knowing what all is involved with it, it's pretty impressive we went through it and came out in good shape.—Mitch

Out of the rubble came *I*. Just a mom who loves her kids, wants to do the best she can, and deals with all these oxymoronic medical conditions with oxymoronic emotions. There isn't a set way or a formula for me, though there seems to be a pattern of rebounding. I try to take my emotional cues from the boys. If they can laugh and smile and joke about this, then so can I, even if it's "fake it till you make it" there in the beginning.—Ramona

The cashier said, "Oh, you have the pendant I always wanted (a necklace symbol of mother and child). You only have one child?" I told her I have two, then showed her my mother rings. Then she asked why I have three rings. When I explained remembering the one I lost, she exclaimed, "Oh, my son means so much to me. I could never survive such a loss. I don't know how you did it. I could never do it." From a great calm distance, I told her that I have learned that we do, we survive what we have to. She didn't believe, but saying the truth to a stranger was a comfort, a validation.—Susan C.

As time passes, life can get easier. Even in the NICU, you can settle in to your parenting role and routine. After homecoming, you and your baby can really come into your own. Over time, outcomes become clearer, and, if necessary, you adjust to any special needs. If you are still in the early months or years of your journey, you can hold on to the hope that it will get more manageable. Know that you'll be able to dust yourself off and that your resilience will shine on. If you hear about outcomes that discourage you, remember that if you do end up traveling that path, your resilience will carry you through.

As my preemies get older, the good does greatly outweigh the bad. When they were infants, life was hard. From feeding issues to sleep deprivation to sensory overload to follow-up clinics to not meeting milestones, it was all so frustrating. When they were toddlers, I was dealing with watching Clare and Emily take off, leaving Jacob behind, and coming to grips with exactly how handicapped Jacob was. When they were kindergartners, I was worrying about learning issues for Clare and Emily and navigating the nightmare of a special education system with Jacob. Things are finally settling in. I love to watch Clare and Emily play with their friends and know that no one has a hint of their early beginnings. Jacob is coming into his own with a wonderful school situation. He's the healthiest he's ever been and is thriving despite his multiple handicaps.—Julie

Personal Growth and Transformation

The NICU experience is something that has changed my life, who I am, and my perspective on life . . . forever.—Corin

Whenever the path you're on is heading uphill, it's daunting at first, but your resilience kicks in and you forge onward. As you get to different vantage points, the view changes accordingly and with it your perspective. Personal growth and adaptation follow.

Having a premature baby, there are a lot of obstacles, there are a lot of things that are going to happen, there's just so much you and your child are going to go through. It's going to make you stronger, even if the outcome is not a favorable one. I've learned so much from this experience.—Betsy

We all do what we have to do. Over the last three and a half years, I have been exposed to many things (prematurity, cerebral palsy) about which I knew nothing before, and circumstances forced us to learn. While I wouldn't wish these experiences on anyone, I know that I am a more patient and compassionate person today because of what we've been through.—Diana

Now I know what it's really like to juggle. At work, I'm juggling clients, but no one's going to die if I screw up. When a big client would come in, I'd worry, but there's no worrying anymore because nobody's going to die. I might get fired or something, but that's it. It takes the pressure off.—Charlie

I guess that my perception of what I considered *fine* five years ago has certainly changed dramatically. Back then, *fine* would have meant having a couple of stitches after my tiring but natural birth of a rather large but healthy full-term baby who is grazing at my breast as I lovingly gaze into the eyes of my husband! Today, *fine* means that my baby has survived another day, Tyrell [my first child] hasn't decided to leave home, and I'm still in one piece and still have a partner!!!—Jo

There were times when I worried that we'd never make it where we are today or times when I just couldn't see far enough into the future to imagine it. I have two beautiful daughters about to enter middle school and puberty. Even their typical preteen theatrics can bring a smile to my face. I have my miracle son who brings me joy every day in his unconditional love and in his zest for life.

I am not the person I was before Jacob, Clare, and Emily were born. I'm richer, I'm fearful, I'm overprotective, I'm fulfilled, I'm amazed, I'm accepting, I'm grieving, I'm intense, I'm grateful, I'm a better person, all because of three tiny babies.—Julie

With hindsight, you can see that you've undergone a personal transformation of sorts. You knew that you felt different as soon as your baby was born, but little did you know you would never be the same again. This experience can hold many lessons for you. As you begin to recognize and accept signs of personal growth, you can see your transformation as another treasure.

I think I came through pretty good. I know that I surprised myself. I now have a little more faith in what I am capable of. If someone had told me beforehand that this was something that I would have made it through, I wouldn't have believed it. I would not have thought that I would have been able to do it. I would've said, "Oh, that's not me. I cannot do that. I will lose my mind and not be able to handle it." And I really think I handled it fairly well, and I think that it has done something permanently to a piece of my self-confidence, so that was a positive thing.—Jaimee

What I now believe is the big miracle is that my daughter has helped me to change. I'm so much more open to people based on their terms or abilities or situations—not mine. And I can now become completely overwhelmed with pride and joy and appreciation when my daughter accomplishes most anything!—Karen

How has a premature birth changed my life? Oh, my. One, I learned how to ask for help. Sounds like such a simple thing. Stan and I are very independent people. It was not an easy lesson. Two, I am thankful for the small things. My daughter chatters constantly. Waking up to her crying means that she's breathing. She is trying to learn how to wink. Those things are pure joy for me. Three, I do not say, "I can hardly wait until she . . . " I enjoy each and every moment as it is. It all passes too quickly. And four, I reach out to those who may need a smile or an encouraging word. I used to be too busy. Not now.—Cindy

Peter probably would have been an involved dad anyway, but as I found the NICU removing more and more of my faith in my ability to be a good mother, it was simultaneously instilling confidence in Peter! He probably does half the caregiving now, from which we all benefit. His priorities changed dramatically, I think. Having a baby who weighs less than two pounds can do that to you! But he went from thinking that work was one of the most important aspects of his life to realizing that his family is what really matters. He's turned down promotions since Neil's birth, and since he wants to be home with us more, he works from home.—Tara

It was not until about two and a half months into Lauren's hospital stay that my priorities changed. . . . Lauren needed me so much more than anyone at work ever would. And no one was going to die if I did not answer my work line, respond to e-mails, or issue settlement checks. My daughter was a different matter. Things were life and death. From that point forward, I've done my best for my company, but I always put Lauren first.—Shanda

I think that my experience has really helped emphasize to me that every child is an individual. I find myself looking at others through a different light now and asking myself, *I wonder what they have had to go through to get to where they are now?*—Stacy

Their b'nai mitzvah, at thirteen, was momentous because when they were still in the hospital, I remember saying that one day we would be celebrating their b'nai mitzvah, and all this would be behind us. It seemed like only a blink in time before that happened. Pay attention and know that this too shall pass. And remember that that holds true for the good things in life as well as the bad. It all passes much more quickly than you can imagine.—Susan B.

Parents who have "regular" pregnancies, deliveries, and newborn periods might also say with a chuckle, "I'll never be the same again," but you know that for you, this is an understatement. Not only will you never be the same again, you have been utterly transformed. Your transformation includes integrating the new and wiser you into your identity as a person and a parent.

I don't think you will ever get over the fact that your baby came early. In time, you accept your situation and grow from it. One thing for sure, you're never the same again, which is good, I think.—Kathy

I don't think you ever feel like yourself again. Too much has changed. . . . If given the choice, I certainly would not ask for a premature baby; however, I think I'm a much better person now. I think I'm stronger and happier. I never appreciated the small things in life. Now I cherish almost every moment.—Laura

I don't think I'll ever be myself again because a part of me passed away with Dominique. But I'm a much better person now than I ever was.—Rosa

Seeing Your Transformation as Healing

Many parents talk about how their babies amaze them. "She is so strong." "He is such a survivor, such a fighter." You may remember witnessing your own baby's mighty determination.

Remember too that *you* made it through an experience you couldn't even have imagined before it happened—and you survived, mustering all you had to give. You've done so much and more: prevailing through complications, unfortunate diagnoses, and separation from your newborn; getting to know and love your tiny baby and growing child; nurturing, protecting, wishing you could take his or her place; making unfathomable decisions; hoping and persevering while living with uncertainty.

But after a year, two years, or twenty, you may worry about how much you are still affected by the traumas and losses. Despite the joy you take in your child, you may worry about the strong feelings that occasionally well up and wonder if this experience has irreparably damaged something in you. You may also feel uneasy, struggling to understand who this new you is, figuring out how you fit into the world you used to inhabit, and deciding how you want to move forward.

When you are struggling, pause for a moment and look back. Think about the way your life used to be—the way *you* used to be. Think about who you were before this pregnancy, before this child. Can you remember? Now review your baby's birth and all that has passed since then. Marvel at yourself. Reflect on the knowledge that you now possess and the lessons that transformed you into the person you are today. You can probably detail your baby's developmental steps, small and large. Have you given yourself the chance to really appreciate your *own* development?

At times you may feel like the walking wounded. It can be a while before you feel settled. But when you recognize and value your own metamorphosis, you can feel robust, accomplished, content even.

Where you are now is not just the result of the NICU experience and its aftermath but also because of your personal growth.

As you move through your life's journey, there are many opportunities to pause, look back, and take stock. Imagine yourself looking out over the path you have traveled, your vantage point high above. You can see the many twists and turns, even the obstacles that you overcame—and those that stopped you cold. And you can truly appreciate how far you've come with your little one and embrace the path that brought you here.

Feeling better (which for me means feeling in control) came when I realized that I didn't have to let the preemie experience, the emotional discoveries, and even the pain fade away.

That I could find peace, even with maintaining a heightened sense of what motherhood means to me based on what I had been through, what my children had been through. That I actually was forever different as a person because of our family journey, and that it was okay, even years later, to still know the hurt intimately, still live with the ache, still feel my breath catch in my throat when I told our stories. That moving on and watching my sons grow into fine, strong children didn't mean that you got over it or that their early arrivals and immense struggles no longer counted. That the past blended into the present, which offered a glimpse of the future. That the journey doesn't always begin with tomorrow, that there doesn't have to be a disconnection to the anguish in order to seek and find and feel and believe the joy.

Surviving my sons' premature births means simply that—that I continue to wake each day wanting the best for them, wanting to protect them, wanting to give them the gift of a loving home and a loving heart, wanting to watch them soar. Surviving it means embracing it.—Maureen

When you embrace the full journey, your life feels enriched, and you can feel more whole. Indeed, as you heal, you may notice that your confidence, ease, joy, and gratitude takes on a brilliance and complexity that sets your life apart from the everyday. You owe this brilliance to where you've been—and to where you're headed.

James starts preschool (four-year-old kindergarten) tomorrow, his first tentative steps into the "big school" system. My boy looked at me and said, "Remember, Mummy, I'm only a little bloke. I might need you to stay. What if I get sad?" Those words knocked me flat—"Remember, I'm only a little bloke." How could I ever forget? Will I ever forget? . . . He's only been my baby for four years. I want some more time.

I'm not ready to hand him over yet. . . . He's mine, we survived together. . . . He held onto my finger when his hand was too small to reach around it all the way, and tomorrow I put his hand into another's . . . I can't. I don't want to . . . "Remember, Mummy, I'm only a little bloke." Oh, but I will.—Leanne

I was asked once, if we knew the end result of our journey to start a family, if we would still go through it all. Without a doubt, I would. Nothing in life comes easy, and while I wish that we had been able to have all healthy children, our experiences have made me a better person and a better mother. I know how blessed I am to have my children.—Corin

The road you are on continues to be different, and the parent you've become is different from the one you had imagined. But different is not the same as damaged. Different doesn't mean that you lack recovery from the NICU experience or its aftermath. True, you haven't recovered the old normal. But you're in possession of a new normal. Different means that you are *transformed*. And that's exactly as it should be.

We spent New Year's at the beach. It was a peaceful few days, and James and I enjoyed a couple of amazing hours together in the water jumping over or running away from the waves. I say amazing [because] it seems that amongst all that sand and water, there was another step in my journey, one that James and I took together.

James loves to run away from the waves. He teases them and laughs at them, but the minute the water reaches his toes he usually turns tail and runs.

This particular day he decided that he didn't want to run away. So my little boy and I stood in the water and let the waves crash around us. When James was frightened and the water seemed to be getting too deep, I lifted him up as he jumped high, and I held him over my head, away from the water, and calmed his fears.

It was odd to be in this water as it rushed in toward the shore and then ran out again, trying to pull us with it. It made me think of childbirth, the contractions like waves rising and falling—an odd connection, perhaps, but it seemed quite right that I was able to lift James out of the water and hold him away from the waves when he was afraid. Being able to protect him in this way and make him feel safe, [being] able to be beside him and do something for him when I hadn't been able to protect him all those years ago.

It was so healing, those couple of hours, watching James move through the water, running and chasing and then standing close as we challenged the ocean together, and together we won.

And the journey continues. Thanks for wanting to share it with me.—Leanne

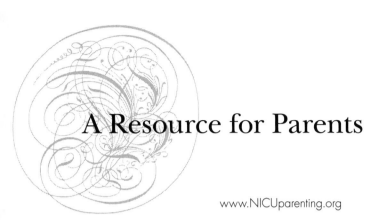

A Resource for Parents

www.NICUparenting.org

On our website you will find additional reassurance and guidance around the emotional aspects of parenting in the NICU and beyond. We also provide information and support to healthcare practitioners to enhance their compassionate care of babies and families like yours. We encourage you to share links and print and distribute these materials.

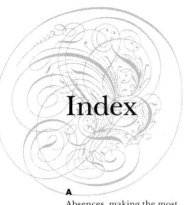

Index

Gray zone, making medical decisions in the, 252–257
Green burial movement, 256
Grief, 31
  anger and, 42, 49–52
  anticipatory, 31
  anxiety and, 40
  catalysts in working through, 298
  center stage, 298
  common feelings of, 41–52
  coping with, 59
  couples and, 52–55
  for death of other babies, 248–250
  failure and, 42, 46–48
  fear and, 41, 43–44
  feeding of baby and, 212–213
  guilt and, 42, 44–46
  letting flow, 65–67
  painful feelings in, 40
  powerless and, 42, 48–49
  process of, 39–52
  sadness and, 41, 42–43
  shock and, 41, 42
  softening of, 306
  yearning and, 41, 44
Grounding, sense of, 39
Guarantees, lack of, in NICU, 43–44
Guilt, grief and, 42, 44–46

H
Healing, 11, 297–319
  evidence of, 298–303
  finding meaning in your journey, 305–308
  finding treasure in adversity, 306–308
  letting go of what might have been, 300–302
  moving on, in the face of uncertainties, 302–303
  talking to your growing child about the NICU, 303–304
  weaving treasures into your tapestry, 308–319
Helplessness, 44
Hesitation, feelings of, 137–138
Holistic nurturing, 104
Home care, feasibility of, 257
Homecoming, 280–282, 313
  anticipating, 2
  feelings associated with, 261–262
Home health care agency, 279
Home monitoring, discharge with, 274–276

Hope(s), 75, 309–312
  balancing fears and, 146, 237–244, 258
  change in direction, 243–244
  dashing of, by medical practitioners, 241–242
  with multiple babies, 244–246
  in NICU, 1, 2–3
  in pregnancy, 2–5
Hopelessness, 39
Hospice care, 254–256
  choosing between intensive care and, 252
Hospital(s)
  doctors in teaching, 111–112
  step-down or transitional unit in, 267
  transfer of baby to larger, 6
  transferring baby back to local, 264–265
Hydration in enhancing milk supply, 206–207
Hypervigilance, 288

I
Infant massage, 186–187
Infection, breast feeding and, 210
Information. *See also* Communication
  as empowering, 115
  strategies for gathering, 118–119
Informed, being, 115–123
Informed consent, 126–127
Innocence, loss of, 39
Intensive care
  babies need for, xix, 1–2, 10, 15–16, 23, 31, 51, 70, 297, 300
  choosing between hospice care and, 252
Interest, sustaining, for baby, 193–194
Internet, use of, 118, 157
Intervention, aggressive, 252, 253
Intuition, trusting your, 61
Isolation, 24–25

J
Journals, keeping, 77

K
Kangaroo care, 180–186
  benefits of, 182
  breast-feeding and, 215
  crying during, 184–185

emotions in, 183–185
  feeding of baby and, 208
  making arrangements for, 185–186
  shared, 183

L
Lactation support, 200–201
  getting referral for, 204
Laughter, 94
Let-down reflex, 204, 209
Letting go of what might have been, 300–302
Long-term care, decisions about, 257
Looking back as evidence of healing, 299
Loss, sense of, 26–27

M
Massage, infant, 186–187
Maternal complications
  during birth, 17
  during pregnancy, 21
Medical barriers, negotiating, 146–149
Medical decisions, making, 126–130
  in the gray zone, 252–257
Medical devices, discharge with, 276–278
Medical equipment, discharge with, 274–280
Medical practitioners. *See also* Collaborative care team; Neonatal nurses; Neonatologists
  choosing pediatrician, 262–264
  dashing of hopes by, 241–242
  discussing feeding options with, 214
  focus on relationships and developmental support as beneficial to, xviii
  getting to know your baby's, 109–112
  joining baby's team, 64, 107–115
  medical experience of, 124
  valuing contributions of, 113–115
Medical procedures, being presence for, 125–26
Meetings
  with neonatologist, 97
  recording, 119
Milestones, importance of each little, 227

About the Authors

Deborah L. Davis, PhD, is a developmental psychologist and writer whose work supports parents who have endured a crisis with their baby during pregnancy or infancy. Her books include *Empty Cradle, Broken Heart: Surviving the Death of Your Baby*; *Loving and Letting Go: For Parents Who Decided to Turn Away from Aggressive Medical Intervention for Their Critically Ill Newborns*; *Parenting Your Premature Baby and Child: The Emotional Journey*; and *A Gift of Time: Continuing Your Pregnancy When Your Baby's Life Is Expected to Be Brief.* She has also written about medical ethics, perinatal bereavement care, and NICU parenting for medical texts and national organizations, informing and supporting the healthcare practitioners who work with these families. She writes a blog for *Psychology Today*.

Mara Tesler Stein, PsyD, is a clinical psychologist in private practice specializing in the emotional aspects of coping with crisis around pregnancy and parenting, parent education, child development, and developmentally supportive care to babies and their families. She presents nationally on these issues and consults to healthcare providers and hospitals, guiding their efforts to improve the level of psychological support and care to families during and after perinatal crisis. She is the coauthor of *Parenting Your Premature Baby and Child: The Emotional Journey*.